Spinal Deformity Surgery

Editors

CHRISTOPHER P. AMES
BRIAN JIAN
CHRISTOPHER I. SHAFFREY

NEUROSURGERY
CLINICS OF NORTH AMERICA

www.neurosurgery.theclinics.com

Consulting Editors
ANDREW T. PARSA
PAUL C. McCORMICK

April 2013 • Volume 24 • Number 2

ELSEVIER

1600 John F. Kennedy Boulevard • Suite 1800 • Philadelphia, Pennsylvania, 19103-2899

http://www.theclinics.com

NEUROSURGERY CLINICS OF NORTH AMERICA Volume 24, Number 2
April 2013 ISSN 1042-3680, ISBN-13: 978-1-4557-7124-0

Editor: Jessica McCool
Developmental Editor: Teia Stone

Neurosurgery Clinics of North America (ISSN 1042-3680) is published quarterly by Elsevier Inc., 360 Park Avenue South, New York, NY 10010-1710. Months of issue are January, April, July, and October. Business and Editorial Offices: 1600 John F. Kennedy Blvd., Suite 1800, Philadelphia, PA 19103-2899. Customer Service Office: 11830 Westline Industrial Drive, St. Louis, MO 63146. Periodicals postage paid at New York, NY, and additional mailing offices. Subscription prices are $360.00 per year (US individuals), $552.00 per year (US institutions), $393.00 per year (Canadian individuals), $674.00 per year (Canadian institutions), $502.00 per year (international individuals), $674.00 per year (international institutions), $177.00 per year (US students), and $243.00 per year (international students). International air speed delivery is included in all *Clinics* subscription prices. All prices are subject to change without notice. **POSTMASTER:** Send address changes to *Neurosurgery Clinics of North America*, Elsevier Periodicals Customer Service, 11830 Westline Industrial Drive, St. Louis, MO 63146. **Customer Service: 1-800-654-2452 (US and Canada). From outside the US and Canada, call: 1-314-453-7041. Fax: 1-314-453-5170. E-mail: JournalsCustomerService-usa@elsevier.com (for print support) and journalsonlinesupport-usa@elsevier.com (for online support).**

Reprints. For copies of 100 or more, of articles in this publication, please contact the Commercial Reprints Department, Elsevier Inc., 360 Park Avenue South, New York, NY 10010-1710. Tel. (212) 633-3812; Fax: (212) 462-1935; E-mail: reprints@elsevier.com.

Neurosurgery Clinics of North America is covered in *MEDLINE/PubMed (Index Medicus), EMBASE/Excerpta Medica,* and *Current Contents/Clinical Medicine (CC/CM).*

Printed and bound by CPI Group (UK) Ltd, Croydon, CR0 4YY

Transferred to digital print 2012

Contributors

CONSULTING EDITORS

ANDREW T. PARSA, MD, PhD
Associate Professor, Principal Investigator, Brain Tumor Research Center, Reza and Georgianna Khatib Endowed Chair in Skull Base Tumor Surgery, Department of Neurological Surgery, University of California, San Francisco, San Francisco, California

PAUL C. McCORMICK, MD, MPH, FACS
Herbert & Linda Gallen Professor of Neurological Surgery, Department of Neurological Surgery, Columbia University Medical Center, New York, New York

EDITORS

CHRISTOPHER P. AMES, MD
Associate Professor, Department of Neurosurgery, Director of Spine Tumor Surgery, Director of Spinal Deformity Surgery, University of California, San Francisco Medical Center, San Francisco, California

CHRISTOPHER I. SHAFFREY, MD, FACS
Harrison Distinguished Professor, Neurological and Orthopaedic Surgery, Department of Neurosurgery, University of Virginia Medical Center, Charlottesville, Virginia

BRIAN JIAN, MD
Department of Neurological Surgery, University of California, San Francisco, San Francisco, California

AUTHORS

MICHAEL AKBAR, MD
Department of Orthopaedic and Trauma Surgery, Spine Center, Heidelberg, Germany

OLAOLU C. AKINBO, MBBS
Department of Neurosurgery, University of California, San Francisco, San Francisco, California

CHRISTOPHER P. AMES, MD
Associate Clinical Professor in Neurological Surgery, Department of Neurological Surgery, Spine Tumor Surgery, Spinal Deformity Surgery, University of California, San Francisco, San Francisco, California

JAMES T. BENNETT, MD
Shriners Hospitals for Children—Philadelphia, Philadelphia, Pennsylvania

SHAY BESS, MD
Rocky Mountain Hospital for Children, Presbyterian/St. Lukes Medical Center, Rocky Mountain Scoliosis and Spine, Denver, Colorado

BENJAMIN BLONDEL, MD
Department of Orthopaedic Surgery, New York University Hospital for Joint Diseases, New York, New York

PATRICK J. CAHILL, MD
Shriners Hospitals for Children—Philadelphia, Philadelphia, Pennsylvania

CHING-JEN CHEN, BA
Department of Neurosurgery, University of Virginia Medical Center, Charlottesville, Virginia

VEDAT DEVIREN, MD
Associate Professor in Clinical Orthopaedics,
Department of Orthopaedic Surgery, Spine
Center, University of California, San Francisco,
San Francisco, California

KAI-MING G. FU, MD, PhD
Department of Neurosurgery, Weill Cornell
College of Medicine, New York, New York

MUNISH C. GUPTA, MD
Department of Orthopaedic Surgery, University
of California Davis, Sacramento, California

RYAN J. HALPIN, MD
Attending Physician, Olympia Orthopaedics
Associates, Division of Neurosurgery, Olympia,
Washington

DAVID KOJO HAMILTON, MD
Oregon Health and Science University,
Portland, Oregon

ROBERT A. HART, MD
Department of Orthopaedic Surgery, Oregon
Health and Sciences University, Portland, Oregon

JANE S. HOASHI, MD, MPH
Shriners Hospitals for Children—Philadelphia,
Philadelphia, Pennsylvania

RICHARD HOSTIN, MD
Department of Orthopaedic Surgery, Baylor
Scoliosis Center, Plano, Texas

ADAM KANTER, MD
Department of Neurosurgery, University
of Pittsburgh Medical Center, Pittsburgh,
Pennsylvania

MANISH K. KASLIWAL, MD, MCh
Department of Neurosurgery, University of
Virginia Medical Center, Charlottesville, Virginia

KHALID KEBAISH, MD
Department of Orthopaedic Surgery, Johns
Hopkins University, Baltimore, Maryland

ERIC KLINEBERG, MD
Department of Orthopaedic Surgery, University
of California Davis, Sacramento, California

TYLER R. KOSKI, MD
Associate Professor, Department of
Neurological Surgery, Northwestern University
Feinberg School of Medicine, Chicago, Illinois

VIRGINIE LAFAGE, PhD
Department of Orthopaedic Surgery, New York
University Hospital for Joint Diseases,
New York, New York

IAN McCARTHY, PhD
Department of Orthopaedic Surgery,
Institute for Health Care Research and
Improvement, Baylor Health Care System;
Southern Methodist University, Dallas,
Texas

PRAVEEN V. MUMMANENI, MD
Professor and Vice-Chairman, Department
of Neurosurgery, University of California,
San Francisco; Co-Director, UCSF Spine
Center Secretary: AANS-CNS Joint
Section - Spine and Peripheral Nerve,
San Francisco, California

GREGORY M. MUNDIS, MD
Co-Director, San Diego Spine Fellowship
Pediatric and Adult Deformity Spine Surgery,
San Diego Center for Spinal Disorder, La Jolla,
California

MICHAEL O'BRIEN, MD
Baylor Scoliosis Center, Plano, Texas

RAJIV SAIGAL, MD
University of California, San Francisco,
San Francisco, California

AMER F. SAMDANI, MD
Shriners Hospitals for Children—Philadelphia,
Philadelphia, Pennsylvania

JUSTIN K. SCHEER, BS
Medical Student, University of California,
San Diego School of Medicine, La Jolla,
California

FRANK SCHWAB, MD
Department of Orthopaedic Surgery, New York
University Hospital for Joint Diseases,
New York, New York

CHRISTOPHER I. SHAFFREY, MD, FACS
Harrison Distinguished Professor, Neurological
and Orthopaedic Surgery, Department of
Neurosurgery, University of Virginia Medical
Center, Charlottesville, Virginia

JUSTIN S. SMITH, MD, PhD
Department of Neurosurgery, University
of Virginia Medical Center, Charlottesville,
Virginia

PATRICK A. SUGRUE, MD
Resident Physician, Department of
Neurological Surgery, Northwestern University
Feinberg School of Medicine, Chicago, Illinois

JAMIE TERRAN, BS
Department of Orthopaedic Surgery, New York
University Hospital for Joint Diseases,
New York, New York

TSUNG-HSI TU, MD
Research Fellow, Department of Neurosurgery,
University of California, San Francisco,
San Francisco, California; Department
of Neurosurgery, Neurological Institute,
Taipei Veterans General Hospital; School
of Medicine, National Yang-Ming University,
Taipei, Taiwan

JOHN E. ZIEWACZ, MD, MPH
Department of Neurosurgery, University
of California, San Francisco, San Francisco,
California

Contents

Among the prevalent forms of adult spinal deformity are residual adolescent idiopathic and degenerative scoliosis, kyphotic deformity, and spondylolisthesis. Clinical evaluation should include a thorough history, discussion of concerns, and a review of comorbidities. Physical examination should include assessment of the deformity and a neurologic examination. Imaging studies should include full-length standing posteroanterior and lateral spine radiographs, and measurement of pelvic parameters. Advanced imaging studies are frequently indicated to assess for neurologic compromise and for surgical planning. This article focuses on clinical and radiographic evaluation of spinal deformity in the adult population, particularly scoliosis and kyphotic deformities.

The goal of any ambulatory patient is to maintain a horizontal gaze with the least amount of energy expenditure. With progressive deformity, and in particular sagittal malalignment, significant compensatory mechanisms must be used to achieve this goal. Each pelvis dictates the amount of lumbar lordosis required through its morphometric parameter pelvic incidence. The pelvis may compensate for decreasing lumbar lordosis (eg, age, flat back deformity) by retroverting and increasing pelvic tilt and decreasing the sacral slope. Underappreciation for these spinopelvic compensatory mechanisms leads to surgical under-correction, iatrogenic flat back and poor clinical outcomes.

Over the past 3 decades the sagittal plane has received increasing attention from the scientific community and spine surgeons alike. There remains a lack of clear and concise methods for incorporating surgical techniques and radiographic parameters to achieve the best possible outcome on a patient-specific level. This article proposes a new method for a treatment approach to sagittal malalignment by incorporating new digital tools for surgical planning. This technique offers a consistent approach to adult spinal deformity with sagittal-plane components, and can permit optimization in consistently achieving proper postoperative spinopelvic alignment.

Adolescent idiopathic scoliosis (AIS) affects up to 3% of the population. It can be stratified by curve type according to the Lenke classification. This classification system incorporates curve magnitude, flexibility, the lumbar modifier, and the sagittal plane. The Lenke classification serves as a guide for selection of levels for surgical treatment of AIS. Surgical treatment of AIS includes anterior and posterior approaches; most AIS is treated through a posterior approach. Surgical goals include maximizing correction in the coronal, sagittal, and axial planes.

Adult spinal deformity (ASD) is a complex disease state that pathologically alters standing upright posture and is associated with substantial pain and disability. This article provides an overview of classification systems for spinal deformity, clarifies the need to differentiate between pediatric and adult classifications, and provides an explanation on the use of the Scoliosis Research Society-Schwab Adult Spinal Deformity Classification (SRS-Schwab ASD Classification). This information allows surgeons, researchers, and health care providers to (1) identify sources of pain and disability in patients with ASD and (2) accurately use the SRSeSchwab ASD Classification to evaluate patients with ASD.

Scoliosis is a broad term encompassing multiple pathologies with different etiologies. Patients may range from the infant with congenital deformity, to the adolescent with idiopathic scoliosis, to the elderly patient with severe degenerative scoliosis. Treatment must be tailored to individual circumstances and the pathoanatomy of each deformity. Various coronal reduction techniques have been described and will be discussed within this article. While scoliosis is generally considered a deformity in the coronal plane, often deformity is present in the sagittal and axial planes also. Treatment of these deformities can require osteotomies or vertebral column resections, techniques further discussed in accompanying articles.

Various osteotomies are useful in making a rigid deformity flexible enough for realignment in coronal and sagittal plane. This article defines the osteotomies and their usefulness in treatment of specific rigid deformities. The pedicle subtraction osteotomy and vertebral column resection used in treating rigid deformities are described in detail.

Proximal junctional failure (PJF) should be distinguished from proximal junctional kyphosis, which is a recurrent deformity with limited clinical impact. PJF includes mechanical failure, and is a significant complication following adult spinal deformity surgery with potential for neurologic injury and increased need for surgical revision. Risk factors for PJF include age, severity of sagittal plane deformity, and extent of operative sagittal plane realignment. Techniques for avoiding PJF will likely require refinements in both perioperative and surgical strategies.

Treatment Algorithms and Protocol Practice in High-Risk Spine Surgery   219

Patrick A. Sugrue, Ryan J. Halpin, and Tyler R. Koski

The practice of appropriate evidence-based medicine should be a goal for all physicians. By using protocols in areas where strong evidence-based medicine exists, physicians have reliably shown they can improve patient outcomes while reducing complications, cost, and hospital stay. Evidence-based protocols in complex spinal care are rare. At Northwestern University the authors have developed a multidisciplinary protocol for the preoperative, intraoperative, and postoperative workup and care of complex spine patients. The rationale and use of the High-Risk Spine Protocol is discussed.

The Role of Minimally Invasive Techniques in the Treatment of Adult Spinal Deformity   231

Praveen V. Mummaneni, Tsung-Hsi Tu, John E. Ziewacz, Olaolu C. Akinbo, Vedat Deviren, and Gregory M. Mundis

Many surgeons use minimally invasive surgery (MIS) approaches for treatment of patients with adult degenerative spinal deformity. The feasibility and efficacy of these techniques in the treatment of certain subtypes of degenerative deformities have been reported. In this article, several MIS techniques are discussed and an established 6-level treatment algorithm (MiSLAT) is presented, to help guide spinal surgeons in the use of MIS techniques for the treatment of patients with degenerative deformity. MIS treatment of MiSLAT level I to IV deformities is recommended, whereas level V and VI deformities require more traditional open approaches for adequate deformity correction.

Assessment and Treatment of Cervical Deformity   249

Justin K. Scheer, Christopher P. Ames, and Vedat Deviren

Cervical deformity is disruption of normal cervical alignment. This article focuses on the varying etiology of cervical deformity, normative data, and evaluation and examination of deformity, and presents various treatment options for the proper management of these debilitating conditions. Surgical treatment may be indicated in patients with severe mechanical neck pain, neurologic compromise, and progressive deformity causing significant disability, such as dysphagia or loss of horizontal gaze.

Management of High-Grade Spondylolisthesis   275

Manish K. Kasliwal, Justin S. Smith, Adam Kanter, Ching-Jen Chen, Praveen V. Mummaneni, Robert A. Hart, and Christopher I. Shaffrey

Management of high-grade spondylolisthesis (HGS) remains challenging and is associated with significant controversies. The best surgical procedure remains debatable. Although the need for instrumentation is generally agreed upon, significant controversies still surround the role of reduction and anterior column support in the surgical management of HGS. Complications with operative management of HGS can be significant and often dictate the selection of surgical approach. This review highlights the pathophysiology, classification, clinical presentation, and management controversies of HGS, in light of recent advances in our understanding of the importance of sagittal spinopelvic alignment and technologic advancements.

NEUROSURGERY CLINICS OF NORTH AMERICA

**DOWNLOAD
Free App!**

Review Articles
THE CLINICS

NOW AVAILABLE FOR YOUR iPhone and iPad

Preface
Spinal Deformity Surgery

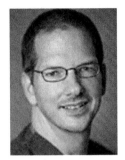

Christopher P. Ames, MD

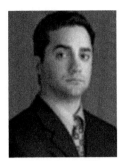

Brian Jian, MD

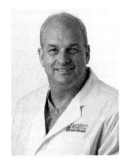

Christopher I. Shaffrey, MD, FACS

Editors

We are delighted to present this issue of *Neurosurgery Clinics of North America* dedicated to the ever expanding role of the neurosurgeon in managing complex adult spinal deformity. Truly, several factors have converged together to create a "perfect storm" of critical educational need in this area.

In the United States we now have an aging population that collectively is demanding improved functionality well into their later years. High prevalence rates of degenerative scoliosis in patients over the age of 65 have been well documented in the literature. Moreover, recently published studies have specifically linked health-related quality of life to specific radiographic thresholds in the sagittal plane. Importantly, neurosurgeons now perform the majority of thoracolumbar surgery in the United States.

Unfortunately, a significant knowledge gap still exists among many spinal surgeons from both neurosurgery and orthopedic surgery on the appropriate preoperative workup and surgical treatment of patients with adult spinal deformity. Commonly, surgeons may report that they do not treat spinal deformity patients and therefore

mastery of these principles is unnecessary. This is however severely flawed logic given the prevalence data and increasingly high rates of revision surgery for iatrogenic deformity. More likely, all neurospinal surgeons are evaluating these patients, but may not be fully appreciating the spinal alignment issues that are already present, nor the alignment goals in fusion surgery.

Over the last 20 years our specialty has progressed tremendously in the realm of complex spinal instrumentation in the areas of trauma, degenerative disease, and spinal oncology. Certainly many spinal neurosurgeons possess the general skill set required to appropriately evaluate and manage adult deformity patients. It is our hope that this work will call further attention to this educational need and serve as a comprehensive and state-of-the-art resource on the topic.

This work in large part represents the combined multidisciplinary efforts of the International Spinal Study Group (ISSG), a group composed of both neurosurgeons and orthopedic surgeons dedicated to high-quality multicenter clinical research and education in adult spinal deformity. The ISSG research work is truly at the forefront of

Neurosurg Clin N Am 24 (2013) xiii–xiv
http://dx.doi.org/10.1016/j.nec.2012.12.013
1042-3680/13/$ – see front matter © 2013 Published by Elsevier Inc.

defining the state-of-the-art treatment and the very latest developments on planning, treatment, and complications are therefore able to be included in this work; for that the editors are deeply grateful and indebted to our colleagues and friends.

Christopher P. Ames, MD
Department of Neurosurgery
Spine Tumor Surgery
Spinal Deformity Surgery
University of California
San Francisco Medical Center
505 Parnassus Avenue, Room M779
San Francisco, CA 94143-0112, USA

Brian Jian, MD
Department of Neurological Surgery
University of California, San Francisco
505 Parnassus Avenue, Room M779
San Francisco, CA 94143-0112, USA

Christopher I. Shaffrey, MD, FACS
Neurological and Orthopaedic Surgery
University of Virginia
P.O. Box 800386
Charlottesville, VA 22908-0386, USA

E-mail addresses:
AmesC@neurosurg.ucsf.edu (C.P. Ames)
brian.jian@gmail.com (B. Jian)
CIS8Z@hscmail.mcc.virginia.edu (C.I. Shaffrey)

Clinical and Radiographic Evaluation of the Adult Spinal Deformity Patient

Justin S. Smith, MD, PhD[a],*, Christopher I. Shaffrey, MD[a],
Kai-Ming G. Fu, MD, PhD[b], Justin K. Scheer, BS[c],
Shay Bess, MD[d], Virginie Lafage, PhD[e], Frank Schwab, MD[e],
Christopher P. Ames, MD[f]

KEYWORDS

- Spine • Deformity • Adult • Imaging • Radiographic • Clinical

KEY POINTS

- Adult spinal deformity encompasses a broad range of conditions. The most common are scoliosis (residual adolescent idiopathic scoliosis, also called adult idiopathic scoliosis, and degenerative or de novo scoliosis), kyphotic deformities with associated positive sagittal malalignment, and spondylolisthesis.
- Clinical evaluation of the adult with spinal deformity should include a thorough history of the condition, discussion of the presenting concerns, and a review of comorbidities. The physical examination should include assessment of the deformity and a complete neurologic examination.
- Imaging studies for adult spinal deformity evaluation should include full-length standing posteroanterior and lateral spine radiographs for assessment of regional and global alignment parameters, as well as measurement of pelvic parameters.
- Advanced imaging studies, including CT, CT myelogram, and MRI, are frequently indicated to assess for neurologic compromise and for surgical planning.

INTRODUCTION

The term adult spinal deformity (ASD) refers to a broad range of spinal conditions that have in common an abnormality of physiologic spinal alignment that may lead to pain, instability, functional disability, cosmetic concerns, neurologic compromise, and/or physiologic dysfunction. A working knowledge of the basic descriptive terminology for ASD is important for those who provide spinal care for these patients. The Scoliosis Research Society (SRS) Terminology Committee and Working Group on Spinal Classification have been proactive in developing and promoting an accurate and accepted nomenclature.[1,2] **Table 1** is a glossary of several frequently used terms, primarily derived from the efforts of the SRS.

Grants, Technical Support, and Corporate Support: No funding was received in support of this study.
IRB: NA (review article).
Disclosures: See last page of the article.
[a] Department of Neurosurgery, University of Virginia, PO Box 800212, Charlottesville, VA 22908, USA; [b] Department of Neurosurgery, Weill Cornell Medical College, 525 East 68th Street, Starr Pavilion 651, New York, NY 10065, USA; [c] University of California San Diego, School of Medicine, 9500 Gilman Dr, La Jolla, CA 92093, USA; [d] Department of Orthopedic Surgery, Rocky Mountain Hospital for Children, 2055 High Street, Suite 130, Denver, CO 80205, USA; [e] Department of Orthopedic Surgery, NYU Hospital for Joint Disease, 333 E 38th Street, 6th Floor, New York, NY 10016, USA; [f] Department of Neurosurgery, University of California San Francisco, 400 Parnassus Avenue, San Francisco, CA 94143, USA
* Corresponding author. Department of Neurosurgery, University of Virginia Health Sciences Center, PO Box 800212, Charlottesville, VA 22908.
E-mail address: jss7f@virginia.edu

neurosurgery.theclinics.com

Table 1
Glossary of descriptive terms for ASD

Term	Definition
Scoliosis	A lateral curvature of the spine on coronal imaging
Kyphosis	A posterior convex angulation of the spine on lateral view with the patient facing rightward. The terms hyperkyphosis and hypokyphosis refer to conditions in which the kyphosis is greater or lesser than the normal range, respectively.
Lordosis	An anterior convex angulation of the spine on lateral view with the patient facing rightward. The terms hyperlordosis and hypolordosis refer to conditions in which the lordosis is greater or less than the normal range, respectively.
Kyphoscoliosis	A scoliosis accompanied by a true hyperkyphosis
Lordoscoliosis	A scoliosis accompanied by a true hyperlordosis
Major Curve	The curve with the largest Cobb angle measurement on upright long cassette radiograph of the spine
Minor Curve	Any curve that does not have the largest Cobb angle measurement on upright long cassette radiograph of the spine
Structural Curve	A measured spinal curve in the coronal plane in which the Cobb measurement fails to correct on supine maximal voluntary lateral side bending radiograph
Compensatory Curve	A minor curve above or below a major curve that may or may not be structural
End Vertebrae	The vertebrae that define the ends of a curve in a coronal or sagittal projection. The cephalad end vertebra is the first vertebra in the cephalad direction from a curve apex whose superior surface is tilted maximally toward the concavity of the curve. The caudal end vertebra is the first vertebra in the caudal direction from a curve apex whose inferior surface is tilted maximally toward the concavity of the curve.
Neutral Vertebra	A vertebra without axial rotation in reference to the most cephalad and caudal vertebrae that are not rotated in a curve
Apical Vertebra	In a curve, the vertebra most deviated laterally from the vertical axis that passes through the patient's sacrum (CSVL)
Apical Disc	In a curve, the disc most deviated laterally from the vertical axis of the patient that passes through the sacrum (CSVL)
Stable Vertebra	The thoracic or lumbar vertebra cephalad to a scoliosis that is most closely bisected by a vertically-directed CSVL, assuming the pelvis is level. Alternatively, both pedicles of this vertebra should lie between vertical reference lines drawn from the sacroiliac joints.
CSVL	The vertical line in a coronal radiograph that passes through the center of the sacrum.
C7 Plumb Line	The vertical line drawn starting from the center of the C7 vertebral body and dropped straight downward. If drawn on a coronal view, the horizontal distance from this line to the central sacral line is a measure of the CA (coronal "balance"), with rightward and leftward deviations designated as positive and negative values, respectively. If drawn on a sagittal view, the horizontal distance from this line to the posterosuperior corner of S1 reflects a measure of the sagittal alignment (SVA), with positive values assigned for C7 plumb lines anterior to the sacrum and negative values assigned for C7 plumb lines that fall behind the sacrum.

Spinal deformity may affect the axial, coronal, and sagittal planes and can involve a combination of abnormalities in multiple planes. Although scoliosis is classically defined based on a lateral curvature of the spine on coronal imaging, it is often a three-dimensional deformity that, in addition to the coronal deformity, may also include a rotational component (axial deformity) and a kyphotic or lordotic component (sagittal deformity). An abnormal sagittal spinal profile (kyphosis or lordosis) may present as a primary deformity or exist in association with other deformities. In uncompensated hyperkyphosis, the normal upright posture of the head over the pelvis and feet (physiologic sagittal alignment) is shifted forward, resulting in positive sagittal malalignment. Spondylolisthesis is a regional abnormality in the sagittal plane in which one vertebra is displaced anteriorly or posteriorly in relation to an adjacent level.

ASD has multiple causes. It may be residual from deformities that presented earlier in life, may result from degenerative conditions, or may be a combination of the two. It may result from unknown factors (eg, adolescent idiopathic scoliosis), congenital anomalies (eg, failure of segmentation), and neuromuscular conditions, including cerebral palsy, spinal cord injury, or spina bifida. ASD may also develop as a consequence of trauma, infection, malignancy, degenerative disease, or iatrogenic causes. Among younger adults, the most common cause for spinal deformity is untreated adolescent idiopathic scoliosis, whereas the most common causes for spinal deformity in middle-aged and older adults include degenerative (de novo) scoliosis, degenerative kyphosis, and iatrogenic causes.

This article focuses on clinical and radiographic evaluation of thoracic and lumbar spinal deformity in the adult population, with a focus on scoliosis and kyphosis.

CLINICAL EVALUATION
Clinical History

Clinical evaluation of the adult with spinal deformity should begin with a thorough history of the condition. For some patients, the initial visit may simply be for education and to establish judicious follow-up of a relatively asymptomatic or incidentally discovered finding. Others may present with pain and disability, neurologic symptoms, or concerns of appearance.[3,4] Establishing the presenting concerns early in the evaluation can be helpful for both the physician and the patient in ensuring that the visit is successful in addressing the needs of the patient.

In contrast to adolescents with spinal deformity, who often present with concerns of cosmesis or progression of deformity, the most common presentation for adults with spinal deformity is pain and disability.[3,5–7] It is important to document the quality, intensity, and location of the pain and whether these have changed over time. Aggravating and ameliorating factors should be elucidated as well. Both leg pain[5,7] and axial back pain[6,7] are common complaints in adults presenting for clinical evaluation of spinal deformity. It should be clarified with patients whether both are present and, if so, the relative severity of each. Aggravating and ameliorating factors should be

elucidated as well. It is also helpful to assess whether nonoperative measures have been used, such as physical therapy, bracing, chiropractic care, medications, or steroid injections, and whether these have been beneficial. For leg pain, it is important to appreciate the distribution of symptoms, whether it is unilateral or bilateral, and whether the symptoms are radicular in nature or more consistent with neurogenic claudication.

Adults with spinal deformity may present with neurologic deficits and care should be taken to elicit a history that may suggest their presence.[4] A history of discrete motor weakness or altered or decreased sensation should be documented, as should symptoms of bowel or bladder dysfunction. Other symptoms of myelopathy should also be discussed, including discoordination and gait unsteadiness. Presence of upper extremity symptoms, such as weakness, numbness, or discoordination, should also be assessed because these may reflect concomitant cervical disease that could affect patient function and treatment approach for thoracolumbar deformity.

The cosmetic appearance of a spinal deformity can be a considerable factor in the psychosocial wellbeing of the patient. The importance of appearance is accepted in the pediatric population, but has yet to be thoroughly evaluated in the adult population.[8,9] Depending on the type and magnitude of the deformity, patients may also report impact on social function. For example, patients with significant positive sagittal malalignment may find it difficult to make eye contact in social interactions. Although pain and disability may dominate the presenting concerns, it is important to also recognize and discuss potential cosmetic and psychosocial issues.

In addition to the clinical history focused on the spinal deformity, it is also important to document other health conditions, previous surgical procedures, and comorbidities. Presence of osteoporosis or osteopenia should be ascertained. In patients with significant thoracic deformity, pulmonary status may need to be addressed. If corrective surgery is considered, a risk-benefit assessment should be performed because adults with deformity, especially older adults, may have significant health issues and surgeries to correct spinal deformity are typically substantial and have inherent risks of complications.[7,10,11] Although presence of comorbidities should not necessarily preclude consideration of surgical treatment, having a thorough appreciation for the patient's global health status is critical to enable effective patient counseling.

It is not uncommon for adults presenting with symptomatic spinal deformity to have had previous spinal surgery, such as limited decompressions, short-segment fusions, or previous surgery for deformity correction.[12] Documenting the previous procedures, including the dates performed and whether they were successful in addressing the symptoms, can be helpful in appreciating the presenting deformity and symptoms, as well as in optimizing subsequent operative and nonoperative management.

Physical Evaluation

Physical examination of the ASD patient should include a global assessment of the deformity. This should be achieved by observing the patient in sequential supine, sitting, and standing postures, and through observing the patient's gait. Rigid thoracic and cervical deformities are readily appreciated in the supine position. Hip flexion contractures can be evaluated by the Thomas test while supine. Sitting removes the effect of the hips and can be used to assess thoracic and lumbar curvature without leg length discrepancy and hip flexion contracture effect.

Standing is the most revealing posture for sagittal and coronal deformity. Trunk shift may be assessed in the coronal plane. Patients should also be assessed with knees extended and locked. In addition, patients with scoliosis should be examined leaning forward at the waist to 90° to reveal rib hump deformities.

Depending on the magnitude, the deformity may be readily apparent on observation (**Figs. 1** and **2**); however, lesser magnitude curves, as are often seen in degenerative lumbar scoliosis, may not be apparent on observation. In both standing and walking postures, the degree to which the patient may be "pitched forward," assume a flattened buttock position, or require knee flexion (crouched posture) can provide indication of positive sagittal malalignment. Camptocormia related to neuromuscular postural disorders such as myopathy and Parkinson disease often become apparent only with gait testing. Coronal imbalance, leg length discrepancy and obliquity of the pelvis may also be apparent.

Sagittal spinal alignment has been strongly correlated with measures of health-related quality

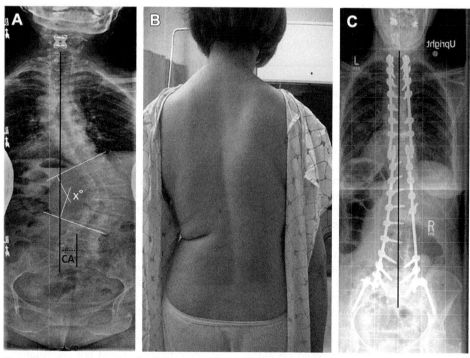

Fig. 1. Clinical photographs and radiographs of a 52-year-old woman presenting with back pain and right lower extremity radicular pain. (*A*) Preoperative posteroanterior radiograph demonstrates a dextroscoliosis with an apex at L1-2. X, coronal Cobb angle measurement. The C7 plumb line and central sacral vertical line are shown in black, and the distance between these (the coronal alignment [CA]) is depicted by the horizontal dashed line. In this case the CA is a negative value (−2.8 cm) because the C7 plumb line falls to the left of CSVL. Findings on clinical assessment are subtle. (*B*). Postoperative full-length posteroanterior radiograph following instrumented correction of the deformity (*C*). The C7 plumb line is shown in black and demonstrates restoration of CA.

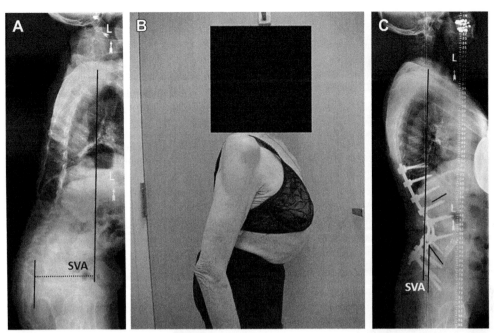

Fig. 2. Clinical photograph and radiographs of a 52-year-old woman presenting with back pain and right lower extremity radicular pain. (*A*) Preoperative full-length lateral radiograph demonstrates positive sagittal malalignment and pelvic retroversion. The C7 plumb line and a vertical line drawn at the posterosuperior aspect of the sacrum are drawn with solid black lines. The horizontal distance between these is shown as a dashed line and is the sagittal vertical axis (SVA). Findings on clinical assessment include a pronounced forward posture and pelvic retroversion on side profile (*B*). Postoperative full-length sagittal radiograph following instrumented correction of the deformity (*C*). Note that the C7 plumb line falls within 2 cm of the posterosuperior aspect of the sacrum, reflecting good restoration of sagittal spinal alignment.

of life.[13–20] Recent studies have demonstrated that the pelvis is a critical component of spinal alignment because the morphology of the pelvis sets the magnitude of lumbar lordosis necessary, which in turn, correlates with thoracic and cervical alignment, in a chain of correlation.[13,18,20–28] Evidence of compensatory mechanisms may also be evident in patients with significant positive sagittal spinopelvic malalignment (**Fig. 3**). In an effort to bring the head into alignment with the pelvis in the sagittal plane, these patients may compensate with pelvic retroversion, which results in the acetabulum assuming a more anterior position. Mild pelvic retroversion may be accompanied by hip extension, whereas more severe or fixed deformities may be accompanied by hip and knee flexion. Patients with chronic positive sagittal malalignment may develop hip flexion contracture that can prevent successful sagittal realignment surgery and should be identified and addressed with physical therapy preoperatively.

Pelvic obliquity may also be evident on clinical and radiographic evaluation and, when present, the radiographic studies should be repeated with a shoe lift (or standing blocks) that approximates the length discrepancy to assess the potential effect on the spinal curve.

A general neurologic assessment of the adult with spinal deformity should include assessment of motor strength and sensation, muscle tone, reflexes (peripheral, abdominal, and pathologic), coordination, and gait. Signs of myelopathy, such as hyperreflexia, clonus, and an impaired gait, may be present in patients with severe thoracic or concomitant cervical disease. This may prompt the need for cervical MRI before lumbar deformity correction.

RADIOGRAPHIC EVALUATION
Conventional Radiographs

Imaging studies are critical to the evaluation of ASD. Initial imaging evaluation typically begins with posteroanterior (PA) and lateral 36-in radiographs to provide assessment of global and regional spinopelvic alignment.[29] For patients able to stand, these radiographs should be obtained in a free-standing posture, with elbows flexed at approximately 45° and fingertips on the clavicles. This position ensures capturing the true degree of deformity

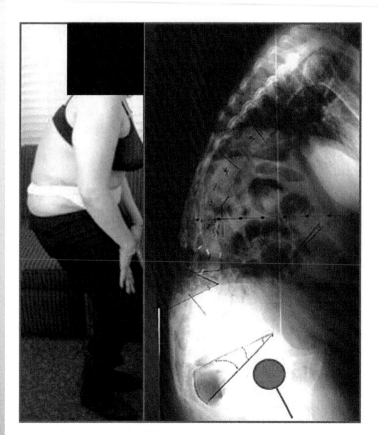

Fig. 3. Compensatory measures of positive sagittal malalignment. A 48-year-old woman with lumbar kyphosis and substantial positive sagittal malalignment shown in clinical photograph (*left panel*) and corresponding lateral standing radiograph (*right panel*) illustrates compensatory pelvic retroversion (increased pelvic tilt) and hip and knee flexion. These compensatory measures are attempts to maintain an upright posture.

and recruitment of compensatory mechanisms without influence from supports. To facilitate radiographic measurements, it is important that the radiographs include visualization of the cervical spine that is at least sufficient to localize the C7 vertebral body and allows for visualization of the bilateral femoral heads.

The PA radiographs should routinely be viewed with the heart on the left side (ie, true-left, true-right) (see **Fig. 1**C). This view enables assessment of the coronal alignment (CA) (**Fig. 4**A). Coronal decompensation is measured as the horizontal distance between a plumb line dropped downward from the center of the C7 (C7PL) vertebral body and the central sacral vertical line (CSVL), which is a line drawn vertically through the center of the sacrum. A C7PL that falls to the left or right of the CSVL is designated with negative or positive values, respectively. A CA of 0 is designated as neutral. Pelvic obliquity can also be measured based on the PA view, as illustrated in **Fig. 4**B. If pelvic obliquity is detected, lower extremity scanograms should be taken to assess limb length discrepancy. Limb length discrepancy may be primary due to congenital length differences or may be secondary due to osteoarthritis or improperly sized lower extremity joint replacements.

The PA view is also used to assess for coronal curvature of the spine (scoliosis). The location of a coronal curvature is defined by the apex of the curve. The apex is typically the disc or vertebra that is maximally displaced from the midline and minimally angulated. A deformity is considered thoracic if it has an apex between T2 and the T11–12 disc, thoracolumbar if the apex lies between T12 and L1 vertebra, and lumbar if the apex is at or distal to the L1–2 disc. In scoliosis the curve is described based on the side of its convexity. A curve convex to the right is designated as dextroscoliosis and a curve convex to the left is designated as levoscoliosis. There are always two or more scoliotic curves in the coronal plane. The largest curve is considered the major curve because it is the primary deformity force in the coronal plane. The smaller curves that are adjacent to the major curve are termed minor curves. Minor curves may be compensatory or structural depending on the flexibility of the curve on side-bending radiographs. Side-bending radiographs should be obtained with the patient in the supine position to eliminate gravity and obtain the greatest amount of correction. Compensatory curves are flexible on side-bending radiographs (typically reduced to <25°), whereas structural

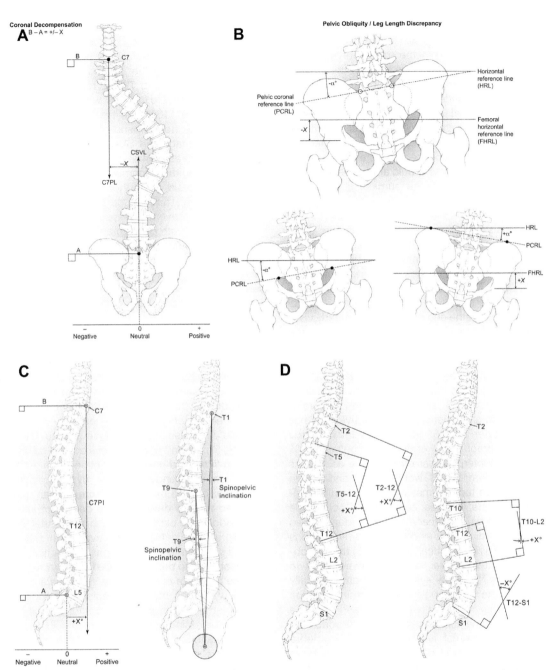

Fig. 4. Spinal radiographic measures and pelvic obliquity. (*A*) Coronal view of the spine illustrating technique to measure CA, which is the horizontal distance "X" between the C7 plumb line (C7PL) and the central sacral vertical line (CSVL). (*B*) Pelvic obliquity and leg length discrepancy. Illustrations of the technique to measure pelvic obliquity. (*C*) Sagittal view of the spine illustrating technique to measure sagittal alignment based on the SVA, which is the horizontal distance ("X") between the posterior superior corner of the sacrum and the C7PL (*left panel*). Also shown are the techniques to measure the T1 and T9 spinopelvic inclinations (T1SPI and T9SPI, respectively), which are alternative measures of global sagittal alignment that do not rely on imaging scaling. (*D*) Drawings showing methods to assess regional sagittal spinal alignment, including T2-T12 TK, T5-T12 TK, T10-L2 thoracolumbar junction alignment, and the lumbar lordosis (T12-S1 angle). PCRL, pelvic coronal reference line; HRL, horizontal reference line; FHRL, femoral horizontal reference line. (*Courtesy of* K.X. Probst/Xavier Studio, 2012; with permission.)

minor curves are rigid (typically >25° on supine side-bending radiographs). Compensatory curves develop in response to the major curve to help maintain the head over the pelvis in the coronal plane and will typically correct spontaneously after surgically correcting the major curve. However, minor curves that are structural are sources of deformity that behave independently from the major curve and, therefore, will not spontaneously correct after correcting the major curve. Therefore, structural minor curves should always be identified and incorporated into the surgical construct to reduce the risk of residual postoperative spinal deformity.

Scoliosis angles are measured via the Cobb method (see **Fig. 1**A). This technique involves selecting the vertebrae maximally tilted into the curve (end vertebra). Lines are drawn parallel to the superior end plate of the cephalad end vertebra and the inferior end plate of the caudal end vertebra. If the end plates are not clearly visualized, an alternative technique is to use the pedicle margins as the basis for these lines. Bisecting perpendicular lines from the endplate lines are drawn, and the angle determined. The Cobb technique is classically thought to have an inherent error of 3° to 5°. Therefore, generally, a change in angle between consecutive films has to be greater than 5° to be considered a true change. Intraobserver error ranges between 1% to 5% and interobserver error can be as high as 10°.[30] Modern PACS workstations and image viewers have tools to measure Cobb angles digitally. To date, studies comparing Cobb angle measurements of primary and secondary curves on digital radiographs and traditional radiographs have shown no statistical difference in the intraobserver or interobserver variance between the two techniques.[31–33] New systems that automatically measure the Cobb angle and determine rotation are currently under development and may be able to reduce intraobserver and interobserver variability. Proximal and distal neutral vertebra (not rotated in axial plane) and stable vertebra (vertebra above and below the end vertebra that is bisected by the CSVL) may also be determined because these are used to help select fusion levels in operative planning.

By convention, the lateral full-length radiograph should be oriented such that the patient faces toward the right (see **Fig. 2**A). This view allows assessment of regional and global sagittal alignment (see **Fig. 4**C–D). The sagittal vertical axis (SVA0 is a global measure of sagittal alignment and is the horizontal distance between the C7PL and the posterior superior corner of the sacrum (see **Fig. 4**C). A C7PL that falls behind or in front

of the posterior superior corner of the sacrum is designated with negative or positive values, respectively. Alternative measures of global sagittal spinal alignment are the T1 and T9 spinopelvic inclinations (T1SPI and T9SPI, respectively) (see **Fig. 4**C). In contrast to the SVA, which is a measure of distance, the T1SPI and the T9SPI are angles and, therefore, not dependent on knowing the scale of the image. An SVA T1SPI, or T9SPI of 0 is designated as neutral.

Regional sagittal alignment measures include thoracic kyphosis (TK), thoracolumbar junction alignment (TLA), and lumbar lordosis (LL) (see **Fig. 4**D). By convention, kyphosis and lordosis are designated with positive and negative values. Common measures of TK are based on the vertebral end plates spanning T2 to T12 or T5 to T12. Assessment of TLA typically reflects the angle spanning the cephalad and caudal endplates of T10 and L2, respectively (see **Fig. 4**D). A common measure of lumbar lordosis is based on the angle between cephalad and caudal endplates of T12 and S1, respectively.

A comparison between the degree of deformity between weight bearing and non-weightbearing films (ie, supine) provides information regarding the rigidity of the deformity. Additional views to help determine stiffness of the deformity can also be helpful. These views include supine lateral bending films, bending films over a bolster, fulcrum bending films, and push and traction views. In the evaluation of spondylolisthesis, dynamic lateral views (flexion and extension) of the lumbar spine are used to help determine the degree of instability. Additional plain radiograph views that can be helpful in spinal deformity evaluation include oblique views to visualize the pars interarticularis, Ferguson view to better visualize the sacral region, and the Stagnara or Leeds view, which is an oblique view through the apical region of a scoliotic curve that accounts for rotation and thus allows better visualization of the pedicles.

Axial rotation on conventional radiograph can be determined using the Nash-Moe method. The Nash-Moe method categorizes vertebral rotation into five grades based on the location of the pedicle in relation to the lateral aspect of the vertebral body.[34] CT imaging may facilitate more accurate measurement of rotation than standard radiograph techniques.[35]

Overall sagittal spinal alignment is substantially affected by relationship of the spine to the pelvis.[13,20,24,26] (Schwab F, Bess S, Blondel B, et al. Combined assessment of pelvic tilt, pelvic incidence or lumbar lordosis mismatch and sagittal vertical axis predicts disability in adult spinal deformity: a prospective analysis. 2012.

Submitted for publication.) An adult patient with thoracic hyperkyphosis or loss of lumbar lordosis will attempt to compensate for positive sagittal malalignment through pelvic retroversion. Key measures of pelvic alignment include pelvic incidence (PI), pelvic tilt (PT), and sacral slope (SS) (**Fig. 5**). The PI is a morphologic parameter that is a fixed angle in each individual once skeletal maturity is reached and does not depend on the position of the pelvis. Although normative mean values for PI range from 50° to 55°, individual reported normative values encountered range broadly, from 28° to 84°.[36] Consistent with the morphologic nature of PI, it does not vary with age. (Blondel B, Schwab F, Ames C, et al. Age-related cervical and spinopelvic parameter

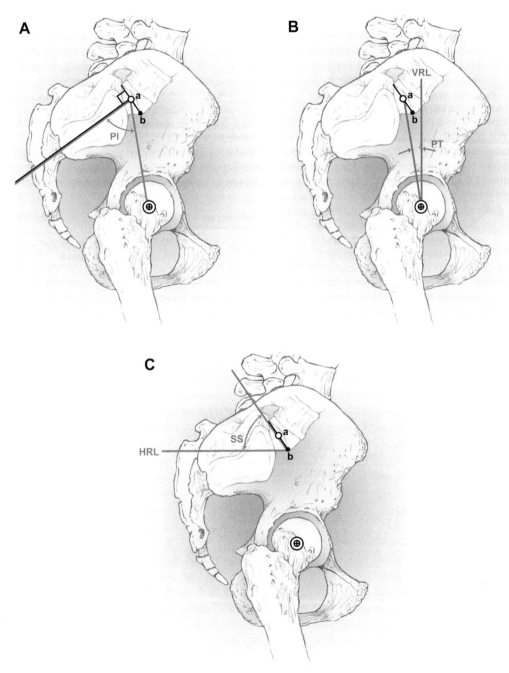

Fig. 5. Measures of sagittal pelvic alignment. PI (*A*), PT (*B*), and SS (*C*). (*Courtesy of* K.X. Probst/Xavier Studio, 2012; with permission.)

variations in a volunteer population. 2012. Submitted for publication.) The PI is measured by determining the angle between a line drawn perpendicular to the sacral end plate at its midpoint and a line from the femoral head axis to this point (see **Fig. 5**). If the femoral heads are not perfectly aligned with each other on lateral radiograph, the femoral head axis location is approximated by the midpoint of a line connecting the geometric center of each femoral head. The PT is a measure of the degree of pelvic retroversion and is a compensatory parameter, such that a patient with positive sagittal malalignment who retroverts the pelvis in an effort to maintain an upright posture will have an increase in the PT. Normative mean values for PT range from 11° to 15°, and individual reported normative values range from −5° to 31°. A PT greater than or equal to 22° has been suggested as a threshold value for moderate disability (Oswestry Disability Index [ODI] score >40) in the setting of ASD. (Schwab F, Blondel B, Bess S, et al. Radiographic spinopelvic parameters and disability in the setting of adult spinal deformity: a prospective multicenter analysis. 2012. Submitted for publication.) The PT is the angle determined between a vertical reference line drawn up from the center of the femoral heads (femoral head axis) and a line drawn from the femoral head axis to the midpoint of the sacral end plate (see **Fig. 5**). The SS is the angle of a line drawn along the sacral end plate relative to a reference horizontal line (see **Fig. 5**). A mathematical relationship exists among these pelvic parameters such that the PI is the sum of the PT and the SS (PI = PT + SS).[21]

Assessment of pelvic parameters can be particularly helpful for surgical planning. Because the PT is a compensatory mechanism, it can mask the degree to which a patient is sagittally malaligned. Thus, a patient may have an SVA that appears to be relatively close to normal but may be maximally compensating by increasing the PT and decreasing the SS. Not taking into account this compensation could lead to continued symptoms due to undercorrection in the sagittal plane. In addition, a relationship between PI and LL has been reported in normal subjects and it can be approximated that the LL should be within 9° of the PI.[13,20,21,26] (Schwab F, Bess S, Blondel B, et al. Combined assessment of pelvic tilt, pelvic incidence or lumbar lordosis mismatch and sagittal vertical axis predicts disability in adult spinal deformity: a prospective analysis. 2012 Submitted for publication.) This relationship can be particularly useful in patients with flat back deformity in determining the magnitude of lumbar lordosis that needs to be recreated with surgical treatment.

Advanced Imaging

Advanced imaging has become nearly standard in the evaluation of adults with spinal deformity. Common modalities include MRI, CT, CT myelography, CT angiography (CTA), and MR angiography (MRA). MRI gives excellent soft tissue detail and is useful in demonstrating disc disease, spondylotic changes, and intraspinal anomalies (**Fig. 6**). MRI should be obtained in all cases with any question of neurologic compromise unless contraindicated. Although CT imaging gives

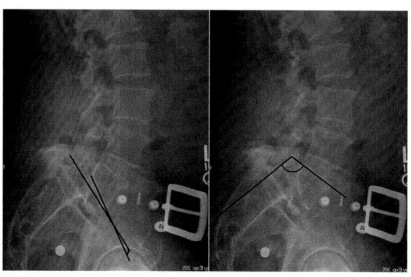

Fig. 6. Lateral radiograph demonstrating measurement of Boxall slip angle (*left*) and Dubousset lumbosacral angle (*right*).

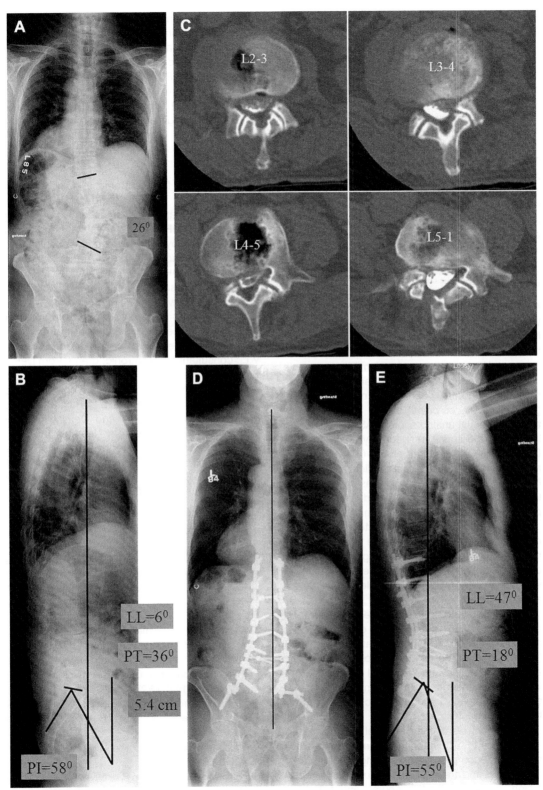

Fig. 7. Imaging studies of a 67-year-old man who presented with severe low back pain when standing, including preoperative PA (*A*) and lateral (*B*) full-length standing radiographs, CT myelogram axial images (*C*), and PA (*D*) and lateral (*E*) full-length standing radiographs at 36 months following surgical correction. See text for clinical details. LL, lumbar lordosis; PI, pelvic incidence; PT, pelvic tilt.

excellent bony detail and is extremely useful in preoperative planning, CT myelography has the added benefit of providing intraspinal information in addition to high-resolution bony detail. CTA and MRA are useful in the evaluation of vascular anatomy, which may have surgical approach implications.

Advances in imaging software such as multiplanar rendering (MPR) allow the surgeon to view multislice CT and MRI data in multiple and adjustable planes. This allows for more accurate preoperative measurement of pedicle diameter and a greater appreciation of the disease process. Three-dimensional reconstructions can easily be created to aid in operative planning (see **Fig. 6**). Thin-cut CT myelography plus MPR provides extremely useful information in operative planning for deformity.

CASE EXAMPLE

A 67-year-old recently retired executive presents with severe low back pain when standing that improves to only a mild ache when sitting that has been present and progressive for the last 5 years. He has symptoms of mild neurogenic claudication but denies any decreased change in radicular symptoms, sensation, motor strength, gait difficulties, or bowel and/or bladder symptoms. His visual analog score (VAS) for back and leg pain are 8 and 2, respectively, on a scale of 0 to 10. His ODI is 48 out of 100 (reflecting high-moderate disability). His past medical and surgical history are significant for hypertension, hypercholesterolemia, appendectomy, and a right L5-S1 posterior hemilaminotomy and microdiscectomy approximately 10 years ago, with resolution of right leg radicular symptoms. He has exhausted nonoperative measures, including multiple trials of physical therapy, narcotics, epidural steroid injections, and facet blocks. He presents for a fourth opinion.

Full-length standing PA and lateral radiographs demonstrate a 26° degenerative dextroscoliosis, measured from T12-L4, with an apex at L3 (**Fig. 7**A) and SVA of 5.4 cm, LL of 6°, PT of 36°, and PI of 58° (see **Fig. 7**B). Axial CT myelogram images demonstrate mild and moderate canal stenosis at the L2-3 and L4-5 disc levels, respectively (see **Fig. 7**C).

The patient elected for surgical treatment and underwent T11-S1 posterior instrumented arthrodesis and decompression, including placement of iliac screws and an L5-S1 anterior lumbar interbody fusion. The postoperative course and follow-up were uncomplicated. At 36-month follow-up, his back and leg pain had resolved (both VAS back and leg pain scores of 0) and his ODI had improved

to 8 (reflecting minimal disability). PA and lateral full-length standing radiographs demonstrated no significant coronal or sagittal spinal malalignment, and radiographic parameters include LL of 47°, PT of 18°, and PI of 55° (see **Fig. 7**D, E). Note that the PI-LL mismatch is now within 9°, the PT is within normal limits (<25°), and the spine is coronally and sagittally aligned.

DISCLOSURES

J.S.: consultant for Medtronic, DePuy, and Biomet; honoraria for teaching from Medtronic, DePuy, Biomet, and Globus; research study group support from DePuy. C.S.: consultant and patent from Biomet; royalties from and consultant for Medtronic; honoraria from DePuy; research support from NIH, DOD, and NACTN; research and fellowship support from AO; consultant for Globus and Nuvasive. K-M.F. and J.S.: none. S.B.: consulting, research support, and speaking for DePuy Spine; consulting for and research support from Medtronic; royalties from Pioneer. V.L.: consultant for Medtronic; grants from DePuy Spine; honoraria from DePuy Spine and K2M; stocks from Nemaris, Inc. F.S.: consultant for DePuy Spine; grants from NIH, DePuy, Medtronic; honoraria from Medtronic and DePuy; royalties from Medtronic; stocks from Nemaris, Inc. C.A.: consultant for DePuy, Medtronic, and Stryker; employment with UCSF; grants from Trans1; patents with Fish & Richardson and PC; royalties from Aesculap and LAWX.

REFERENCES

1. Lenke L. SRS terminology committee and working group on spinal classification revised glossary terms. 2000. Available at: http://www.srs.org/professionals/glossary/glossary.php. (Accessed on November 30, 2012).
2. Stokes IA. Three-dimensional terminology of spinal deformity. A report presented to the Scoliosis Research Society by the Scoliosis Research Society Working Group on 3-D terminology of spinal deformity. Spine 1994;19(2):236–48.
3. Bess S, Boachie-Adjei O, Burton D, et al. Pain and disability determine treatment modality for older patients with adult scoliosis, while deformity guides treatment for younger patients. Spine 2009;34(20): 2186–90.
4. Smith JS, Fu KM, Urban P, et al. Neurological symptoms and deficits in adults with scoliosis who present to a surgical clinic: incidence and association with the choice of operative versus nonoperative management. J Neurosurg Spine 2008;9(4):326–31.

5. Smith JS, Shaffrey CI, Berven S, et al. Operative versus nonoperative treatment of leg pain in adults with scoliosis: a retrospective review of a prospective multicenter database with two-year follow-up. Spine 2009;34(16):1693–8.

6. Smith JS, Shaffrey CI, Berven S, et al. Improvement of back pain with operative and nonoperative treatment in adults with scoliosis. Neurosurgery 2009; 65(1):86–93 [discussion: 93–4].

7. Smith JS, Shaffrey CI, Glassman SD, et al. Risk-benefit assessment of surgery for adult scoliosis: an analysis based on patient age. Spine 2011;36(10): 817–24.

8. Koch KD, Buchanan R, Birch JG, et al. Adolescents undergoing surgery for idiopathic scoliosis: how physical and psychological characteristics relate to patient satisfaction with the cosmetic result. Spine 2001;26(19):2119–24.

9. Smith PL, Donaldson S, Hedden D, et al. Parents' and patients' perceptions of postoperative appearance in adolescent idiopathic scoliosis. Spine 2006;31(20):2367–74.

10. Smith JS, Kasliwal MK, Crawford A, et al. Outcomes, expectations, and complications overview for the surgical treatment of adult and pediatric spinal deformity. Spine Deformity 2012;(Preview Issue):4–14.

11. Fu KM, Smith JS, Sansur CA, et al. Standardized measures of health status and disability and the decision to pursue operative treatment in elderly patients with degenerative scoliosis. Neurosurgery 2010;66(1):42–7 [discussion: 47].

12. Kasliwal MK, Smith JS, Shaffrey CI, et al. Does prior short-segment surgery for adult scoliosis impact perioperative complication rates and clinical outcome among patients undergoing scoliosis correction? J Neurosurg Spine 2012;17(2):128–33.

13. Ames CP, Smith JS, Scheer JK, et al. Impact of spinopelvic alignment on decision making in deformity surgery in adults: a review. J Neurosurg Spine 2012; 16(6):547–64.

14. Blondel B, Schwab F, Ungar B, et al. Impact of magnitude and percentage of global sagittal plane correction on health-related quality of life at 2-years follow-up. Neurosurgery 2012;71(2):341–8.

15. Glassman SD, Berven S, Bridwell K, et al. Correlation of radiographic parameters and clinical symptoms in adult scoliosis. Spine 2005;30(6): 682–8.

16. Glassman SD, Bridwell K, Dimar JR, et al. The impact of positive sagittal balance in adult spinal deformity. Spine 2005;30(18):2024–9.

17. Jackson RP, McManus AC. Radiographic analysis of sagittal plane alignment and balance in standing volunteers and patients with low back pain matched for age, sex, and size. A prospective controlled clinical study. Spine 1994;19(14):1611–8.

18. Lafage V, Smith JS, Bess S, et al. Sagittal spino-pelvic alignment failures following three column thoracic osteotomy for adult spinal deformity. Eur Spine J 2012;21(4):698–704.

19. Schwab F, Farcy JP, Bridwell K, et al. A clinical impact classification of scoliosis in the adult. Spine 2006;31(18):2109–14.

20. Schwab F, Lafage V, Patel A, et al. Sagittal plane considerations and the pelvis in the adult patient. Spine 2009;34(17):1828–33.

21. Boulay C, Tardieu C, Hecquet J, et al. Sagittal alignment of spine and pelvis regulated by pelvic incidence: standard values and prediction of lordosis. Eur Spine J 2006;15(4):415–22.

22. Klineberg E, Schwab F, Ames C, et al. Acute reciprocal changes distant from the site of spinal osteotomies affect global postoperative alignment. Adv Orthop 2011;2011:415946.

23. Lafage V, Ames C, Schwab F, et al. Changes in thoracic kyphosis negatively impact sagittal alignment after lumbar pedicle subtraction osteotomy: a comprehensive radiographic analysis. Spine 2012;37(3):E180–7.

24. Lafage V, Bharucha NJ, Schwab F, et al. Multicenter validation of a formula predicting postoperative spinopelvic alignment. J Neurosurg Spine 2012;16(1): 15–21.

25. Schwab FJ, Patel A, Shaffrey CI, et al. Sagittal realignment failures following pedicle subtraction osteotomy surgery: are we doing enough?: clinical article. J Neurosurg Spine 2012;16(6):539–46.

26. Smith JS, Bess S, Shaffrey CI, et al. Dynamic changes of the pelvis and spine are key to predicting postoperative sagittal alignment after pedicle subtraction osteotomy: a critical analysis of preoperative planning techniques. Spine 2012;37(10): 845–53.

27. Smith JS, Shaffrey CI, Lafage V, et al. Spontaneous improvement of cervical alignment after correction of global sagittal balance following pedicle subtraction osteotomy. J Neurosurg Spine 2012;17(4):300–7.

28. Schwab F, Bess S, Blondel B, et al. Combined assessment of pelvic tilt, pelvic incidence or lumbar lordosis mismatch, and sagittal vertical axis predicts disability in adult spinal deformity: a prospective analysis. Spine 2012.

29. Angevine PD, Kaiser MG. Radiographic measurement techniques. Neurosurgery 2008;63(Suppl 3): 40–5.

30. Morrissy RT, Goldsmith GS, Hall EC, et al. Measurement of the Cobb angle on radiographs of patients who have scoliosis. Evaluation of intrinsic error. J Bone Joint Surg Am 1990;72(3):320–7.

31. Gstoettner M, Sekyra K, Walochnik N, et al. Inter- and intraobserver reliability assessment of the Cobb angle: manual versus digital measurement tools. Eur Spine J 2007;16(10):1587–92.

32. Kuklo TR, Potter BK, Schroeder TM, et al. Comparison of manual and digital measurements in adolescent idiopathic scoliosis. Spine 2006;31(11):1240–6.

33. Mok JM, Berven SH, Diab M, et al. Comparison of observer variation in conventional and three digital radiographic methods used in the evaluation of patients with adolescent idiopathic scoliosis. Spine 2008;33(6):681–6.

34. Nash CL Jr, Moe JH. A study of vertebral rotation. J Bone Joint Surg Am 1969;51(2):223–9.

35. Lam GC, Hill DL, Le LH, et al. Vertebral rotation measurement: a summary and comparison of common radiographic and CT methods. Scoliosis 2008; 3:16.

36. Schwab F, Patel A, Ungar B, et al. Adult spinal deformity-postoperative standing imbalance: how much can you tolerate? An overview of key parameters in assessing alignment and planning corrective surgery. Spine 2010;35(25): 2224–31.

Sagittal Spinal Pelvic Alignment

Eric Klineberg, MD[a],*, Frank Schwab, MD[b],
Justin S. Smith, MD, PhD[c], Munish C. Gupta, MD[a],
Virginie Lafage, PhD[b], Shay Bess, MD[d]

KEYWORDS

• Spine • Deformity • Adult • Radiographic • Pelvic • Sagittal

KEY POINTS

- The spine and pelvis have robust compensatory mechanisms to achieve a globally well-aligned spine (center of mass over pelvis, horizontal eye gaze) to allow for minimum energy expenditure.
- Pelvic incidence is a morphometric parameter and is both constant and dictates the amount of lumbar lordosis needed to achieve a globally aligned spine.
- Pelvic tilt and sacral slope are compensatory mechanisms that reflect pelvic rotation in space (sagittal) and reflect efforts to maintain global alignment in the setting of spinal deformity.
- Pelvic parameters play a critical role in heath-related quality of life outcome measures and must be accounted for when planning spinal surgery.
- Underappreciation of the compensatory mechanisms in the pelvis may lead surgeons to poor surgical planning and corresponding poor clinical outcomes.

INTRODUCTION

Adult spinal deformity is a broad category that encompasses a diverse group of spinal malalignment patterns. The range of diseases extends from simple biplanar deformity to a more complex three-dimensional deformity with significant loss of coronal and sagittal alignment. With an aging population, the prevalence of adult spinal deformity is increasing in the United States and may be approaching rates as high as 70% among elderly individuals.[1] Although most patients are able to tolerate mild to moderate deformities without significant dysfunction, there is a subset of patients who experience significant back pain, root compression, and loss of acceptable standing global alignment.[2] Whereas historically, treatment focused on scoliosis correction and coronal plane deformity, more recent data have shown the impact of the sagittal plane, and lumbopelvic parameters on health-related quality of life (HRQoL).[3–6] These parameters are therefore critical to understand and integrate for successful surgical planning in the setting of adult spinal deformity.[3,4,7,8]

CONE OF ECONOMY

The ability to maintain an upright posture and horizontal eye gaze is fundamental to normal activities

Grants, Technical Support, and Corporate Support: No funding was received in support of this study.
IRB: NA (review article).
[a] Department of Orthopaedic Surgery, University of California – Davis, 4860 Y Street, Suite 3800, Sacramento, CA 95817, USA; [b] Department of Orthopaedic Surgery, NYU Hospital for Joint Diseases, 306 East 15th Street, Suite 1F, New York, NY 10003, USA; [c] Department of Neurosurgery, University of Virginia, PO Box 800212, Charlottesville, VA 22908, USA; [d] Rocky Mountain Hospital for Children, 2055 High Street, Suite 130, Denver, CO 80205, USA
* Corresponding author. Department of Orthopaedic Surgery, University of California – Davis, 4860 Y Street, #3800, Sacramento, CA 95817.
E-mail address: eric.klineberg@ucdmc.ucdavis.edu

Neurosurg Clin N Am 24 (2013) 157–162
http://dx.doi.org/10.1016/j.nec.2012.12.003
1042-3680/13/$ – see front matter © 2013 Elsevier Inc. All rights reserved.

of daily living. Spinal deformity creates suboptimal spinal alignment, and may result in increased energy requirements to maintain appropriate posture and balance. The spine is not the only structure that is involved in the standing axis, and any analysis that attempts to understand global alignment must involve the pelvis and lower extremities.[9–15] Dubousset[16] was the first surgeon to consider the pelvis as a critical structure in the setting of global alignment and introduced the concept of a cone of economy (**Fig. 1**). The cone is defined as originating from the feet and projected upwards to define the range of mobility that the body can achieve with a minimum of energy expenditure, without external support. If the spinal alignment is ideal, the patient is able to maintain an upright posture in the zone of economy and allow for painless upright posture at rest and during motion.[9] If the body is forced out of this cone (spinal deformity), the energy expenditure increases with the need for compensatory mechanisms (ie, bending of the knee, or pelvic retroversion). The patient may require assistive devices if internal compensation is insufficient

or requires excessive energy.[16] The degree of global alignment can be determined by radiographic parameters that assess the patient in a static position. Such an approach allows the physician to determine where the trunk is in relation to the pelvis and to determine some of the compensatory mechanisms that are being used. For optimal radiographic analysis, it is essential that patients stand upright in a free-standing position[17] and then 91.44-cm (36-in) cassette films are obtained in both the coronal and sagittal planes.

SAGITTAL VERTICAL AXIS

Global spinal alignment is most often assessed by determining the sagittal vertical axis (SVA). The SVA is determined by measuring the horizontal distance from the C7 plumb line and the posterior superior aspect of the S1 vertebral body (**Fig. 2**). Positive and negative values are defined depending whether the C7 plumb line falls anterior or posterior, respectively. Normative values have been established as being less then 5 cm. The C7 plumb serves as a surrogate for where the

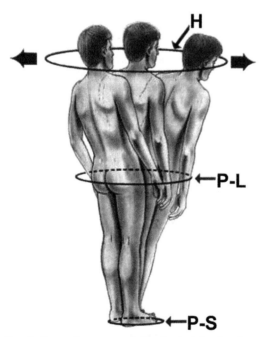

Fig. 1. Cone of economy defined as originating from the feet and projected upwards to define the range of mobility that the body can achieve with a minimum of energy expenditure, without external support. H, Head; P-L, Pelvic Level; and P-S, Polygon of Sustentation. (*From* Dubousset J. Three-dimensional analysis of the scoliotic deformity. In: Weinstein SL (ed): The Pediatric Spine: Principles and Practice. New York: Raven Press, 1994; with permission.)

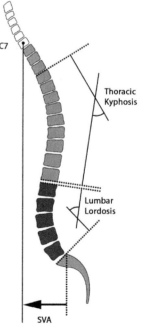

Fig. 2. Sagittal spinal parameters. The SVA is determined by measuring the horizontal distance from the C7 plumb line and the posterior superior aspect of the S1 vertebral body. Lumbar lordosis is measured from the superior end plate of L1 to the superior end plate of S1. Thoracic kyphosis can be determined by measuring the angle of the thoracic spine from the superior vertebral end plate of T2 and the inferior end plate of T12.

head falls in space but ignores the cervical alignment. Similarly, the S1 vertebral body serves as a surrogate for where the feet are in space but ignores the contribution of the foot, knees, hips, and pelvis. Although this global assessment gives the surgeon a general idea of the global sagittal deformity, it underappreciates the role of the pelvis and compensatory mechanisms used.

SPINAL ALIGNMENT

Global spinal alignment may be subdivided into its component parts, namely the thoracic kyphosis (TK) and lumbar lordosis (LL). LL is measured from the superior end plate of L1 to the superior end plate of S1 and plays an important role in maintenance of upright posture (see **Fig. 2**).[14] Normative values of 40° to 60° have been described in the adult population; however, that number seems to decrease with aging. Decreasing lordosis or flatback deformity has been associated with inability to maintain spinal balance, and resultant pain and disability.[18] In addition, TK can be determined by measuring the angle of the thoracic spine from the superior vertebral end plate of T2 and the inferior end plate of T12. TK also increases with age and influences global spinal alignment.

THE PELVIS

The pelvis is the base of the spine. Its morphology determines the foundation on to which the spine is seated. Although the morphology is relatively constant in adulthood, the mobile spine may adapt to the sacral position, adjusting the degree of curvature to achieve a mechanically efficient posture.[19] In order for the body to achieve an efficient upright posture, the spine must be in harmony with the pelvis. This harmony has been coined the spinopelvic alignment[20] to describe the synergistic relationship between pelvic morphology and spinal curvature. To understand the spinopelvic alignment, it is critical to understand the static morphometric pelvic parameters (pelvic incidence [PI]) and the dynamic parameters (sacral slope [SS], pelvic tilt [PT]), and how these interact with spinal regional curvatures (LL, TK).

PI

PI is defined as the angle subtended by a line drawn between the center of the femoral heads and the sacral end plate and a line drawn perpendicular to the sacral end plate (**Fig. 3**).[21] This angle represents the sacral relationship to the acetabulum and assumes limited motion through the sacroiliac joints. PI normative values of 50 to 55 are typically found; however, the individual reported range

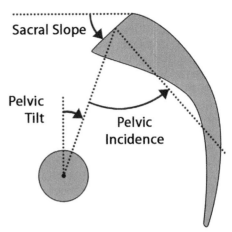

Fig. 3. Pelvic parameters. PI is described as an angle subtended by a line that is drawn from the center of the femoral heads to the midpoint of the sacral end plate and a line perpendicular to the center of the sacral end plate. PT is defined as the angle created by a line from the midpoint of the sacral end plate to the center femoral heads and a vertical plumb line. The sacral slope is the angle between the superior sacral end plate and a horizontal reference line.

may vary substantially from 28 to 84.[6] PI is therefore a static morphologic parameter that is consistent throughout a patient's life time, with only slight changes that occur during growth.[22] After this time, PI is a fixed parameter (minimal sacroiliac motion), which reliably reproduces the relationship of the sacrum to the pelvis.[22] The constant PI has a profound effect on the spinal parameters. With a large PI, the sacrum is more vertical and thus requires a larger LL to maintain proper global sagittal alignment of the trunk. Conversely, with a low PI, the more horizontal sacrum requires a smaller LL to achieve a balanced posture. Schwab and colleagues[14] reported on the role of PI in determining the degree of LL and developed a formula, based on the work of Boulay and colleagues,[23] in which ideal $LL = PI + 9° (±9°)$.

PT

PT is defined as the angle created by a line from the midpoint of the sacral end plate to the center femoral heads and a vertical plumb line (see **Fig. 3**).[4] This is a dynamic pelvic parameter, which can increase or decrease through rotation about the hip axis and can also change over time.[4,14] With age, the hip joints may become arthritic, and thereby lose range of motion, most notably the ability to recruit hip extension in the setting of spinal deformity. This situation may in turn limit the ability for a patient to augment pelvic retroversion (PT). In addition, as individuals age, the LL may decrease because of disk settling, adding the need to increase PT to maintain global alignment. Increasing PT retroverts the pelvis and requires hip extension and has limitations. As the PT increases, it represents a compensatory mechanism that requires both effort and energy. Schwab and colleagues[14] found a significant correlation between HRQoL outcome measures and PT. With increasing PT, HRQoL deteriorates, and an ideal pelvis version (surgical goal) of PT of less than 20° has been established.[6] Normative values may range from –5° to 30°, with a mean of 11° to 15°. However; unlike PI, PT changes with aging and has been found to increase, because of lost lordosis and increasing TK, reflecting the recruitment of a compensatory mechanism.[22]

SS

SS is defined as the angle created by a line drawn parallel to the end plate of the sacrum to a horizontal reference line (see **Fig. 3**).[24] By performing simple geometry, PI is defined as the sum of PT and SS (PI = PT + SS).[4,6,8,9,24] According to the formula, as PT increases (pelvic retroversion), the SS decreases and the sacral end plate becomes more horizontal.[14]

SPINOPELVIC ALIGNMENT

Historically, the focus of surgical treatment of scoliosis has been on the coronal alignment and less on the sagittal parameters. However, several studies[3,6,25] have shown that proper sagittal alignment is the single most important factor that determines the outcome for adults undergoing spinal deformity surgery. Patients with spinal deformity and undercorrected sagittal alignment with decreased LL have significantly worse HRQoL scores for physical and social function, self-image, and pain.[3] Several recent studies[10,11,13,26,27] have emphasized the relevance of LL and corresponding influence of pelvic parameters on the standing alignment in normal adults and children.

The pelvis exerts significant influence on the spine, and vice versa PI determines the optimal LL, and is different for each individual.[13,22,24,28] Boulay and colleagues[23] determined the optimal LL to achieve a harmonious balance and created a mathematical formula to predict the ideal LL for a given PI. Compensatory mechanisms can allow the pelvis to retrovert and increase the PT as the LL decreases, and in so doing, achieve a globally aligned trunk. However, this abnormal PT is often a marker of disability and underlying spinal malalignment and underscores the importance of the pelvis in determining overall alignment.[12]

SURGICAL PLANNING

Understanding and measuring the global spinal parameters, as well as the regional specific parameters, allows the surgeon to plan more effectively when determining the amount of correction necessary to achieve a good outcome. A high PT indicates pelvic retroversion, which is caused by an attempt to compensate for decreased LL.[14] Correction of deformity requires correction of not only the LL but must do so in the context of understanding the impact on PT. Failure to recognize an elevated PT leads to a fixed deformity, with inadequate correction and persistent clinical symptoms of global sagittal malalignment.[9] The optimal surgical goal should be to return the PT to a more physiologically normal value of less than 20°.[6] Proper version of the pelvis allows for more efficient standing and locomotion. Restoration of PT independently correlates with walking tolerance.[4,14,29]

Recently, a new classification system has been developed for adult deformity, the Scoliosis Research Society (SRS)-Schwab classification, which incorporates spinal and pelvic parameters with high interobserver and intraobserver reliability and is useful for classifying patients.[30] This classification system groups patients by their primary deformity and uses SVA, PT, and PI-LL mismatch as modifiers. Recent unpublished data from Smith and colleagues[31] evaluated 341 patients with adult deformity and assessed their improvement in spinopelvic parameters using the SRS-Schwab classification at 1 year. These investigators found significant correlation with improvement in PT or PI-LL modifiers with HRQoL outcomes. Schwab and colleagues[5] found that failure to achieve successful realignment occurred most in patients with large SVA, PT, PI, and greater mismatch. This finding suggests that even for experienced deformity surgeons, spinal realignment for sagittal plane deformity requires meticulous analysis and planning to customize treatment on a patient-specific level.

SUMMARY

Many of the current sagittal plane radiographic parameters (SVA, TK, LL) do not account for compensatory mechanisms above and below the measured segments. Compensation may occur through the feet, knees, hips, pelvis, and cervical spine to restore horizontal eye gaze and maintain proper truncal posture. Excessive compensation leads to pain and disability. The pelvis plays a critical role in the maintenance of global spinal alignment. Restoration of spinopelvic harmony allows the spine and pelvis to use minimal energy expenditure to maintain the patient within the ideal zone of the cone of economy. Matching the pelvic and spinal parameters allows the surgeon to achieve a properly aligned spine. Apparently normal SVA is insufficient in assessing global spinal alignment, because significant pelvic compensatory mechanisms can be in recruitment. The most relevant is the PT, which increases to compensate for regional malalignment in the lumbar or thoracic spine. Underappreciation of the dynamic pelvic parameters (PT, SS) leads to undercorrection of spinal deformity and poor patient outcomes.

REFERENCES

1. Schwab F, Dubey A, Pagala M, et al. Adult scoliosis: a health assessment analysis by SF-36. Spine (Phila Pa 1976) 2003;28(6):602–6.

2. Smith JS, Fu KM, Urban P, et al. Neurological symptoms and deficits in adults with scoliosis who present to a surgical clinic: incidence and association with the choice of operative versus nonoperative management. J Neurosurg Spine 2008;9(4):326–31.

3. Glassman SD, Bridwell K, Dimar JR, et al. The impact of positive sagittal balance in adult spinal deformity. Spine (Phila Pa 1976) 2005;30(18):2024–9.

4. Lafage V, Schwab F, Patel A, et al. Pelvic tilt and truncal inclination: two key radiographic parameters in the setting of adults with spinal deformity. Spine 2009;34(17):E599–606.

5. Schwab FJ, Patel A, Shaffrey CI, et al. Sagittal realignment failures following pedicle subtraction osteotomy surgery: are we doing enough?: Clinical article. J Neurosurg Spine 2012;16(6):539–46.

6. Schwab F, Patel A, Ungar B, et al. Adult spinal deformity-postoperative standing imbalance: how much can you tolerate? An overview of key parameters in assessing alignment and planning corrective surgery. Spine (Phila Pa 1976) 2010;35(25): 2224–31.

7. Bridwell KH, Glassman S, Horton W, et al. Does treatment (nonoperative and operative) improve the two-year quality of life in patients with adult symptomatic lumbar scoliosis: a prospective multicenter evidence-based medicine study. Spine 2009;34(20):2171–8.

8. Lafage V, Bharucha NJ, Schwab F, et al. Multicenter validation of a formula predicting postoperative spinopelvic alignment. J Neurosurg Spine 2012;16(1): 15–21.

9. Ames CP, Smith JS, Scheer JK, et al. Impact of spinopelvic alignment on decision making in deformity surgery in adults: a review. J Neurosurg Spine 2012; 16(6):547–64.

10. Labelle H, Roussouly P, Berthonnaud E, et al. The importance of spino-pelvic balance in L5-s1

developmental spondylolisthesis: a review of pertinent radiologic measurements. Spine (Phila Pa 1976) 2005;30(Suppl 6):S27–34.

11. Legaye J, Duval-Beaupere G. Sagittal plane alignment of the spine and gravity: a radiological and clinical evaluation. Acta Orthop Belg 2005;71(2):213–20.

12. Neal CJ, McClendon J, Halpin R, et al. Predicting ideal spinopelvic balance in adult spinal deformity. J Neurosurg Spine 2011;15(1):82–91.

13. Roussouly P, Gollogly S, Berthonnaud E, et al. Classification of the normal variation in the sagittal alignment of the human lumbar spine and pelvis in the standing position. Spine (Phila Pa 1976) 2005;30(3):346–53.

14. Schwab F, Lafage V, Patel A, et al. Sagittal plane considerations and the pelvis in the adult patient. Spine 2009;34(17):1828–33.

15. Schwab F, Lafage V, Boyce R, et al. Gravity line analysis in adult volunteers: age-related correlation with spinal parameters, pelvic parameters, and foot position. Spine 2006;31(25):E959–67.

16. Dubousset J. Three-dimensional analysis of the scoliotic deformity. In: Weinstein S, editor. The pediatric spine: principles and practice. New York: Raven Press; 1994. p. 479–96.

17. Horton WC, Brown CW, Bridwell KH, et al. Is there an optimal patient stance for obtaining a lateral 36" radiograph? A critical comparison of three techniques. Spine 2005;30(4):427–33.

18. Lu DC, Chou D. Flatback syndrome. Neurosurg Clin N Am 2007;18(2):289–94.

19. Labelle H, Roussouly P, Berthonnaud E, et al. Spondylolisthesis, pelvic incidence, and spinopelvic balance: a correlation study. Spine 2004;29(18):2049–54.

20. Vaz G, Roussouly P, Berthonnaud E, et al. Sagittal morphology and equilibrium of pelvis and spine. Eur Spine J 2002;11(1):80–7.

21. Legaye J, Duval-Beaupere G, Hecquet J, et al. Pelvic incidence: a fundamental pelvic parameter for three-dimensional regulation of spinal sagittal curves. Eur Spine J 1998;7(2):99–103.

22. Mac-Thiong JM, Berthonnaud E, Dimar JR 2nd, et al. Sagittal alignment of the spine and pelvis during growth. Spine 2004;29(15):1642–7.

23. Boulay C, Tardieu C, Hecquet J, et al. Sagittal alignment of spine and pelvis regulated by pelvic incidence: standard values and prediction of lordosis. Eur Spine J 2006;15(4):415–22.

24. Berthonnaud E, Dimnet J, Roussouly P, et al. Analysis of the sagittal balance of the spine and pelvis using shape and orientation parameters. J Spinal Disord Tech 2005;18(1):40–7.

25. Glassman SD, Carreon L, Dimar JR. Outcome of lumbar arthrodesis in patients sixty-five years of age or older. Surgical technique. J Bone Joint Surg Am 2010;92(Suppl 1 Pt 1):77–84.

26. Lowe T, Berven SH, Schwab FJ, et al. The SRS classification for adult spinal deformity: building on the

King/Moe and Lenke classification systems. Spine 2006;31(Suppl 19):S119–25.

27. Benner B, Ehni G. Degenerative lumbar scoliosis. Spine (Phila Pa 1976) 1979;4(6):548–52.

28. Mac-Thiong JM, Labelle H, Berthonnaud E, et al. Sagittal spinopelvic balance in normal children and adolescents. Eur Spine J 2007;16(2):227–34.

29. Skalli W, Zeller RD, Miladi L, et al. Importance of pelvic compensation in posture and motion after posterior spinal fusion using CD instrumentation for idiopathic scoliosis. Spine (Phila Pa 1976) 2006; 31(12):E359–66.

30. Schwab F, Ungar B, Blondel B, et al. Scoliosis Research Society-Schwab adult spinal deformity classification: a validation study. Spine (Phila Pa 1976) 2012;37(12):1077–82.

31. Scoliosis Research Society, Podium Presentation. Chicago, 2012.

Use of Surgimap Spine in Sagittal Plane Analysis, Osteotomy Planning, and Correction Calculation

Michael Akbar, MD[a], Jamie Terran, BS[b],
Christopher P. Ames, MD[c], Virginie Lafage, PhD[b],*,
Frank Schwab, MD[b]

KEYWORDS

• Sagittal deformity • Sagittal balance • Osteotomy • Surgimap

KEY POINTS

• Poor sagittal alignment has been shown to correlate highly with poor preoperative and postoperative patient-reported outcomes.
• Surgical techniques exist to correct sagittal alignment, including osteotomies; however, there is a lack of a clear standardized methodology for planning and executing surgical corrections.
• New digital tools can make surgical planning, in particular osteotomy planning, more effective and accurate.
• This article offers a logical and thoughtful process in surgical planning with regard to the use of corrective osteotomy in the adult patient with spinal deformity.

INTRODUCTION
Sagittal Plane Deformity: A Growing Problem

Over the past 3 decades the scientific community and spine surgeons have shown an increased interest in sagittal-plane deformity, ultimately acknowledging the complexity of this problem. The term, initially restricted to abnormalities such as "flat back syndrome" or "failed back," is gaining applicability as it now refers to any condition with an abnormal spinopelvic alignment in the sagittal plane: from degenerative conditions,[1,2] to pediatric abnormalities such as adolescent idiopathic scoliosis[3–5] or spondylolisthesis,[6,7] and including a broad range of deformity in the adult spine.[8–10] The general principles of realignment procedures are well accepted,[11] although the

systematic analysis of patients remains challenging and poorly implemented. The lack of implementation can be easily explained by the limited availability of formal training in the relevance of sagittal parameters and by the historical emphasis given to the coronal Cobb angle. However, a shift in perspective is necessary, as coronal Cobb angle has been proved to poorly correlate with patient-reported outcomes in the adult population.[12]

Why Should We Plan?

Identification of the sagittal plane as a major driver of poor clinical outcomes has given way for science to delve deeper into the concept and, ultimately, offer better clinical approaches to sagittal

[a] Department of Orthopaedic and Trauma Surgery, Spine Center, University of Heidelberg, Schlierbacher Landstrasse 200a, 69118, Heidelberg, Germany; [b] Department of Orthopaedic Surgery, NYU Hospital for Joint Diseases, 301 E 17th Street, New York, NY 10003, USA; [c] Department of Neurosurgery, University of California, Spine Center, 400 Parnassus Ave., 3rd Floor, San Francisco, CA 94143, USA
* Corresponding author. Spine Division, Hospital for Joint Diseases, New York University, New York.
E-mail address: virginie.lafage@gmail.com

Neurosurg Clin N Am 24 (2013) 163–172
http://dx.doi.org/10.1016/j.nec.2012.12.007
1042-3680/13/$ – see front matter © 2013 Elsevier Inc. All rights reserved.

malalignment and associated methods of compensation. Acknowledging the influence of sagittal alignment on health-related quality of life (HRQoL) forces a clear change in surgeons' perspectives; to improve clinical outcomes, we must correct sagittal malalignment. Several studies have proved that proper restoration of the sagittal profile is critical to postoperative patient-perceived improvement as quantified through HRQoL scores.[13,14]

Acknowledging the impact of sagittal alignment on patient outcomes is critical; however, a systematic approach to quantifying sagittal parameters and planning optimal correction is lacking. Through multicenter studies it is emerging that a reasonably sizable number of patients are ultimately undercorrected after surgery. In one such study examining patients who underwent lumbar pedicle subtraction osteotomy (PSO), it was determined that 23% of realignment procedures failed.[15] Similarly, 22% of thoracic PSO patients were found to have poor postoperative spinopelvic alignment.[16] Realignment failure has been associated with not only poor functional outcome but also major complications, such as pseudarthrosis and rod breakage, which often ultimately result in addition surgical procedures. Smith and colleagues[17] evaluated symptomatic rod fracture after posterior instrumented fusion for adult spinal deformity, and found rod breakage in up to 8.6% of adult patients with deformity and 15.6% of PSO patients. The investigators concluded that remaining sagittal malalignment may increase the risk for rod breakage. It is clear that this issue must be addressed, and a method for determining the ideal amount of sagittal correction on a patient-by-patient basis is essential to attaining favorable postoperative outcomes.

How Much Correction is Necessary to Achieve Good Postoperative Results?

The question of the required amount of correction in the setting of deformity is not simple. A proper response requires measuring key spinopelvic parameters, and classifying the extent of compensation. It is necessary to accept that surgical planning starts with measurement of the spinopelvic parameter.[18] The objective of this article is to propose a systematic clinical approach for surgeons through a step-by-step analysis based on a patient presenting with sagittal-plane deformity. For each key radiographic parameter, the clinical relevance of the measurements are discussed in light of the recent literature, and a new method for surgical planning using Surgimap Spine software (Nemaris Inc, New York, NY) is offered as a tool. This case presentation aims to

illustrate how a complex spinopelvic alignment can be broken down into simple key numbers to differentiate the primary drivers of the deformity from the compensatory mechanisms.

STEP-BY-STEP ANALYSIS
Case Presentation

The patient is a 73-year-old man complaining of low back pain for about 7 years. The patient feels he also has marked truncal shift anteriorly. He underwent spine surgery with an interspinous device in 2008 and experienced mild relief of some leg pain, but over time, particularly the last 4 years, he has noted increasing low back pain (7 out of 10 on a visual analog scale), with fatigue to the lower extremities and loss of standing and ambulatory endurance. The patient denies any neurologic deficits such as leg numbness, weakness, or paresthesias. Past treatment included pharmacologic management, physical therapy, and steroid injections.

On physical examination the patient's standing posture is with marked positive truncal inclination and an ability to stand fully erect. The patient demonstrates paravertebral lumbar tenderness, and discomfort with range of motion of the lumbar spine. Neurologic examination of the lower extremities reveals no deficits.

Evaluation of the Coronal Plane

Historically, evaluation of the coronal plane has been extrapolated from the Lenke classification of adolescent idiopathic scoliosis (AIS)[19,20]; however, recent studies have demonstrated that adult spinal deformity should not be considered an "adult version" of AIS. One of the first studies to closely examine the clinical impact of coronal deformity demonstrated that the obliquity of lumbar vertebrae (but not Cobb angle) correlate with pain scores.[21] Subsequently, multicenter studies[12,22] have revealed that apical level of a scoliotic deformity,[12] intervertebral subluxation, and coronal imbalance are also correlated with outcomes scores.[23] In light of these findings, a systematic evaluation of the coronal plane in the setting of adult spinal deformity should include the quantification of local (ie, intervertebral subluxation), regional (ie, identification of the apex), and global deformities (ie, global coronal malalignment). It appears that coronal C7 to center of the sacrum (central sacral vertical line) offset up to 4 to 5 cm is well tolerated, and that rotatory subluxations become mostly significant above 7 mm.[12]

As illustrated **Fig. 1** (left), preoperatively the patient did not present any coronal deformity (local, regional, or global).

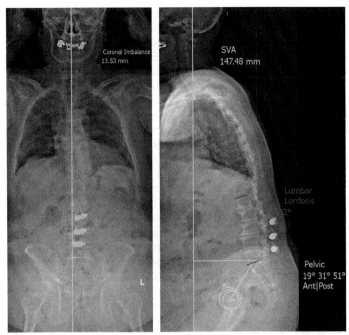

Fig. 1. Preoperative coronal and sagittal radiographs demonstrating a severe sagittal-plane deformity in association with previously placed interspinous devices (sagittal vertical axis [SVA] = 14.7 cm, PT = 31°, and PI-LL mismatch = 49°).

Evaluation of the Sagittal Plane

Global spinopelvic alignment

One of the most commonly used radiographic parameters in the setting of sagittal-plane evaluation is the sagittal vertical axis (SVA). This global parameter is defined as the linear offset between a plumb line dropped from C7 and the posterosuperior corner of S1. A possible substitution of the SVA is the T1 spinopelvic inclination (T1SPI), defined as the angle between a vertical and the line from T1 to the center of the bicoxofemoral axis.[8] T1SPI demonstrates almost perfect correlation with SVA and carries the advantage of being an angular measurement, which avoids the error inherent in measuring offsets in noncalibrated radiographs.[8] Global spinal realignment should attempt to obtain a postoperative SVA of less than 50 mm, or T1SPI of less than 0°.[8] Restoration of global alignment facilitates level gaze and achievement of a physiologic standing posture. From a clinical point of view, both parameters correlate with HRQoL (pain and disability),[8] and restoration of these parameters within normative values correlates with an increased likelihood of reaching a minimal clinically important difference.[13,14]

As illustrated in **Fig. 1** (right), preoperatively the patient had an SVA measured at 14.7 cm. According to the Scoliosis Research Society Schwab classification of adult spinal deformity,[24] this level of SVA identifies the patient as "severe sagittal deformity" with an SVA grade of ++.

Compensatory mechanisms

In addition to the evaluation of global spinopelvic alignment, it is of primary importance to also identify and quantify the use of compensatory mechanisms used in an effort to maintain the trunk as vertical as possible.[18] From a physiologic point of view several mechanisms have been reported in the literature,[1] such as changes of spinal curvatures (eg, hyphokyphosis of the thoracic spine, flexion of the knee, or retroversion of the pelvis). Changes in spinal curvatures are very common across the spectrum of spinal pathology (eg, increase of segmental lumbar lordosis above spondylolisthesis); they require not only a flexible spine but also the muscular ability to maintain those changes. Because of the nature of standard scoliosis films, knee flexion is difficult to evaluate on radiographs; a surrogate measurement can be the quantification of the femoral angulation with the vertical.[25,26]

Among the possible compensatory mechanisms to sagittal-plane malalignment, pelvic retroversion is probably the most commonly measured parameter. Pelvic retroversion is defined as a backward rotation of the pelvis; it is quantified by an elevated pelvic tilt (PT): the angle between the vertical and the line from the center of the bicoxofemoral axis to the middle of the superior endplate of S1. Jean Dubbouset[27] introduced the concept of "pelvic vertebra," considering the pelvis as the pedestal[28] of the spine where pelvic retroversion aims at "bringing back" the spine into a vertical position. From a physiologic point of view, an increase in PT is not energy efficient, and correlates with increased pain and disability.[8,18]

As illustrated in **Fig. 2**A, preoperatively the patient had a PT of 31°, illustrating a pelvic retroversion in an effort to compensate for the sagittal deformity. From a hypothetical point of view, if the patient was able to further increase his pelvic retroversion (physiologic limit of pelvic retroversion = horizontal sacral endplate), the SVA would be within normative values (**Fig. 2**B; PT = 48°, SVA = 2.5 cm). From a pragmatic point of view, this illustrates that measurement of SVA alone does not permit accurate quantification of the sagittal plane, as it does not integrate how much of the "true SVA" is compensated for by increased retroversion. Using the same analogy, if the patient was not using any pelvic compensation (ie, PT = normative value [~20°]), the projected SVA would be even more severe than the one measured on standing radiographs (**Fig. 2**C; PT = 20°, SVA = 22 cm).

The ability of a patient to compensate for a spinal malalignment via an increase of pelvic retroversion is of primary importance in the clinical evaluation. Nevertheless, one should keep in mind that pelvic retroversion may also be the primary cause of sagittal malalignment if a patient presents with some specific soft-tissue[8] or lower-extremity disorder (shortening of the hamstring, hip-flexion contracture, hip deformity).[8] It is also interesting that a small number of patients have a mismatch between PT and SVA and do not compensate through the pelvis for their sagittal-plane malalignment. Ames and colleagues[18] reported that patients with an elevated SVA and a low PT (lack of pelvic compensation for a high SVA) represent a distinct subgroup in which surgical realignment procedures are at risk of postoperative failure. This relation may be seen in (1) patients with pre-existing hip flexion contracture, (2) patients with degenerative flat back with primary extensor muscle abnormality, (3) globally decompensated patients with secondary extensor muscle weakness, and (4) patients leaning forward to compensate for severe lumbar stenosis.[18] All patients for whom corrective surgery is being considered should undergo clinical evaluation of the lower extremities to rule out hip-flexion contracture.[18]

Lumbar lordosis

Lumbar lordosis is probably the most commonly used sagittal radiographic parameter across all spinal abnormalities. The analysis of reported normative values[29–35] revealed an average lumbar lordosis of 60° on asymptomatic adult volunteers.

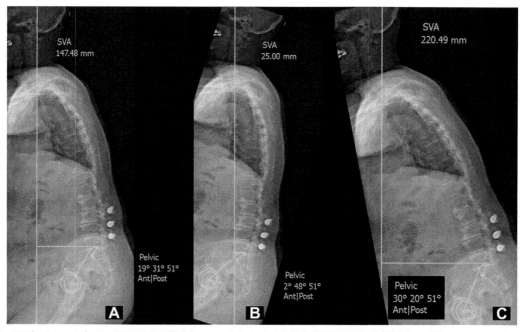

Fig. 2. The impact that pelvic version (PT) has on global alignment. Preoperatively (*A*), the patient presented with a sagittal vertical axis (SVA) of 14.7 cm and a pelvic tilt (PT) of 31°. A hypothetical further increase of pelvic retroversion (eg, PT = 48°; *B*) would drastically reduce the projected SVA. On the other hand, a reduction of pelvic tilt (PT = 20°; *C*) would increase the projected SVA.

It is important to note the extremely wide range of lumbar lordosis values contributing to that average. Vialle and colleagues,[36] in their review of 300 asymptomatic subjects, reported a lumbar lordosis ranging from 30° to 89°. These large variations reflect that each subject requires his or her own amount of lumbar lordosis. As reported by numerous investigators, the lumbar lordosis for a given subject should be proportional to the observed pelvic incidence (PI). PI is a morphologic parameter defined as the angle between the perpendicular to the sacral plate at its midpoint and a line connecting the same point to the center of the bicoxofemoral axis. The intrinsic relationship between PI and lumbar lordosis can easily be explained by the strong relationship between PI and sacral slope (ie, inclination of the sacral endplate with the horizontal).

- *Small PI* is associated with a vertical sacrum and, therefore, a horizontal sacral endplate. Because the spine originates at the sacrum, a horizontal sacral endplate is associated with an almost horizontal L5 vertebra. As a result, a small lumbar lordosis is sufficient to maintain the head over the pelvis.
- *Large PI* is associated with a more horizontal sacrum and therefore a titled sacral endplate and L5 vertebra. As a result, a large lumbar lordosis is required to maintain the head over the pelvis.

While the optimal lordosis specific for a particular subject is still a debatable question, the analysis of normative data demonstrates that 80% of subjects have a lumbar lordosis within 10° of their measured PI. Based on this finding, a new parameter has recently been introduced to evaluate the mismatch between PI and lumbar lordosis (PI minus lumbar lordosis, or PI-LL mismatch) rather than each parameter independently. The analysis of HRQoL in the setting of adult spinal deformity also demonstrates that an increase in PI-LL mismatch was associated with higher level of pain and disability. In terms of surgical realignment planning, the PI-LL mismatch can thus be a simplified way to assess the degree of realignment necessary. The caveat is that this applies only when the sagittal plane deformity is isolated to the lumbar spine and does not account for abnormal thoracic or thoracolumbar alignment. In addition, such a simplified realignment planning does not account for changes in unfused portions of the spine that can occur (eg, reciprocal increased kyphosis following lumbar realignment).

As illustrated **Fig. 1** (right), preoperatively the patient had a PI-LL mismatch of 49° (PI = 51°, LL = 2°). From a planning point of view, a 40° increase in lumbar lordosis would be necessary to reach a PI-LL of less than 10° (if LL = 40° + 2°, PI-LL = 51°–42° = 9°).

Surgical Planning

Mathematical planning

In an attempt to optimize postoperative spinopelvic alignment, several investigators have proposed mathematical formulas to assist surgical planning. These formulas[37–42] vary in their level of complexity, as some simply provide a target postoperative lumbar lordosis/thoracic kyphosis relationship, whereas others estimate the degree of osteotomy resection needed to restore an acceptable global sagittal alignment. The predictive accuracy of these formulas has recently been analyzed in a large database of 3-column osteotomies, which revealed that only formulas integrating pelvic parameters preoperatively were able to correctly predict postoperative global alignment (SVA) and pelvic version (PT).[43] Lafage and colleagues[44] reported on the formula with the highest accuracy in predicting postoperative SVA after PSO. A limitation of the aforementioned formulas are the lack of full consideration of the position of the lower extremities and the head.[43] When planning spinal reconstructive procedures, it is important to acknowledge that preoperative planning formulas that do not evaluate pelvic parameters, especially PI and PT, may be inaccurate and may increase the risk for postoperative undercorrection. Although these formulas clearly represent an advancement in predicting the postoperative outcome, they may be too complex for routine clinical use.[37–42]

Graphical planning

Existing methods In addition to published mathematical formulas, several investigators have proposed graphical methods for surgical planning of osteotomy procedures. Ondra and colleagues[39] used a trigonometric method to calculate the angle of correction needed to achieve neutral alignment for PSO procedures. One shortcoming of this method, however, is that the contribution of the pelvis to sagittal alignment is neglected; the use of this method will probably lead to undercorrection. The FBI technique[25] is a more comprehensive graphical method integrating the pelvis and the lower extremities in the geometric calculation. The technique is based on a global analysis of the full body. The amount of correction is geometrically calculated using appropriate radiographic measurements. To determine the amount of correction required, the FBI technique applies 3 distinct angle measurements. The integration of the femoral shaft to represent knee flexion on long cassette radiograph films is an important parameter for analyzing the patient's posture in the standing position, avoiding postoperative undercorrection and residual sagittal malalignment. A limitation of the FBI graphical technique is that the femoral shaft needs to be visualized and that the exact extent of pelvic retroversion (PT) is not integrated, as the investigators propose a generic solution (increase of correction by 5° in the setting of any pelvic retroversion).

Surgimap Spine Surgimap Spine, a free computer program (http://www.surgimap.com; Nemaris Inc, New York, NY) that integrates spine-related measurement and tools for surgical planning in combination with knowledge gained from the published literature, offers a pragmatic graphical method for the surgical planning of osteotomies. This method integrates not only global malalignment but also the spinopelvic parameters, and enables the user to simulate the sagittal correction and its influence on the spinopelvic parameters and global alignment. After import of preoperative digital radiographs into a Surgimap Spine customizable database, realignment planning can be executed in 4 simple phases (**Figs. 3–6**).

1. Measurement of preoperative sagittal radiographs (see **Fig. 3**). As described previously,

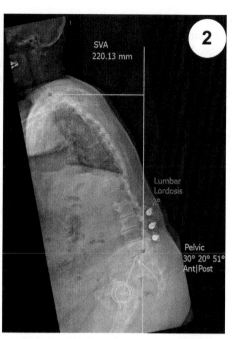

Fig. 4. The second phase of the graphical surgical planning consists in rotating (in this case counterclockwise) the sagittal radiograph until a desired planned pelvic tilt is reached (here 20°).

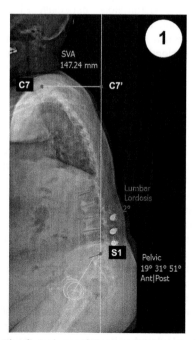

Fig. 3. The first phase of the graphical surgical planning consists in the identification of the pelvic parameters, lumbar lordosis, and global alignment. SVA, sagittal vertical axis.

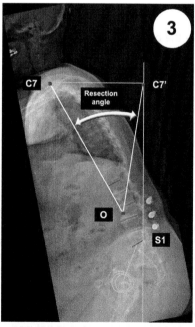

Fig. 5. The third phase of the graphical surgical planning consists in the identification of the resection angle based on the osteotomy site (O), the current location of C7, and the desired postoperative location of C7 (C7').

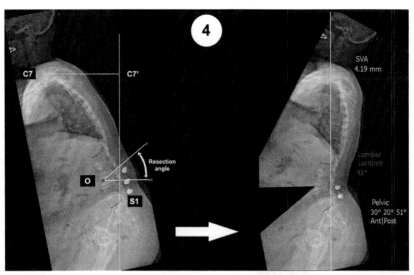

Fig. 6. The fourth and last phase of the graphical surgical planning consists in drawing the resection matched to the angle from O to C7 and C7′, followed by (wedge osteotomy) simulation of the osteotomy. On the left is the planning scheme and on the right the activated planning simulation, with transition indicated by the arrow.

the minimum set of measurements required for sagittal-plane analysis include pelvic parameters, lumbar lordosis, and global alignment (SVA or T1SPI). Surgimap Spine offers dedicated tools for each of these measurements. The pelvic parameters are automatically calculated on identification of the sacral endplate and the 2 femoral heads. The lumbar lordosis measure requires the identification of the cranial endplate of L1 in addition to the sacral endplate. Finally, in the context of the proposed method, the SVA is constructed in a reverse fashion, by dropping a plumb line from the posterosuperior corner of S1 and by the identification of C7. Using this specific construction of the SVA, the overall objective of the method consists in "bringing C7 in line with the posterosuperior corner of S1" (ie, moving C7 over C7′ as illustrated in **Fig. 3**).

2. Rotation of the image to reach desired postoperative PT (see **Fig. 4**). Surgimap Spine offers the ability to rotate images (degree by degree) while monitoring the impact of the rotation on existing measurements (instant recalculation). In an effort to take into account the pelvic compensation, this second phase consists of turning the entire image until PT reaches the planned, or ideal postoperative PT (20° in this case presentation).

3. Quantification of the resection needed (see **Fig. 5**). After identification of the osteotomy site (point O in **Fig. 5**), the third phase consists in calculating the amount of resection needed to superimpose C7 and C7′. As for other

graphical techniques of osteotomy planning, this angle is defined as the angle between OC7 and OC7′, and can be measured via Surgimap Spine using the generic "angle" tool.

4. Simulation of the osteotomy (see **Fig. 6**). The fourth and final phase consists in applying a resection angle at the intended osteotomy site using the "Wedge Osteotomy" tool and graphically tracing the osteotomy directly on the radiographic image. Of note, this tool offers the ability to adjust the ratio of rotation between the trunk and the pelvis. Surgimap depicts this ratio via a third line. In the proposed realignment approach described here, the ratio line should be shifted to directly over the lower resection line of the osteotomy (ratio set at 100%). In other methods, if the PT is not adjusted first through image rotation, one can use the ratio line of the osteotomy to adjust for variable correction of PT or SVA.

Of note, this graphical technique does not necessarily represent the exact amount of resection needed but rather of amount of change in lumbar lordosis needed to correct the global alignment and pelvic retroversion. One of limitations of the method is that it does not take into account the possible reciprocal changes that may occur in the unfused segments of the spine.

As illustrated in **Fig. 7**, using the proposed technique with a grade 3 osteotomy[45] applied at L3, the sagittal plane of the patient was corrected to reach an SVA of 0.9 cm, PT of 22°, and lumbar lordosis of 44°.

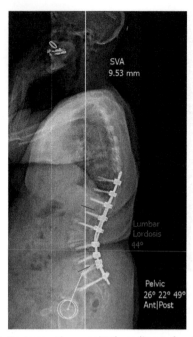

Fig. 7. Postoperative sagittal radiograph demonstrating correction of the deformity (PT = 22°, SVA = 0.9 cm, and PI-LL mismatch = 5°) according to plan.

Surgical tools

Schwab and colleagues[45] proposed an osteotomy classification system based on 6 anatomic grades of resection (1 through 6) corresponding to the extent of bone resection and the increasing degree of destabilizing potential. The classification provides a comprehensive description of the various osteotomies performed in spinal deformity correction surgery (Surgimap tools offer openings and various methods of resections and vertebrectomy reflecting the range of osteotomies from grades 1 through 6). Its use may allow a common framework for osteotomy description and comparative analysis. Ames and colleagues[18] reported that the location of the osteotomy along the spine needs to be considered when attempting to normalize PT. PT reduction is greater when the osteotomy performed is more caudal. It is also important to consider that spinal segments not incorporated within the fusion may become more kyphotic after lumbar PSO.

SUMMARY

Surgical planning should not be simply an academic or purely theoretical exercise. It is critical that surgeons adopt planning tools to encourage better outcomes for their patients. This article offers a pragmatic and systematic approach involving measurement of the key spinopelvic parameters, evaluation if the compensatory mechanisms, identification of the amount of correction needed, and selection of surgical tools needed to achieve outlined objectives.

Depending on the severity of sagittal deformity, spinopelvic parameters, and compensatory mechanism (high preoperative PT), there is the possibility to select the most adapted type and extent of osteotomy, pursue a simulated correction, and assess its direct influence on spinopelvic parameters. The surgeon-developed surgical planning software Surgimap Spine can be a tremendously helpful tool in assessing various approaches and strategies to combat spinal deformity, with the goal of optimal treatment for patients (http://www.surgimap.com, Nemaris, New York, NY).

REFERENCES

1. Barrey C, Roussouly P, Perrin G, et al. Sagittal balance disorders in severe degenerative spine. Can we identify the compensatory mechanisms? Eur Spine J 2011;20(Suppl 5):626–33.
2. Barrey C, Jund J, Noseda O, et al. Sagittal balance of the pelvis-spine complex and lumbar degenerative diseases. A comparative study about 85 cases. Eur Spine J 2007;16(9):1459–67.
3. Blondel B, Lafage V, Farcy JP, et al. Influence of screw type on initial coronal and sagittal radiological correction with hybrid constructs in adolescent idiopathic scoliosis. Correction priorities. Orthop Traumatol Surg Res 2012;98(8):873–8.
4. Ilharreborde B, Vidal C, Skalli W, et al. Sagittal alignment of the cervical spine in adolescent idiopathic scoliosis treated by posteromedial translation. Eur Spine J 2012. [Epub ahead of print].
5. Roussouly P, Labelle H, Rouissi J, et al. Pre- and post-operative sagittal balance in idiopathic scoliosis: a comparison over the ages of two cohorts of 132 adolescents and 52 adults. Eur Spine J 2012. [Epub ahead of print].
6. Labelle H, Roussouly P, Berthonnaud E, et al. Spondylolisthesis, pelvic incidence, and spinopelvic balance: a correlation study. Spine 2004;29(18):2049–54.
7. Roussouly P, Gollogly S, Berthonnaud E, et al. Sagittal alignment of the spine and pelvis in the presence of L5-s1 isthmic lysis and low-grade spondylolisthesis. Spine 2006;31(21):2484–90.
8. Lafage V, Schwab F, Patel A, et al. Pelvic tilt and truncal inclination: two key radiographic parameters in the setting of adults with spinal deformity. Spine 2009;34(17):E599–606.
9. Schwab F, Bess S, Blondel B, et al. Combined assessment of pelvic tilt, pelvic incidence/lumbar lordosis mismatch and sagittal vertical axis predicts

disability in adult spinal deformity: a prospective analysis. Louisville (KY): Scoliosis Research Society (SRS); 2011.

10. Sanchez-Mariscal F, Gomez-Rice A, Izquierdo E, et al. Correlation of radiographic and functional measurements in patients who underwent primary scoliosis surgery in adult age. Spine 2012;37(7):592–8.

11. Schwab F, Patel A, Ungar B, et al. Adult spinal deformity-postoperative standing imbalance: how much can you tolerate? An overview of key parameters in assessing alignment and planning corrective surgery. Spine 2010;35(25):2224–31.

12. Schwab F, Farcy JP, Bridwell K, et al. A clinical impact classification of scoliosis in the adult. Spine 2006;31(18):2109–14.

13. Blondel B, Schwab F, Ungar B, et al. Impact of magnitude and percentage of global sagittal plane correction on health-related quality of life at 2-years follow-up. Neurosurgery 2012;71(2):341–8.

14. Smith J, Klineberg E, Schwab F, et al. Change in classification grade by the Schwab-SRS Adult Spinal Deformity (ASD) classification predicts impact on Health Related Quality of Life (HRQOL) measures: prospective analysis of operative and nonoperative treatment. Paper presented at: Scoliosis Research Society (SRS). Chicago, September 7, 2012.

15. Schwab FJ, Patel A, Shaffrey CI, et al. Sagittal realignment failures following pedicle subtraction osteotomy surgery: are we doing enough?: clinical article. J Neurosurg Spine 2012;16(6):539–46.

16. Lafage V, Smith JS, Bess S, et al. Sagittal spinopelvic alignment failures following three column thoracic osteotomy for adult spinal deformity. Eur Spine J 2012;21(4):698–704.

17. Smith JS, Shaffrey CI, Ames CP, et al. Assessment of symptomatic rod fracture following posterior instrumented fusion for adult spinal deformity. Neurosurgery 2012;71(4):862–7.

18. Ames CP, Smith JS, Scheer JK, et al. Impact of spinopelvic alignment on decision making in deformity surgery in adults: a review. J Neurosurg Spine 2012; 16(6):547–64.

19. Lenke LG, Edwards CC 2nd, Bridwell KH. The Lenke classification of adolescent idiopathic scoliosis: how it organizes curve patterns as a template to perform selective fusions of the spine. Spine 2003;28(20): S199–207.

20. Lenke LG, Betz RR, Harms J, et al. Adolescent idiopathic scoliosis: a new classification to determine extent of spinal arthrodesis. J Bone Joint Surg Am 2001;83-A(8):1169–81.

21. Schwab FJ, Smith VA, Biserni M, et al. Adult scoliosis: a quantitative radiographic and clinical analysis. Spine 2002;27(4):387–92.

22. Glassman SD, Berven S, Bridwell K, et al. Correlation of radiographic parameters and clinical symptoms in adult scoliosis. Spine 2005;30(6):682–8.

23. Glassman SD, Bridwell K, Dimar JR, et al. The impact of positive sagittal balance in adult spinal deformity. Spine 2005;30(18):2024–9.

24. Schwab F, Ungar B, Blondel B, et al. SRS-Schwab adult spinal deformity classification: a validation study. Spine (Phila Pa 1976) 2012;37(12):1077–82.

25. Le Huec JC, Leijssen P, Duarte M, et al. Thoracolumbar imbalance analysis for osteotomy planification using a new method: FBI technique. Eur Spine J 2011;20(Suppl 5):669–80.

26. Obeid I, Hauger O, Aunoble S, et al. Global analysis of sagittal spinal alignment in major deformities: correlation between lack of lumbar lordosis and flexion of the knee. Eur Spine J 2011;20(Suppl 5):681–5.

27. Dubousset J. Importance de la vertèbre pelvienne dans l'équilibre rachidien. Application à la chirurgie de la colonne vertébrale chez l'enfant et l'adolescent. In: Villeneuve P, editor. Pied équilibre et rachis. Paris: Frison-Roche; 1998. p. 141–9.

28. Le Huec JC, Saddiki R, Franke J, et al. Equilibrium of the human body and the gravity line: the basics. Eur Spine J 2011;20(Suppl 5):558–63.

29. Bernhardt M, Bridwell KH. Segmental analysis of the sagittal plane alignment of the normal thoracic and lumbar spines and thoracolumbar junction. Spine 1989;14(7):717–21.

30. Berthonnaud E, Dimnet J, Roussouly P, et al. Analysis of the sagittal balance of the spine and pelvis using shape and orientation parameters. J Spinal Disord Tech 2005;18(1):40–7.

31. During J, Goudfrooij H, Keessen W, et al. Toward standards for posture. Postural characteristics of the lower back system in normal and pathologic conditions. Spine 1985;10(1):83–7.

32. Gelb DE, Lenke LG, Bridwell KH, et al. An analysis of sagittal spinal alignment in 100 asymptomatic middle and older aged volunteers. Spine 1995;20(12):1351–8.

33. Jackson RP, Kanemura T, Kawakami N, et al. Lumbopelvic lordosis and pelvic balance on repeated standing lateral radiographs of adult volunteers and untreated patients with constant low back pain. Spine 2000;25(5):575–86.

34. Vaz G, Roussouly P, Berthonnaud E, et al. Sagittal morphology and equilibrium of pelvis and spine. Eur Spine J 2002;11(1):80–7.

35. Schwab F, Lafage V, Boyce R, et al. Gravity line analysis in adult volunteers: age-related correlation with spinal parameters, pelvic parameters, and foot position. Spine 2006;31(25):E959–67.

36. Vialle R, Levassor N, Rillardon L, et al. Radiographic analysis of the sagittal alignment and balance of the spine in asymptomatic subjects. J Bone Joint Surg Am 2005;87(2):260–7.

37. Boulay C, Tardieu C, Hecquet J, et al. Sagittal alignment of spine and pelvis regulated by pelvic incidence: standard values and prediction of lordosis. Eur Spine J 2006;15(4):415–22.

38. Kim YJ, Bridwell KH, Lenke LG, et al. An analysis of sagittal spinal alignment following long adult lumbar instrumentation and fusion to L5 or S1: can we predict ideal lumbar lordosis? Spine 2006;31(20): 2343–52.

39. Ondra SL, Marzouk S, Koski T, et al. Mathematical calculation of pedicle subtraction osteotomy size to allow precision correction of fixed sagittal deformity. Spine 2006;31(25):E973–9.

40. Rose PS, Bridwell KH, Lenke LG, et al. Role of pelvic incidence, thoracic kyphosis, and patient factors on sagittal plane correction following pedicle subtraction osteotomy. Spine 2009;34(8):785–91.

41. Schwab F, Lafage V, Patel A, et al. Sagittal plane considerations and the pelvis in the adult patient. Spine 2009;34(17):1828–33.

42. Yang BP, Ondra SL. A method for calculating the exact angle required during pedicle subtraction osteotomy for fixed sagittal deformity: comparison with the trigonometric method. Neurosurgery 2006; 59(4 Suppl 2):ONS458–63 [discussion: ONS463].

43. Smith JS, Bess S, Shaffrey CI, et al. Dynamic changes of the pelvis and spine are key to predicting postoperative sagittal alignment after pedicle subtraction osteotomy: a critical analysis of preoperative planning techniques. Spine 2012;37(10): 845–53.

44. Lafage V, Schwab F, Vira S, et al. Spino-pelvic parameters after surgery can be predicted: a preliminary formula and validation of standing alignment. Spine 2011;36(13):1037–45.

45. Schwab F, Blondel B, Chay E, et al. The Comprehensive Anatomical Spinal Osteotomy Classification. Paper presented at: international Meeting on Advanced Spine Techniques (IMAST). Istanbul, July 18-21, 2012.

Adolescent Scoliosis Classification and Treatment

Jane S. Hoashi, MD, MPH, Patrick J. Cahill, MD,
James T. Bennett, MD, Amer F. Samdani, MD*

KEYWORDS

- Adolescent idiopathic scoliosis • Lenke classification • Scoliosis • Pediatric spine deformity
- Pedicle screws

KEY POINTS

- Adolescent idiopathic scoliosis (AIS) can be classified according to the Lenke classification system, which incorporates curve magnitude, flexibility, the lumbar modifier, and the sagittal plane.
- The Lenke classification serves as a guide with respect to level selection in patients with AIS.
- The widespread use of pedicle screws has resulted in most AIS being treated through a posterior approach.

INTRODUCTION

Adolescent idiopathic scoliosis (AIS) is a spinal condition causing deformity of the spine in 3 dimensions: the coronal, sagittal, and axial planes. AIS is defined as any curve equal to or greater than 10° in the coronal plane[1,2] in patients 10 to 18 years old.[3] It is a diagnosis of exclusion after congenital, neuromuscular, neural, or syndromic causes of scoliosis have been ruled out. Preoperative magnetic resonance imaging is useful for ruling out neural causes of scoliosis, such as syringomyelia or Chiari malformation, although its use as a preoperative screening tool is controversial.[4,5] A genetic component has been described regarding the cause of AIS.[6–11] With an incidence of 11% among first-degree relatives,[12] it is not uncommon for a health care provider to manage multiple members of a family with scoliosis.

AIS affects approximately 2% to 3% of the adolescent population, but fewer than 10% of patients with AIS need treatment.[13] The higher the curve magnitude, the lower the prevalence and the higher the female/male ratio. Curves greater than 30° have a 0.1% to 0.3% prevalence and affect females 10 times more than males.[14]

For years, the King-Moe classification was the most widely used system for guiding treatment in AIS. Its shortcomings included classifying curves based only on the coronal plane and showing low interobserver reliability.[15] Also, only variants of the thoracic curve were described, leaving some other curve types such as thoracolumbar or lumbar curves unable to be classified by this system. The Lenke classification[16] addresses these shortcomings and is now considered the gold standard for classifying AIS and guiding treatment. In this article, the Lenke classification is used to describe the AIS types and the treatment options.

Treatment of scoliosis includes nonoperative management such as bracing of curves measuring 20° to 40° or progressing more than 5° per year. Larger curve magnitude, younger chronologic age, and Risser sign are associated with curve progression.[17] The literature has shown bracing to be more effective in patients with earlier Risser scores (0–1) and open triradiate cartilages.[18–20] The goal of bracing is to maintain curve magnitude throughout a patient's growth period, although conflicting evidence of its effectiveness have been reported.[18,19]

No funding was received in support of this work.

Department of Orthopaedic Surgery, Shriners Hospitals for Children—Philadelphia, 3551 North Broad Street, Philadelphia, PA 19140, USA

* Corresponding author.

E-mail address: amersamdani@gmail.com

neurosurgery.theclinics.com

Surgery is indicated when a curve is progressive despite bracing and generally when the curve reaches 45° to 50°. The main goal is to stop the curve from progressing, leading to potentially severe complications from an untreated curve, including pulmonary function and back pain. Other goals driven by the patients themselves are improvement of cosmesis. Quality of life studies as measured by the SRS-22 (Scoliosis Research Society 22) questionnaire have shown that patients with AIS have lower self-image and are more self-conscious about their general appearance than the general population.[21,22] This finding can be related to a shoulder imbalance, rib prominence, or trunk asymmetry. Thus, the psychological impact of the deformity must also be taken into account when considering surgery.

The goals of surgery are to restore coronal and sagittal balance, reduce the rib prominence, and achieve shoulder balance. However, another important goal is to leave as many unfused segments as possible to preserve motion in the lumbar spine. The specific treatment options are discussed further in this article.

Two approaches to AIS surgery exist: the anterior approach and the posterior approach; a combination of the 2 is also used. Some potential advantages to the anterior approach are saving fusion levels,[23,24] decreased prominence of instrumentation, and decreased risk of crankshaft phenomenon in a skeletally immature adolescent.[16,25] However, some studies have indicated morbidity related to decreased pulmonary function,[26,27] which seems to improve at 2-year follow-up.[28] The anterior approach can be used to fuse simple thoracic curves and can also be used to perform anterior release and fusion combined with posterior spinal fusion in stiffer and larger (>90°) curves, although similar curve correction can be achieved in these larger curves by the posterior approach alone.[29]

Since the development of pedicle screws, the posterior-only approach has become the mainstay of treatment of AIS. Pedicle screws provide a 3-column fixation that permits greater curve correction and improved derotation.[30] Even in the more severe (>90°) and stiffer curves, pedicle screw constructs with osteotomies render good correction,[29] thereby reducing the need for combined anterior and posterior approaches. The crankshaft phenomenon may also be reduced by using pedicle screws.[31]

However, pedicle screw placement has a learning curve, especially with the free hand technique.[32] With surgeon experience, the accuracy of pedicle screw placement improves, and the medial breach rate decreases.[33,34] Reported breach rates range from 1.6% to as high as 58%.[33–38] However, rates for neurologic and visceral injuries despite these breaches are low. Although hypokyphosis has been observed with posterior-only pedicle screw constructs,[39,40] long-term follow-up has shown good maintenance of correction and coronal and sagittal alignment.[31,41]

LENKE CLASSIFICATION
Overview

The Lenke classification for AIS was developed as a tool to help surgeons classify curve types and guide them in operative treatment.[16] The curve type (the major curve), lumbar modifier (A, B, and C, depending on the location of the center sacral vertical line [CSVL] in relation to the apical lumbar vertebra), and the sagittal profile (–, N, +) is used to determine a specific curve pattern. Although there are 6 Lenke curve types, a total of 42 curve patterns can be observed.

The basis of surgical treatment is to fuse only the structural curves. The curve with the largest Cobb magnitude is defined as the major curve, which, by definition, is structural. Curves with lesser magnitude (minor curves) can be structural or nonstructural, depending on the degree of their flexibility seen on bending films. Generally, minor curves are not considered part of the arthrodesis if they bend out to less than 25°. Focal kyphosis is also a criterion for considering a curve to be structural.

The Lenke classification differentiates King-Moe type 2 curves into Lenke types 1 and 3, helping surgeons select which curves are amenable to selective fusions (Lenke type 1) and those that require an extended fusion in the lumbar spine (Lenke type 3). Unlike the King-Moe classification, which considers only the coronal plane, the Lenke classification accounts for both coronal and sagittal planes and has been shown to have good interobserver reliability. However, the axial plane (a reflection of vertebral body rotation) is still not included in the Lenke classification. Moreover, some curve types such as curves with C lumbar modifiers are subject to controversy regarding selective versus nonselective fusion. The following section on the specific Lenke curve types includes some of the controversies and current recommendations for treatment.

Treatment of Lenke Curve Types

Lenke 1: single thoracic curve
For single thoracic curves (**Fig. 1**), it is generally accepted to perform selective fusions of the main thoracic curve, unless there is a kyphosis of more than 20° in the thoracolumbar area, in which case, the lumbar curve is also included in the

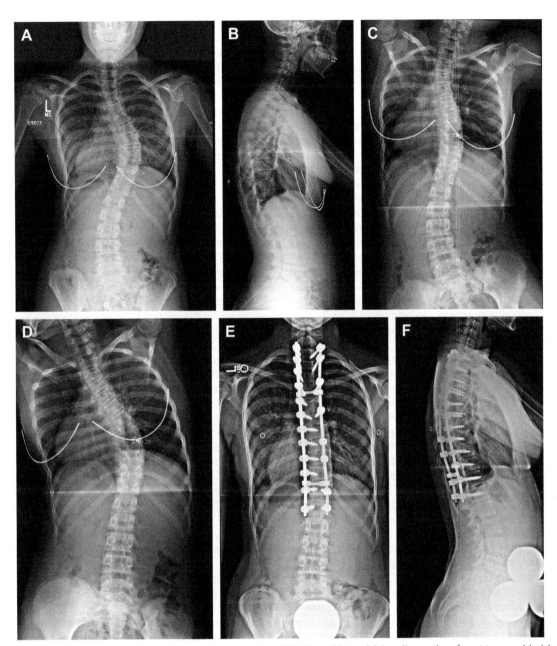

Fig. 1: Lenke 1. Preoperative standing posteroanterior (PA) (*A*) and lateral (*B*) radiographs of an 11-year-old girl with a right 50° main thoracic curve and a 25° left lumbar curve. Right (*C*) and left (*D*) bend films show that the main thoracic curve bends down to 28° and the lumbar curve bends down to 4°. Two-year follow-up PA (*E*) and lateral (*F*) radiographs show correction of the main thoracic curve to 15° and correction of the lumbar curve to 3° with posterior pedicle screws from T2 to L1.

fusion.[16] The unfused lumbar curve is nonstructural and usually spontaneously corrects itself after thoracic fusion.[42–46] It is important to note any preoperative shoulder height discrepancy, because this often determines the upper fusion levels. Shoulder height can be determined clinically as well as radiographically using the clavicle angle or T1 tilt.[47]

Three different scenarios exist regarding shoulder height. The first and most common scenario is a right main thoracic curve, with the right shoulder being higher than the left. In this case, correction of the thoracic spine also brings down the right shoulder, usually achieving equal shoulder height. In these cases, the upper instrumented level is usually T4 or T5.[48] If the left shoulder is elevated, the compensatory proximal thoracic curve is usually included in the fusion (to T2) to oppose the corrective forces being placed on the main thoracic curve, which would otherwise continue to drive the left shoulder up. If both shoulders are equal in height preoperatively, T3 is usually the upper level of fusion.

For single thoracic curves with minor flexible lumbar curves (Lenke 1A and 1B), selective thoracic fusions are generally indicated. For distal fusion levels, it is important to choose the appropriate lowest instrumented vertebra (LIV) so as to leave good coronal balance and avoid lumbar decompensation or progression of the primary curve (adding-on). Conventional guidelines have used the stable vertebra, or the most proximal vertebra with pedicles most closely bisected by the CSVL as the LIV.[15] However, this guideline was based on Harrington instrumentation, in which the corrective forces were uniplanar. With 3-column fixation using pedicle screws, an additional 1 or 2 distal motion segments can be saved, instead of fusing to the stable vertebra.[49]

The neutral vertebra is also used to determine the distal fusion level.[49,50] The relation between the neutral vertebra and the end vertebra can be used to ascertain the LIV. If there is no more than 1 level between the end vertebra and the neutral vertebra, then fusion to the neutral vertebra is sufficient. This level corresponds to 1 level proximal to the stable vertebra. However, if the neutral vertebra is 2 or more levels distal to the end vertebra, then the LIV is NV-1. If the neutral vertebra is the end vertebra, then it is adequate to fuse to the distal end vertebra. A 2-year follow-up by Suk and colleagues[49] in patients treated using these guidelines showed satisfactory results with good coronal balance, compensatory lumbar straightening, and no adding-on.

With regard to adding-on, Miyanji and colleagues[51] differentiated 2 types of Lenke 1 curves, depending on the L4 tilt: 1A-L (tilted to the left) and 1A-R (tilted to the right). 1A-R curves have been shown to have a higher risk of adding-on because of the overhanging curve pattern, requiring a more distal fusion, approximately 2 levels more distal than a 1A-L curve.[51,52]

Lenke 1C curves have been subject to ongoing controversy regarding their fusion levels because often they behave like double major curves. In the 1C pattern, the nonstructural lumbar curve is flexible (side-bending to <25°), in which the apex completely crosses the midline. A study by Lenke and colleagues[53] showed that selective thoracic fusion was performed in 62% of patients with 1C curves, implying that the remaining 38% had nonselective fusions. Newton and colleagues[54]

reported that larger preoperative lumbar curve magnitude, greater lumbar apical vertebra displacement from the CSVL, and smaller thoracic/lumbar magnitude ratio were factors associated with nonselective fusion. Lenke and colleagues[55] reported that for a selective fusion to be successful for 1B and 1C curves, the thoracic/lumbar ratios for Cobb magnitude, apical vertebral translation, and apical vertebral rotation should be greater than 1.2.

Lenke 2: double thoracic curves

In treating double thoracic curves (**Fig. 2**), it is important to not overlook a structural proximal thoracic curve. Both the main thoracic and the structural proximal thoracic curves must be included in the fusion, according to the Lenke criteria for structural curves. Inappropriate distinction of a structural proximal thoracic curve leading to exclusion of the proximal curve from the fusion, especially in the context of a preoperative elevated left shoulder, can lead to severe worsening of shoulder imbalance and patient dissatisfaction. Suk and colleagues[56] reported improved results when both proximal and main thoracic curves were fused in patients with level shoulders or a higher shoulder on the side of the proximal thoracic curve. In patients with an elevated left shoulder, fusing to T2 as the upper instrumented level is usually sufficient to gain good correction of the proximal thoracic curve and achieve adequate shoulder alignment. In patients with level shoulders preoperatively, the upper level of fusion can be T2 or T3, depending on the correction and shoulder balance achieved intraoperatively. In general, fusion of both proximal and main thoracic curves is recommended for Lenke type 2 curves. Suk and colleagues[56] found that the proximal thoracic curve can be left unfused if the left shoulder is lower than the right by a difference greater than 12 mm.

To select the LIV, the distal fusion rules used for Lenke 1 curves can be applied to Lenke 2 curves. Using the NV and EV as landmarks, the LIV is generally the stable vertebra (the most proximal vertebra intersected by the CSVL).[48–50] Recommendations for selective fusions for type 2C are the same for 1C curves, where the ratio of the main thoracic/thoracolumbar/lumbar curves for Cobb magnitude, apical vertebral translation (AVT), and apical vertebral rotation (AVR) must be 1.2 or greater in curves lacking a focal thoracolumbar kyphosis 10° or greater.[55]

Lenke 3: double major curves

Lenke type 3 curves (**Fig. 3**) are those in which both thoracic and lumbar curves are structural,

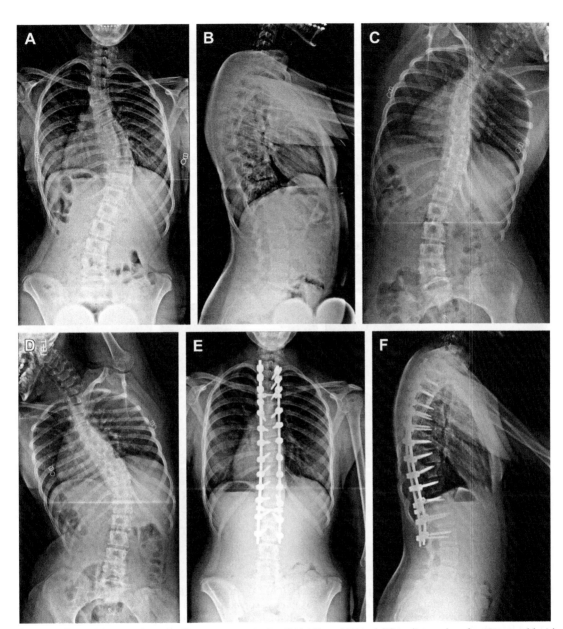

Fig. 2: Lenke 2. Preoperative standing posteroanterior (PA) (*A*) and lateral (*B*) radiographs of a 12-year-old girl with a right 45° main thoracic curve and a left 38° proximal thoracic curve. Right (*C*) and left (*D*) bend films show that the main thoracic curve bends down to 30° and the proximal thoracic curve bends down to 27°. One-month follow-up PA (*E*) and lateral (*F*) radiographs show correction of the main thoracic curve to 16° and correction of the proximal thoracic curve to 17° with posterior pedicle screws from T2 to L2.

so both curves are generally included in the fusion. Some confusion exists between Lenke 1C and Lenke 3 curves, because they can behave similarly, especially Lenke 1C curves with lumbar curves with a borderline nonstructural criterion (bending to slightly <25°).

The goals for double major curves include obtaining adequate correction and balance of both curves. Preoperatively, it is important to note any waist asymmetry or trunk shift in these patients, because the goal is to restore coronal balance. This balance is attained by centralizing and neutralizing the LIV. Also crucial in achieving coronal balance is making the LIV disk as horizontal as possible. It is also not uncommon to find hyperkyphosis in the thoracolumbar area (T10-L2), which should be corrected to achieve normal sagittal alignment. The upper instrumented

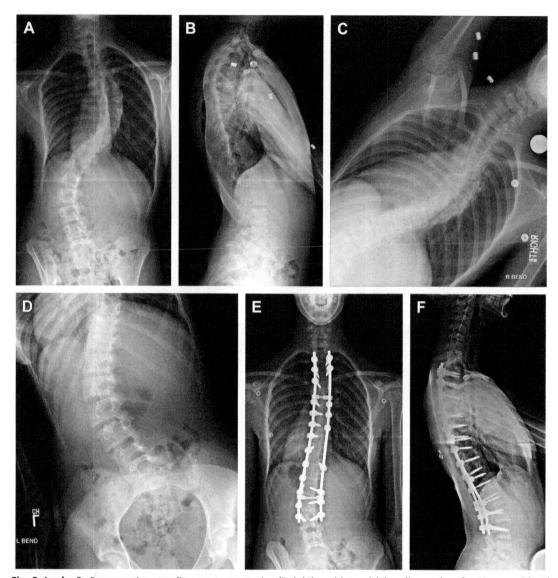

Fig. 3: Lenke 3. Preoperative standing posteroanterior (PA) (*A*) and lateral (*B*) radiographs of a 12-year-old girl with a right 72° main thoracic curve and a left 56° lumbar curve. Right (*C*) and left (*D*) bend films show that the main thoracic curve bends down to 56°, and the lumbar curve bends down to 40°. Two-year follow-up PA (*E*) and lateral (*F*) radiographs show correction of the main thoracic curve to 16° and correction of the lumbar curve to 18° with posterior pedicle screws from T3 to L4.

vertebra (UIV) is determined first by the magnitude and characteristics of the thoracic curve, but shoulder asymmetry and characteristics of the proximal nonstructural thoracic curve must also be considered before deciding the proximal level of fusion. This level usually corresponds to T3 to T5.

As a general guideline for the distal fusion level, the most proximal lumbar vertebra intersected by the CSVL is usually the LIV,[48] either L3 or L4. On posteroanterior standing films, if the apex of the thoracolumbar/lumbar curve is L2 or distal, the L3 to L4 disk space opens on the convexity, and if the rotation of L4 is Nash-Moe grade I or greater,[57] then the fusion should extend to L4. However, if the apex is the L1 to 2 disk or proximal, the L3 to L4 disk space closes or is neutral on the convexity, and the rotation of L3 is grade 1.5 or less, then the fusion can stop at L3.[57] Side-bending films can also be useful for deciding whether to fuse to L3 or L4. For a typical right-sided thoracic and left-sided lumbar curve, Suk and colleagues[49,50] recommend fusing to L3, if L3 crosses the CSVL in the left bending radiograph, or if the rotation of L3 in the right bending radiograph is less than Nash-Moe grade II. Fusion to L4 is recommended if L3 does not cross the CSVL on left bending films, or if L3 rotation is grade II or higher on the right bending films.

Selective thoracic fusion can be considered in some 3C curves in which the main thoracic curve is larger than the thoracolumbar/lumbar curve and there is an absence of thoracolumbar kyphosis from T10 to L2 of 10° or greater. The same main thoracic/thoracolumbar/lumbar ratio criteria of more than 1.2 described for 1C and 2C curves amenable to selective thoracic fusions is used for 3C curves as well.[55,57]

Lenke 4: triple major curves

Lenke 4 curves are those in which the proximal thoracic, main thoracic, and thoracolumbar/lumbar curves are all structural. All 3 curves should be included in the arthrodesis by means of

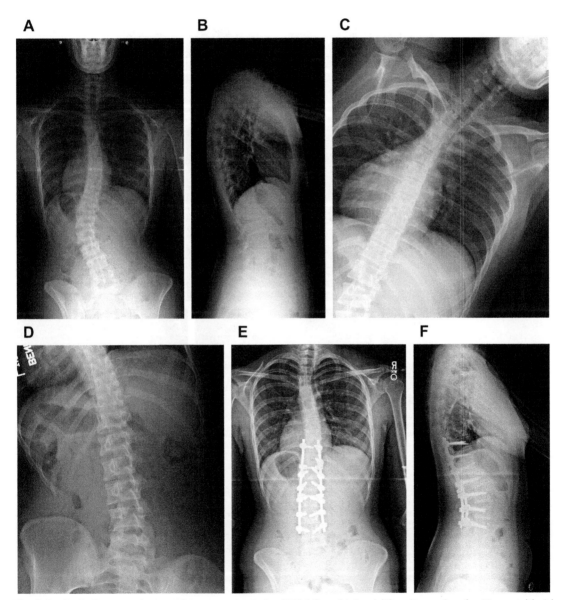

Fig. 4: Lenke 5. Preoperative standing posteroanterior (PA) (*A*) and lateral (*B*) radiographs of a 17-year-old girl with a left 45° main lumbar curve and a right 28° thoracic curve. Right (*C*) and left (*D*) bend films show that the main lumbar curve bends down to 7° and the thoracic curve bends down to 14°. One-year follow-up PA (*E*) and lateral (*F*) radiographs show correction of the main lumbar curve to 10° and correction of the thoracic curve to 6° with posterior pedicle screws from T10 to L4.

a posterior spinal fusion. The choice of the UIV is the same as for double thoracic curves, and is T2 or T3, depending on curve flexibility and shoulder height discrepancy. Selection of LIV is in accordance with the rules for double major curves.

Lenke 5: thoracolumbar/lumbar

For Lenke 5 curves (**Fig. 4**), generally, only the major thoracolumbar/lumbar curve is fused using an anterior or posterior approach. Traditionally, the anterior approach was often used because of its ability to save fusion levels compared with the posterior approach using hooks and rods.[58–64] The fusion levels for the anterior approach included only the thoracolumbar/lumbar curve from the proximal end vertebra to the distal end vertebra. With the use of pedicle screws, studies have shown that fusion levels through the posterior approach can be equivalent to those using the anterior approach, as well as the ability to achieve correction without having to violate the thoracic cavity.[65–69]

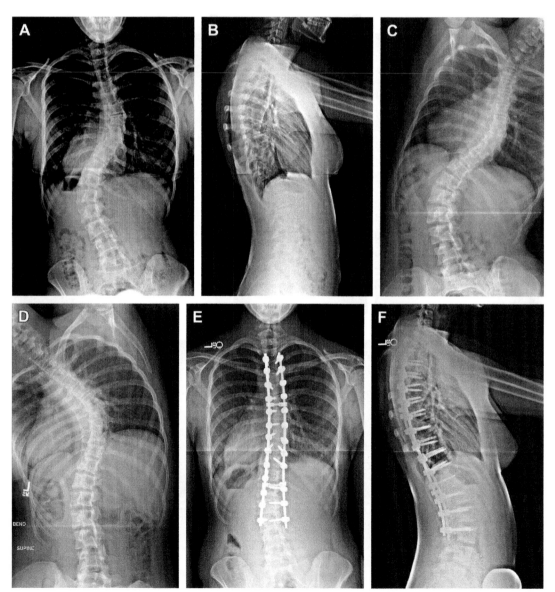

Fig. 5: Lenke 6. Preoperative standing posteroanterior (PA) (*A*) and lateral (*B*) radiographs of a 14-year-old girl with a left 52° main thoracolumbar curve and a right 42° thoracic curve. Right (*C*) and left (*D*) bend films show that the main thoracolumbar curve bends down to 27° and the thoracic curve bends down to 29°. One-month follow-up PA (*E*) and lateral (*F*) radiographs show correction of the main thoracolumbar curve to 19° and correction of the thoracic curve to 17° with posterior pedicle screws from T2-L3.

Similar to recommendations for selective thoracic fusions, for selective thoracolumbar/lumbar fusions to be successful, the ratio criteria of thoracolumbar/lumbar/main thoracic Cobb magnitude, AVT and AVR should be greater than 1.2, and the main thoracic curve should be more flexible than the thoracolumbar/lumbar curve.[55] In cases in which the main thoracic curves are not flexible, and thus have a high probability for postoperative residual curve, the UIV of the fused thoracolumbar/lumbar curve should be left tilted to achieve good balance between the fused curve and unfused main thoracic curve. A relative contraindication for a selective thoracolumbar/lumbar fusion is if a major left thoracolumbar/lumbar curve was accompanied by a depressed left shoulder, because correction of the curve would further accentuate the shoulder imbalance by pulling the left shoulder down.[55]

Lenke 6: thoracolumbar/lumbar/main thoracic

Lenke 6 curves (**Fig. 5**) can be treated similarly to double major curves, because both the major thoracolumbar/lumbar curve and the minor main thoracic curve are structural. Both curves should be included in the fusion. In choosing UIV levels, the upper limits of the main thoracic curve and shoulder alignment should be considered, similar to treating type 3 curves. Treatment guidelines for the LIV are similar to types 3, 4, and 5, in which the most proximal lumbar vertebra crossing the CSVL is used. Suk and colleagues' rules for choosing L3 or L4 using lumbar bending films are also applicable for Lenke 6 curves.[49,56]

SUMMARY

The Lenke classification is a general guideline for the operative treatment of AIS. Since the original classification was proposed, some controversies have arisen, especially for indications for selective fusions. In an era of pedicle screw use, the posterior-only approach is becoming the mainstay of treatment of all Lenke curve types. Further studies on AIS will better define the specific indications and exceptions to the Lenke guidelines to optimize treatment.

REFERENCES

1. Bunnell WP. The natural history of idiopathic scoliosis before skeletal maturity. Spine (Phila Pa 1976) 1986;11(8):773–6.
2. Cobb JR. Outline for the study of scoliosis. Instr Course Left 1948;5:261–75.
3. James JI. Idiopathic scoliosis: the prognosis, diagnosis, and operative indications related to curve patterns and the age at onset. J Bone Joint Surg Br 1954;36(1):36–49.
4. Diab M, Landman Z, Lubicky J, et al. Use and outcome of MRI in the surgical treatment of adolescent idiopathic scoliosis. Spine (Phila Pa 1976) 2011;36(8):667–71.
5. Do T, Fras C, Burke S, et al. Clinical value of routine preoperative magnetic resonance imaging in adolescent idiopathic scoliosis. A prospective study of three hundred and twenty-seven patients. J Bone Joint Surg Am 2001;83(6):577–9.
6. Ogilvie JW, Braun J, Argyle V, et al. The search for idiopathic scoliosis genes. Spine (Phila Pa 1976) 2006;31:679–81.
7. Carr AJ. Adolescent idiopathic scoliosis in identical twins. J Bone Joint Surg Br 1990;72(6):1077.
8. Kesling KL, Reinker KA. Scoliosis in twins: a meta-analysis of the literature and report of six cases. Spine (Phila Pa 1976) 1997;22(17):2009–14.
9. Gao X, Gordon D, Zhang D, et al. CHD7 gene polymorphisms are associated with susceptibility to idiopathic scoliosis. Am J Hum Genet 2007; 80(5):957–65.
10. Kulkarni S, Nagarajan P, Wall J, et al. Disruption of chromodomain helicase DNA binding protein 2 (CHD2) causes scoliosis. Am J Med Genet A 2008; 146A(9):1117–27.
11. Gurnett CA, Alaee F, Bowcock A, et al. Genetic linkage localizes an adolescent idiopathic scoliosis and pectus excavatum gene to chromosome 18 q. Spine (Phila Pa 1976) 2009;34(2):E94–100.
12. Risser JC, Norquist DM, Cockrell BR Jr, et al. The effect of posterior spine fusion on the growing spine. Clin Orthop Relat Res 1966;46:127–39.
13. Lonstein JE. Scoliosis: surgical versus nonsurgical treatment. Clin Orthop Relat Res 2006;443:248–59.
14. Weinstein SL. Adolescent idiopathic scoliosis: prevalence and natural history. Instr Course Lect 1989; 38:115–28.
15. King HA, Moe JH, Bradford DS, et al. The selection of fusion levels in thoracic idiopathic scoliosis. J Bone Joint Surg Am 1983;65(9):1302–13.
16. Lenke LG, Betz RR, Harms J, et al. Adolescent idiopathic scoliosis: a new classification to determine extent of spinal arthrodesis. J Bone Joint Surg Am 2001;83(8):1169–81.
17. Lonstein JE, Carlson JM. The prediction of curve progression in untreated idiopathic scoliosis during growth. J Bone Joint Surg Am 1984;66(7):1061–71.
18. Katz DE, Herring A, Browne RH, et al. Brace wear control of curve progression in adolescent idiopathic scoliosis. J Bone Joint Surg Am 2010;92(6):1343–52.
19. Nachemson AL, Peterson LE. Effectiveness of treatment with a brace in girls who have adolescent idiopathic scoliosis. A prospective, controlled study based on data from the Brace Study of the Scoliosis

Research Society. J Bone Joint Surg Am 1995;77(6): 815–22.

20. Rowe DE, Bernstein SM, Riddick MF, et al. A meta-analysis of the efficacy of non-operative treatments for idiopathic scoliosis. J Bone Joint Surg Am 1997;79(5):664–74.

21. Fowles JV, Drummond DS, L'Ecuyer S, et al. Untreated scoliosis in the adult. Clin Orthop Relat Res 1978;134:212–7.

22. Asher M, Min Lai S, Burton D, et al. Discrimination validity of the Scoliosis Research Society-22 patient questionnaire: relationship to idiopathic scoliosis curve pattern and curve size. Spine (Phila Pa 1976) 2003;28(1):74–8.

23. Kuklo TR, O'Brien MF, Lenke LG, et al. Comparison of the lowest instrumented, stable, and lower end vertebrae in "single overhang" thoracic adolescent idiopathic scoliosis: anterior versus posterior spinal fusion. Spine (Phila Pa 1976) 2006;31(19): 2232–6.

24. Turi M, Johnston CE II, Richards BS. Anterior correction of idiopathic scoliosis using TSRH instrumentation. Spine (Phila Pa 1976) 1993;18:417–22.

25. Betz RR, Shufflebarger H. Anterior versus posterior instrumentation for the correction of thoracic idiopathic scoliosis. Spine (Phila Pa 1976) 2001;26: 1095–100.

26. Kim YJ, Lenke LG, Bridwell KH, et al. Pulmonary function in adolescent idiopathic scoliosis relative to the surgical procedure. J Bone Joint Surg Am 2005;87(7):1534–41.

27. Lenke LG, Newton PO, Marks MC, et al. Prospective pulmonary function comparison of open versus endoscopic anterior fusion combined with posterior fusion in adolescent idiopathic scoliosis. Spine (Phila Pa 1976) 2004;29(18):2055–60.

28. Graham EJ, Lenke LG, Lowe TG, et al. Prospective pulmonary function evaluation following open thoracotomy for anterior spinal fusion in adolescent idiopathic scoliosis. Spine (Phila Pa 1976) 2000; 25(18):2319–25.

29. Dobbs MB, Lenke LG, Kim YJ, et al. Anterior/posterior spinal instrumentation versus posterior instrumentation alone for the treatment of adolescent idiopathic scoliotic curves more than 90 degrees. Spine (Phila Pa 1976) 2006;31(20): 2386–91.

30. Hwang SW, Samdani AF, Lonner B, et al. Impact of direct vertebral body derotation on rib prominence. Are preoperative factors predictive of changes in rib prominence? Spine (Phila Pa 1976) 2012;37(2): E86–9.

31. Suk SI, Lee SM, Chung ER, et al. Selective thoracic fusion with segmental pedicle screw fixation in the treatment of thoracic idiopathic scoliosis: more than 5-year follow-up. Spine (Phila Pa 1976) 2005; 30(14):1602–9.

32. Kim YJ, Lenke LG, Bridwell KH, et al. Free hand pedicle screw placement in the thoracic spine: is it safe? Spine (Phila Pa 1976) 2004;29(3):333–42.

33. Samdani AF, Ranade A, Sciubba DM, et al. Accuracy of free-hand placement of thoracic pedicle screws in adolescent idiopathic scoliosis: how much of a difference does surgeon experience make? Eur Spine J 2010;19(1):91–5.

34. Samdani AF, Ranade A, Saldanha V, et al. Learning curve for placement of thoracic pedicle screws in the deformed spine. Neurosurgery 2010;66(2): 290–4.

35. Suk SI, Kim WJ, Lee SM, et al. Thoracic pedicle screw fixation in spinal deformities: are they really safe? Spine (Phila Pa 1976) 2001;26(18):2049–57.

36. Lehman RA Jr, Lenke LG, Keeler KA, et al. Computed tomography evaluation of pedicle screws placed in the pediatric deformed spine over an 8-year period. Spine (Phila Pa 1976) 2007;32(24): 2679–84.

37. Belmont PJ Jr, Klemme WR, Robinson M, et al. Accuracy of thoracic pedicle screws in patients with and without coronal plane spinal deformities. Spine (Phila Pa 1976) 2002;27(14):1558–66.

38. Guzey FK, Emel E, Hakan Seyithanoglu M, et al. Accuracy of pedicle screw placement for upper and middle thoracic pathologies without coronal plane spinal deformity using conventional methods. J Spinal Disord Tech 2006;19(6):436–41.

39. Newton PO, Yaszay B, Upasani VV, et al. Preservation of thoracic kyphosis is critical to maintain lumbar lordosis in the surgical treatment of adolescent idiopathic scoliosis. Spine (Phila Pa 1976) 2010;35(14): 1365–70.

40. Hwang SW, Samdani AF, Tantorski M, et al. Cervical sagittal plane decompensation after surgery for adolescent idiopathic scoliosis: an effect imparted by postoperative thoracic hypokyphosis. J Neurosurg Spine 2011;15(5):491–6.

41. Lehman RA Jr, Lenke LG, Keeler KA, et al. Operative treatment of adolescent idiopathic scoliosis with posterior pedicle screw-only constructs: minimum three-year follow-up of one hundred fourteen cases. Spine (Phila Pa 1976) 2008;33(14):1598–604.

42. Lenke LG, Betz RR, Bridwell KH, et al. Spontaneous lumbar curve coronal correction after selective anterior or posterior thoracic fusion in adolescent idiopathic scoliosis. Spine (Phila Pa 1976) 1999; 24(16):1663–71.

43. McCance SE, Denis F, Lonstein JE, et al. Coronal and sagittal balance in surgically treated adolescent idiopathic scoliosis with the King II curve pattern. A review of 67 consecutive cases having selective thoracic arthrodesis. Spine (Phila Pa 1976) 1998; 23(19):2063–73.

44. Winter RB, Lonstein JE. A meta-analysis of the literature on the issue of selective thoracic fusion for

the King-Moe type II curve pattern in adolescent idiopathic scoliosis. Spine (Phila Pa 1976) 2003; 28(9):948–52.

45. Jansen RC, van Rhijn LW, Duinkerke E, et al. Predictability of the spontaneous lumbar curve correction after selective thoracic fusion in idiopathic scoliosis. Eur Spine J 2007;16(9):1335–42.

46. Peelle MW, Boachie-Adjei O, Charles G, et al. Lumbar curve response to selective thoracic fusion in adult idiopathic scoliosis. Spine J 2008;8(6): 897–903.

47. Kuklo TR, Lenke LG, Graham EJ, et al. Correlation of radiographic, clinical, and patient assessment of shoulder balance following fusion versus nonfusion of the proximal thoracic curve in adolescent idiopathic scoliosis. Spine (Phila Pa 1976) 2002; 27(18):2013–20.

48. Rose PS, Lenke LG. Classification of operative adolescent idiopathic scoliosis: treatment guidelines. Orthop Clin North Am 2007;38(4):521–9.

49. Suk SI, Lee SM, Chung ER, et al. Determination of distal fusion level with segmental pedicle screw fixation in single thoracic idiopathic scoliosis. Spine (Phila Pa 1976) 2003;28(5):484–91.

50. Suk SI. Pedicle screw instrumentation for adolescent idiopathic scoliosis: the insertion technique, the fusion levels and direct vertebral rotation. Clin Orthop Surg 2011;3(2):89–100.

51. Miyanji F, Pawelek JB, Van Valin SE, et al. Is the lumbar modifier useful in surgical decision making? Defining two distinct Lenke 1A curve patterns. Spine (Phila Pa 1976) 2008;33(23):2545–51.

52. Cho RH, Yaszay B, Bartley CE, et al. Which Lenke 1A curves are at greatest risk for adding-on and why? Spine (Phila Pa 1976) 2012;37:1384–90.

53. Lenke LG, Betz RR, Clements D, et al. Curve prevalence of a new classification of operative adolescent idiopathic scoliosis: does classification correlate with treatment? Spine (Phila Pa 1976) 2002;27:604–11.

54. Newton PO, Faro FD, Lenke LG, et al. Factors involved in the decision to perform a selective versus nonselective fusion of Lenke 1B and 1C (King-Moe II) curves in adolescent idiopathic scoliosis. Spine (Phila Pa 1976) 2003;28(20):S217–23.

55. Lenke LG, Edwards CC II, Bridwell KH. The Lenke classification of adolescent idiopathic scoliosis: how it organizes curve patterns as a template to perform selective fusions of the spine. Spine (Phila Pa 1976) 2003;28(20):S199–207.

56. Suk SI, Kim WJ, Lee CS, et al. Indications of proximal thoracic curve fusion in thoracic adolescent idiopathic scoliosis. Recognition and treatment of double thoracic curve pattern in adolescent idiopathic

scoliosis treated with segmental instrumentation. Spine (Phila Pa 1976) 2000;25(18):2342–9.

57. Lenke LG. The Lenke classification system of operative adolescent idiopathic scoliosis. Neurosurg Clin North Am 2007;18(2):199–206.

58. Baumann R, Brown H, Johnston C, et al. Selective anterior lumbar fusion in King I curves. Scoliosis Research Society Annual Meeting. San Diego, CA, September 22-25, 1999.

59. Bernstein RM, Hall JE. Solid short segment anterior fusion in thoracolumbar scoliosis. J Pediatr Orthop B 1998;7(2):124–31.

60. Dwyer AF, Newton NC, Sherwood AA. Anterior approach to scoliosis: A preliminary report. Clin Orthop Relat Res 1969;62:192–202.

61. Dwyer AF, Schafer MF. Anterior approach to scoliosis. Results of treatment in fifty-one cases. J Bone Joint Surg Br 1974;56(2):218–24.

62. Hsu LC, Zucherman J, Tang SC, et al. Dwyer instrumentation in the treatment of adolescent idiopathic scoliosis. J Bone Joint Surg Br 1982;64(5):536–41.

63. Kaneda K, Fujiya N, Satoh S. Results with Zielke instrumentation for idiopathic thoracolumbar and lumbar scoliosis. Clin Orthop Relat Res 1986;205: 195–203.

64. Kelly DM, McCarthy RE, McCullough FL, et al. Long-term outcomes of anterior spinal fusion with instrumentation for thoracolumbar and lumbar curves in adolescent idiopathic scoliosis. Spine (Phila Pa 1976) 2010;35(2):194–8.

65. Geck MJ, Rinella A, Hawthorne D, et al. Comparison of surgical treatment in Lenke 5C adolescent idiopathic scoliosis: anterior dual rod versus posterior pedicle fixation surgery: a comparison of two practices. Spine (Phila Pa 1976) 2009;34(18):1942–51.

66. Hee HT, Yu ZR, Wong HK. Comparison of segmental pedicle screw instrumentation versus anterior instrumentation in adolescent idiopathic thoracolumbar and lumbar scoliosis. Spine (Phila Pa 1976) 2007; 32(14):1533–42.

67. Kim YJ, Lenke LG, Kim J, et al. Comparative analysis of pedicle screw versus hybrid instrumentation in posterior spinal fusion of adolescent idiopathic scoliosis. Spine (Phila Pa 1976) 2006; 31(3):291–8.

68. Li M, Ni J, Fang X, et al. Comparison of selective anterior versus posterior screw instrumentation in Lenke 5C adolescent idiopathic scoliosis. Spine (Phila Pa 1976) 2009;34(11):1162–6.

69. Shufflebarger HL, Geck MJ, Clark CE. The posterior approach for lumbar and thoracolumbar adolescent idiopathic scoliosis: posterior shortening and pedicle screws. Spine (Phila Pa 1976) 2004;29(3):269–76.

Classifications for Adult Spinal Deformity and Use of the Scoliosis Research Society–Schwab Adult Spinal Deformity Classification

Shay Bess, MD[a],*, Frank Schwab, MD[b],
Virginie Lafage, PhD[b], Christopher I. Shaffrey, MD[c,d],
Christopher P. Ames, MD[a]

KEYWORDS

- Adult spinal deformity • Classification • Schwab Adult Spinal Deformity Classification • Disability

KEY POINTS

- Classification systems should describe important features of disease states and provide clinical information regarding the classified disease state.
- Previous classifications for adult spinal deformity (ASD) neglected evaluation of sagittal spinopelvic parameters.
- Pelvic incidence/lumbar lordosis mismatch (PI-LL), increased sagittal vertical axis (SVA), and increased pelvic tilt (PT) correlate strongly with pain and disability in patients with ASD.
- The Scoliosis Research Society (SRS)–Schwab ASD Classification describes the location of the scoliotic curve and uses 3 sagittal modifiers (PI-LL, SVA, and PT) to evaluate the sagittal plane and correlate spinal deformity with patient pain and disability.
- Greater spinal deformity grade on the SRS-Schwab ASD Classification predicts patient disability.

Disclosures: Dr Bess consults for Alphatec, Allosource, DePuy Spine, and Medtronic; receives royalties from Pioneer Spine; receives research support from DePuy Spine, Medtronic, Orthopaedic Research and Education Foundation; and is on the Scientific Advisory Board for Allosource. Dr Schwab consults for Medtronic, DePuy Spine; receives royalties from Medtronic; is a shareholder of Nemaris Inc.; receives research support from DePuy Spine, NIH; and provides educational communication for Medtronic, DePuy Spine. Dr Lafage consults for Medtronic; receives research support from the Scoliosis Research Society; is a shareholder of Nemaris Inc.; and provides educational communication for Medtronic, K2M, and DePuy Spine. Dr Shaffrey consults for Biomet, DePuy-Synthes, Globus, Medtronic, and Nuvasive; receives royalties from Biomet, and Medtronic; receives research support from AO, DePuy-Synthes, Department of Defense, Medtronic, NACTN, and NIH. Conflicts of interest: None.

[a] Departments of Orthopedics, Rocky Mountain Hospital for Children, Presbyterian/St Lukes Medical Center, Rocky Mountain Scoliosis and Spine, 2055 High Street, Suite 130, Denver, CO 80205, USA; [b] Departments of Orthopedics, NYU Hospital for Joint Diseases, 306 East 15th Street, New York, NY 10003, USA; [c] Department of Neurological Surgery, University of Virginia, Box 800212, Charlottesville, VA 22908, USA; [d] Department of Orthopaedic Surgery, University of Virginia, Box 800212, Charlottesville, VA 22908, USA
* Corresponding author.
E-mail address: shay_bess@hotmail.com

Neurosurg Clin N Am 24 (2013) 185–193
http://dx.doi.org/10.1016/j.nec.2012.12.008
1042-3680/13/$ – see front matter © 2013 Elsevier Inc. All rights reserved.

INTRODUCTION

Classification systems are created to provide organization to pathologic conditions and provide treatment options for disease states that share a common theme. A classification ideally provides a cohesive approach to the disease state that (1) identifies different severities of the disease state (often in a hierarchical manner), (2) facilitates communication between health care providers and researchers to assure accuracy and reproducibility in describing the disease state, (3) allows for comparison of different treatment methods and, as a consequence, (4) allows for creation of accurate treatment recommendation guidelines. From a statistical standpoint, a classification system should have high construct validity (the extent to which classification accurately measures the disease state) and high reliability as shown by high intrarater reliability (consistent grading by 1 rater at different time points) and inter-rater reliability (consistent grading by different raters). The classification should also have high reproducibility (the degree of agreement between measurements on replicate specimens in different locations by different observers). This article provides an overview of existing classification systems for spinal deformity and highlights the challenges of creating an effective classification for adult spinal deformity (ASD). This article then focuses on the Scoliosis Research Society (SRS)–Schwab ASD Classification, including the rationale behind the development of the SRS-Schwab ASD Classification, guidelines for use of the SRS-Schwab ASD Classification, and initial data on use of the classification.

BACKGROUND ON SPINAL DEFORMITY CLASSIFICATION SYSTEMS

Most classifications traditionally used to describe spinal deformity have been oriented toward pediatric spinal deformities. In the past, the King-Moe Classification for Adolescent Idiopathic Scoliosis (AIS) has been the standard to describe scoliosis.[1] The principle benefit of the King-Moe classification was that it provided a treatment algorithm based on curve type that allowed surgeons to determine the appropriate curves and vertebral levels for spinal fusion. Five types of curves were described in detail including type I, a double major curve, in which the thoracic and lumbar curves are considered structural and both curves should be included in the fusion; type II, a single major curve, in which the thoracic and lumbar curves cross the midline (center sacral vertical line [CSVL]), but the thoracic curve is larger and more rigid than the lumbar curve and therefore the thoracic curve is structural and only the thoracic curve should be included in the fusion; type III, in which only the thoracic curve crosses the midline, and only the thoracic curve should be included in the fusion; type IV, a long, sweeping thoracic curve in which L4 is titled toward the thoracic curve and L5 is centered over the sacrum, distal fusion level recommended to be the first vertebra bisected by the CSVL; type V, a double thoracic curve pattern in which the proximal and main thoracic curves are considered structural and are included in the fusion (**Fig. 1**).

The King-Moe system remained the principal classification for AIS for more than 20 years, guiding evaluation and treatment; however, several limitations of the King-Moe system have been highlighted. First, the King-Moe system is not comprehensive, because isolated thoracolumbar and triple major curves were not described. All patients in the King and colleagues[1] series received Harrington rod instrumentation that solely corrected deformity in the coronal plane via distraction, therefore the deformities were evaluated only in the coronal plane, failing to recognize scoliosis as a three-dimensional deformity and the need to assess the coronal, sagittal, and axial planes. The King-More system has also shown fair to poor interobserver and intraobserver validity, reliability, and reproducibility by 2 separate studies.[2,3] In response to these shortcomings, Lenke and colleagues[4] developed a classification system for the operative treatment of AIS. This classification was designed to be (1) comprehensive, to include all AIS curve types; (2) provide two-dimensional analysis with increased emphasis on evaluation of the sagittal plane; (3) treatment based, advocating selective arthrodesis only of the structural curves; and (4) provide objective criteria to differentiate individual curve types and provide guidelines for fusion. The Lenke classification describes 3 curve regions (proximal thoracic [PT], apex at T3, T4, or T5; main thoracic [MT], apex between T6 and the T11–T12 disc; and thoracolumbar/lumbar [TL/L], apex at T12 or L1 for thoracolumbar curves, and between the L1–L2 disc and L4 for lumbar curves) and 2 curve types (major curve, the largest measured curve; minor curve, the smaller curves). The minor curves are then established as structural or nonstructural by evaluating curve flexibility and sagittal alignment. Structural curves show coronal plane rigidity (do not reduce less than 25° on side bending radiographs) and/or are focally kyphotic in the sagittal plane (focal kyphosis >20°). Focal kyphosis for the described curve regions is measured in the following areas: PT, T2 to T5; MT, T10 to L2; and TL/L, T10 to L2. Using the

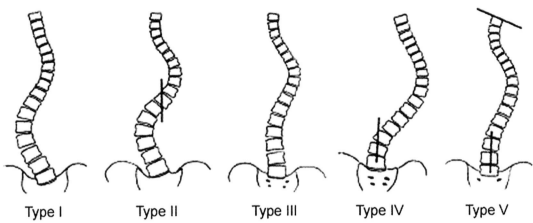

| Type I | Type II | Type III | Type IV | Type V |

Fig. 1. King-Moe Classification for Thoracic Idiopathic Scoliosis. (*Adapted from* King HA, Moe JH, Bradford DS, et al. The selection of fusion levels in thoracic idiopathic scoliosis. J Bone Joint Surg Am 1983;65:1302–13; with permission.)

Lenke classification, 6 curve types can be assigned according to the identified major and minor structural curves, and are named according to the identified structural curves: type 1, MT curve (structural); type 2, double thoracic (PT and MT curves are structural); type 3, double major (MT and TL/L curves are structural, MT is larger on standing radiographs); type 4, triple major (PT, MT, and TL/L curves are structural); type 5, thoracolumbar/lumbar (TL/L curve structural); and type 6 (MT and TL/L are structural, TL/L is larger on standing radiographs). Treatment guidelines recommend selective fusion, advocating fusion only of those curves that are structural as per the classification guidelines (**Fig. 2**).

The Lenke classification has been widely adopted for evaluation and treatment of AIS, with excellent success. However, despite the initial usefulness of the King-Moe and, subsequently, the Lenke classifications to describe AIS, there have been attempts to apply many of these same classification guidelines to ASD. The error in applying AIS and/or pediatric spinal deformity assessment guidelines to creating an ASD classification lies in heterogeneity of the clinical and radiographic presentation of ASD. Although cosmetic deformity and coronal malalignment are the most common reasons for presentation and treatment of pediatric patients with spinal deformity, especially AIS, pain is the primary complaint for patients with ASD.[5–8] Effective AIS classifications have therefore focused on strategies to evaluate and treat scoliosis and coronal malalignment; however, classifications for ASD must quantify the major predictors of pain in the ASD population. Early attempts at developing ASD classifications by Aebi[10] and by the SRS failed to integrate this clinical component of pain in the ASD population,

and therefore, despite being descriptive of the cause and observed radiographic parameters, these classifications lacked clinical relevance.[9,10] Scoliosis and coronal plane deformities are common for both AIS and ASD; however, it has been repeatedly shown that sagittal malalignment is a fundamental component of ASD, and that sagittal malalignment is a primary determinant of pain and disability in the ASD population.[6,11–14] One advantage of the Lenke classification is that it calls for greater attention to the sagittal plane, although it does so within the confines of defining the structural behavior of a coronal deformity (idiopathic scoliosis) rather than purely quantifying the amount of sagittal plane deformity. Based on these concepts, initial work by Schwab and colleagues[8] established a foundation for a clinical impact classification for ASD that integrated radiographic parameters correlating with poor health-related quality of life (HRQOL) parameters.[15–17] This initial classification by Schwab and colleagues[17] described 5 types of scoliosis based on the apical level of the curve: type I, thoracic only; type II, upper thoracic major (apex T4–T8); type III, lower thoracic major (apex T9–T10); type IV, thoracolumbar major curve (apex T11–L1); type V, lumbar major curve (apex L2–L4). Two radiographic parameters were then added as modifiers to the curve type: lumbar lordosis and intervertebral subluxation. Loss of lumbar lordosis and increased intervertebral subluxation correlated with poor HRQOL scores, so it is these modifiers that denoted the clinical impact of this classification. Soon after publication, it was recognized that global sagittal malalignment, measured by sagittal vertical axis (SVA; distance from the C7 plumb line to the posterior, superior corner of S1) is an equally important predictor of poor HRQOL

Curve Type

Type	Proximal Thoracic	Main Thoracic	Thoracolumbar/ Lumbar	Curve Type
1	Non-Structural	Structural (Major*)	Non-Structural	Main Thoracic (MT)
2	Structural	Structural (Major*)	Non-Structural	Double Thoracic (DT)
3	Non-Structural	Structural (Major*)	Structural	Double Major (DM)
4	Structural	Structural (Major*)	Structural	Triple Major (TM)
5	Non-Structural	Non-Structural	Structural (Major*)	Thoracolumbar/Lumbar (TL/L)
6	Non-Structural	Structural	Structural (Major*)	Thoracolumbar/Lumbar— Main Thoracic (TL/L–MT)

STRUCTURAL CRITERIA
(Minor Curves)

Proximal Thoracic: —Side Bending Cobb ≥ 25°
—T2–T5 Kyphosis ≥ +20°

Main Thoracic: —Side Bending Cobb ≥ 25°
—T10–L2 Kyphosis ≥ +20°

Thoracolumbar/Lumbar: —Side Bending Cobb ≥ 25°
—T10–L2 Kyphosis ≥ +20°

*Major = Largest Cobb Measurement, always structural
Minor = all other curves with structural criteria applied

LOCATION OF APEX
(SRS definition)

CURVE	APEX
THORACIC	T2–T11-12 DISC
THORACOLUMBAR	T12–L1
LUMBAR	L1-2 DISC–L4

Modifiers

Lumbar Spine Modifier	CSVL to Lumbar Apex
A	CSVL Between Pedicles
B	CSVL Touches Apical Body(ies)
C	CSVL Completely Medial

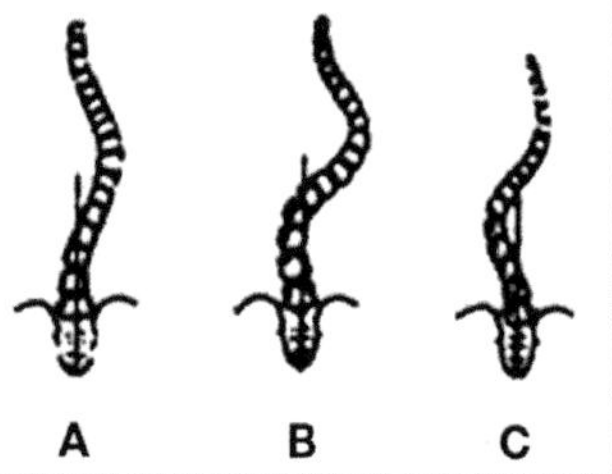

A   B   C

	Thoracic Sagittal Profile T5–T12	
−	(Hypo)	<10°
N	(Normal)	10°–40°
+	(Hyper)	>40°

Curve Type (1–6) + Lumbar Spine Modifier (A, B, or C) + Thoracic Sagittal Modifier (−, N, or +)

Classification (e.g. 1B+): _____

Fig. 2. Lenke Classification for Adolescent Idiopathic Scoliosis. (*Adapted from* Lenke LG, Betz RR, Harms J, et al. Adolescent idiopathic scoliosis: a new classification to determine extent of spinal arthrodesis. J Bone Joint Surg Am 2001;83:1169–81; with permission.)

scores as regional sagittal malalignment (loss of lumbar lordosis). Therefore the classification added a third modifier, termed the global balance modifier, as a final component to describe the radiographic deformity and predict the associated disability (**Box 1**).

SRS-SCHWAB ASD CLASSIFICATION

The Schwab Clinical Impact Classification represented an advance in the manner by which ASD is classified because it highlighted radiographic parameters that correlate with pain and disability in ASD. However, further research has shown that lumbar lordosis (LL) and SVA alone do not provide a complete picture of the disorders leading to sagittal malalignment.[18–20] The importance of pelvic alignment to the maintenance of upright posture has been increasingly emphasized, leading to the concept of spinopelvic alignment as a more complete description of the physiologic mechanisms used to maintain standing upright posture.[21–24] Pelvic measurements include pelvic incidence (PI), which is a fixed, morphologic parameter, and 2 dynamic parameters that reflect compensatory changes within the pelvis to maintain upright posture: pelvic tilt (PT) and sacral slope (SS; **Fig. 3**). Pelvic retroversion is a compensatory mechanism used to maintain upright posture in the setting of sagittal malalignment. Increased PT indicates pelvic retroversion, and has been shown to correlate with poor HRQOL.[12] PT has also been described to normalize (relaxation of pelvic retroversion) in conjunction with improved SVA following lumbar osteotomy procedures.[25] PI is a morphologic

---

Box 1
Schwab Clinical Impact Classification for ASD

Type: location of the deformity (apical level of the major curve or sagittal plane only)

   Type I: thoracic-only scoliosis (no thoracolumbar or lumbar component)

   Type II: upper thoracic major, apex T4 to T8 (with thoracolumbar or lumbar curve)

   Type III: lower thoracic major, apex T9 to T10 (with thoracolumbar/lumbar curve)

   Type IV: thoracolumbar major curve, apex T11 to L1 (with any other minor curve)

   Type V: lumbar major curve, apex L2 to L4 (with any other minor curve)

   Type K: deformity in the sagittal plane only

Lordosis modifier: sagittal Cobb angle from T12 to S1

   A: marked lordosis greater than 40°

   B: moderate lordosis 0°–40°

   C: no lordosis present Cobb less than 0°

Subluxation modifier: frontal or sagittal plane (anterior or posterior), maximum value

   0: no subluxation

   +: subluxation 1 to 6 mm

   + +: subluxation greater than 7 mm

Global balance modifier: sagittal plane C7 offset from posterior superior corner S1

   N: normal (0–4 cm)

   P: positive (4–9.5 cm)

   VP: very positive (>9.5 cm)

Adapted from Schwab F, Lafage V, Farcy JP, et al. Surgical rates and operative outcome analysis in thoracolumbar and lumbar major adult scoliosis: application of the new adult deformity classification. Spine 2007;32:2723–30; with permission.

---

parameter, and therefore, as an isolated measure, PI provides limited information; however, the relationship of PI to LL provides valuable information regarding the patient's sagittal spinopelvic alignment and provides surgeons with reconstructive requirements to restore a physiologic sagittal profile. In line with these findings, work by Lafage and colleagues[12] and Schwab and colleagues[13,14,26] has led to the discovery of threshold spinopelvic parameters for pain and severe disability. Values including PT greater than 22°, PI-LL greater than 11°, and SVA greater than 46 mm have been shown to correlate with Oswestry Disability Index (ODI) scores greater than

40 (severe disability) in a prospective cohort of patients with ASD.[26] The Schwab classification, in conjunction with efforts through the SRS, was consequently updated to reflect these data and create the SRS-Schwab ASD Classification.[27]

RADIOGRAPHIC ANALYSIS AND CLASSIFICATION

Accurate radiographic analysis of ASD requires full-length frontal and lateral radiographs that visualize C7 and the bilateral femoral heads. As an overview of the SRS-Schwab ASD Classification, the 2 primary components of the classification include (1) coronal curve type (assessment of the frontal plane deformity by denoting the location and magnitude of scoliotic curves) and (2) sagittal modifiers (assessment of the sagittal plane deformity via PI-LL, SVA, and PT as referenced earlier). The sagittal modifiers are then graded by the severity of the deformity (**Fig. 4**).[12–14,22,26]

The curve type is assigned based on the location and Cobb angle of the scoliotic curve(s). Only curves greater than 30° are considered for classification. Curve types include type T (isolated major thoracic curve >30°, curve apex at T9 or cranial), type L (isolated thoracolumbar or lumbar curve >30°, curve apex at T10 or caudal), type D (double major curve in which the thoracic and thoracolumbar/lumbar curves are >30°), and type N (normal; no scoliotic curve >30°).

The first sagittal modifier, PI-LL modifier, measures the PI/LL mismatch, providing an assessment of the amount of disharmony between the patient's morphologic PI and corresponding LL. LL should be within 10° of PI, consequently patients with PI-LL less than 10° are assigned a PI-LL modifier of 0. Patients with PI-LL between 10° and 20° are assigned PI-LL modifier of +, and patients with PI-LL greater than 20° are assigned PI-LL modifier of ++.

Global alignment is the second sagittal modifier and is assessed by SVA. As indicated earlier, SVA should be greater than 40 mm of PI, consequently patients with SVA less than 40 mm are assigned the global alignment modifier 0. Patients with SVA between 40 and 95 mm are assigned global alignment modifier +, and patients with SVA greater than 95 mm are assigned global alignment modifier ++.

Pelvic tilt is the third sagittal modifier. As indicated earlier, PT greater than 20° reflects compensatory pelvic retroversion to maintain upright posture, and has also correlated with pain and disability. Patients with PT less than 20° are assigned PT modifier 0. Patients with PT between 20° and 30° are assigned PT modifier +, and

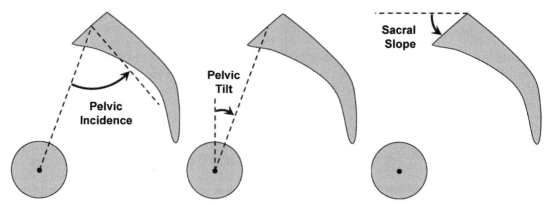

Fig. 3. Sagittal spinopelvic parameters. PI, the angle between the line drawn perpendicular to the sacral end plate at its midpoint and the line drawn from the midpoint of the sacral end plate to the midpoint of the bicoxofemoral axis; PT, the angle between the line connecting the midpoint of the sacral end plate to the midpoint of the bicoxofemoral axis and the vertical; and SS, the angle between the horizontal and the upper sacral endplate. (*Adapted from* Schwab F, Patel A, Ungar B, et al. Adult spinal deformity-postoperative standing imbalance: how much can you tolerate? An overview of key parameters in assessing alignment and planning corrective surgery. Spine (Phila Pa 1976) 2010;35:2224–31; with permission.)

patients with PT greater than 30° are assigned PT modifier ++ (**Figs. 5 and 6**).

In addition to correlating with pain and disability, the sagittal modifiers can be used as a guideline for surgical planning, because the modifiers provide an objective measure for the amount of sagittal spinopelvic deformity. Patients with a PI-LL modifier ++, by definition, require an addition of at least 10° of LL to restore the normal physiologic relationship between PI and LL. The global alignment and PT modifiers, together, also provide a guide for surgical planning, by denoting the amount of sagittal plane deformity and compensatory mechanisms the patient is using to maintain

upright posture. Patients with a high SVA and high pelvic tilt have a greater sagittal deformity and require larger sagittal plane correction than patients with high SVA and normal pelvic tilt, because effective correction for the patient with high SVA and high PT requires not only reduction of SVA but also normalization of PT. Evaluation of patients having lumbar pedicle subtraction osteotomy (PSO) showed that PT reduces following PSO procedures; however, high PT is also a risk factor for residual sagittal deformity following PSO.[28] Patients with high PT and high SVA consequently require a greater degree of osteotomy resection at the PSO site and/or a combination

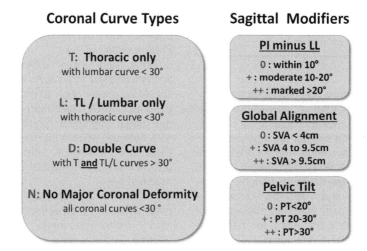

Fig. 4. SRS-Schwab ASD Classification. (*Adapted from* Schwab F, Ungar B, Blondel B, et al. Scoliosis Research Society-Schwab Adult Spinal Deformity Classification: a validation study. Spine 2012;37:1077–82; with permission.)

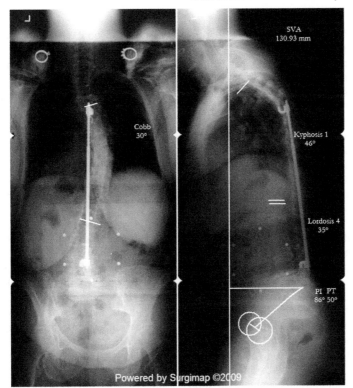

Fig. 5. Example of SRS-Schwab ASD Classification. Patient has a thoracic curve of 30°, a PI-LL of 51° (PI = 86°, LL = 35°), a pelvic tilt of 50°, and an SVA of 13.1 cm. The patient therefore has a classification grade of T, PI-LL++, PT++, SVA++.

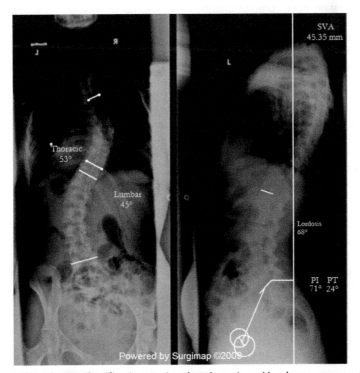

Fig. 6. Example of SRS-Schwab ASD Classification. Patient has thoracic and lumbar curves greater than 30°, a PI-LL of 26° (PI = 71°, LL = 68°), a pelvic tilt of 24°, and an SVA of −4.5 cm. The patient therefore has a classification grade of D, PT+.

of other corrective techniques to prevent residual postoperative sagittal deformity.

In order to have practical value, a classification must balance information provided, ease of use, and ability to generate consistent classification ratings for the same user and between users. Initial data on the use of the SRS-Schwab ASD Classification reported good to excellent intrarater reliability (mean kappa score range 0.88–0.97 for curve type and sagittal modifiers; mean kappa total grade 0.87) and good to excellent inter-rater reliability (mean kappa score range 0.75–0.98 for curve type and sagittal modifiers; mean kappa total grade 0.70–0.79), reflecting relative ease of use and consistent user scores.[27] As a consequence of the methodology used to create the classification, the classification has been shown to predict patient disability and patient preference for operative versus nonoperative treatment. Prospective evaluation of a consecutive cohort of operatively and nonoperatively treated patients with ASD using the SRS-Schwab Classification showed that operatively treated patients had worse HRQOL scores and worse sagittal modifier grades on all sagittal modifier categories than patients treated nonoperatively.[29] The classification has also been shown to be responsive to change in disability and disease state as a result of treatment. Smith and colleagues[30] evaluated whether the classification could predict changes in HRQOL values following treatment using a prospective, consecutive cohort of operatively treated patients with ASD. Change in SVA modifier at 1 year was associated with changes in ODI, Short Form 36 (SF-36) physical component score (PCS), and SRS-22 questionnaire total and all subscores. Change in PI-LL modifier at 1 year was associated with changes in SF-36 PCS and SRS-22 total score and subscores. Changes in SVA and PI-LL modifiers were associated with likelihood of achieving minimal clinically important difference for ODI and SRS subscores.

SUMMARY

Classifications for spinal deformity provide a common language for surgeons, health care providers, and researchers to effectively identify and communicate details regarding specific subsets of the disease state. Most existing spinal deformity classifications are rooted in pediatric spinal deformity, and, more specifically, AIS. Although these classifications have improved care for pediatric patients, the fundamental concepts behind these classifications do not effectively evaluate ASD, and therefore cannot fully describe the diverse disease states of ASD.

A primary goal when treating pediatric spinal deformity is preventing scoliosis progression, therefore the classifications have focused on identifying structural curves most at risk for progression and requiring treatment. Relief of pain and disability is the primary treatment goal for ASD, therefore classifications that describe ASD should identify features most predictive of pain and disability. The clinical impact classifications developed first by Schwab and colleagues and then collaboratively between Schwab and the SRS represent an attempt to communicate these clinical aspects of ASD.

Sagittal spinopelvic alignment has emerged as a critically important concept for ASD, because sagittal spinopelvic malalignment has repeatedly been shown to correlate with pain and disability in ASD. Assessment of sagittal spinopelvic parameters and integration of these parameters into a classification for ASD are consequently as fundamentally important as scoliosis assessment is for AIS classification. The SRS-Schwab ASD Classification assesses deformity in the coronal and sagittal plane, but the distinctive feature of the classification is the use of the sagittal modifiers (PI-LL, SVA, and PT) to both quantify the deformity and correlate with patients' pain. This HRQOL predictive component of the classification has been demonstrated in a prospective cohort of patients with ASD.[29] The classification has also shown responsiveness to changes in disease state, because improvement in sagittal modifiers following deformity correction has been shown to correlate with improvement in HRQOL scores.[30] Further research using the SRS-Schwab ASD Classification will focus on widespread adoption of the classification and further validating the clinical usefulness of the classification by identifying the deformity parameters that are most responsive to different treatment modalities.

REFERENCES

1. King HA, Moe JH, Bradford DS, et al. The selection of fusion levels in thoracic idiopathic scoliosis. J Bone Joint Surg Am 1983;65:1302–13.
2. Cummings RJ, Loveless EA, Campbell J, et al. Interobserver reliability and intraobserver reproducibility of the system of King et al. for the classification of adolescent idiopathic scoliosis. J Bone Joint Surg Am 1998;80:1107–11.
3. Lenke LG, Betz RR, Bridwell KH, et al. Intraobserver and interobserver reliability of the classification of thoracic adolescent idiopathic scoliosis. J Bone Joint Surg Am 1998;80:1097–106.
4. Lenke LG, Betz RR, Harms J, et al. Adolescent idiopathic scoliosis: a new classification to determine

extent of spinal arthrodesis. J Bone Joint Surg Am 2001;83:1169–81.

5. Bess S, Boachie-Adjei O, Burton D, et al. Pain and disability determine treatment modality for older patients with adult scoliosis, while deformity guides treatment for younger patients. Spine (Phila Pa 1976) 2009;34:2186–90.

6. Glassman SD, Berven S, Bridwell K, et al. Correlation of radiographic parameters and clinical symptoms in adult scoliosis. Spine (Phila Pa 1976) 2005; 30:682–8.

7. Schwab F, Dubey A, Pagala M, et al. Adult scoliosis: a health assessment analysis by SF-36. Spine 2003; 28:602–6.

8. Schwab FJ, Smith VA, Biserni M, et al. Adult scoliosis: a quantitative radiographic and clinical analysis. Spine (Phila Pa 1976) 2002;27:387–92.

9. Lowe T, Berven SH, Schwab FJ, et al. The SRS classification for adult spinal deformity: building on the King/Moe and Lenke classification systems. Spine (Phila Pa 1976) 2006;31:S119–25.

10. Aebi M. The adult scoliosis. Eur Spine J 2005;14: 925–48.

11. Glassman SD, Bridwell K, Dimar JR, et al. The impact of positive sagittal balance in adult spinal deformity. Spine 2005;30:2024–9.

12. Lafage V, Schwab F, Patel A, et al. Pelvic tilt and truncal inclination: two key radiographic parameters in the setting of adults with spinal deformity. Spine (Phila Pa 1976) 2009;34:E599–606.

13. Schwab F, Lafage V, Patel A, et al. Sagittal plane considerations and the pelvis in the adult patient. Spine (Phila Pa 1976) 2009;34:1828–33.

14. Schwab F, Patel A, Ungar B, et al. Adult spinal deformity-postoperative standing imbalance: how much can you tolerate? An overview of key parameters in assessing alignment and planning corrective surgery. Spine (Phila Pa 1976) 2010;35:2224–31.

15. Schwab F, el-Fegoun AB, Gamez L, et al. A lumbar classification of scoliosis in the adult patient: preliminary approach. Spine (Phila Pa 1976) 2005;30: 1670–3.

16. Schwab F, Farcy JP, Bridwell K, et al. A clinical impact classification of scoliosis in the adult. Spine (Phila Pa 1976) 2006;31:2109–14.

17. Schwab F, Lafage V, Farcy JP, et al. Surgical rates and operative outcome analysis in thoracolumbar and lumbar major adult scoliosis: application of the new adult deformity classification. Spine 2007;32: 2723–30.

18. Sarwahi V, Boachie-Adjei O, Backus SI, et al. Characterization of gait function in patients with postsurgical sagittal (flatback) deformity: a prospective study of 21 patients. Spine (Phila Pa 1976) 2002; 27:2328–37.

19. Yang BP, Chen LA, Ondra SL. A novel mathematical model of the sagittal spine: application to pedicle subtraction osteotomy for correction of fixed sagittal deformity. Spine J 2008;8:359–66.

20. Angevine PD, McCormick PC. The importance of sagittal balance: how good is the evidence? J Neurosurg Spine 2007;6:101–3 [discussion: 3].

21. Duval-Beaupere G, Robain G. Visualization on full spine radiographs of the anatomical connections of the centres of the segmental body mass supported by each vertebra and measured in vivo. Int Orthop 1987;11:261–9.

22. Lafage V, Schwab F, Skalli W, et al. Standing balance and sagittal plane spinal deformity: analysis of spinopelvic and gravity line parameters. Spine (Phila Pa 1976) 2008;33:1572–8.

23. Legaye J, Duval-Beaupere G. Sagittal plane alignment of the spine and gravity: a radiological and clinical evaluation. Acta Orthop Belg 2005;71:213–20.

24. Legaye J, Duval-Beaupere G, Hecquet J, et al. Pelvic incidence: a fundamental pelvic parameter for three-dimensional regulation of spinal sagittal curves. Eur Spine J 1998;7:99–103.

25. Schwab F, Lafage V, Patel A, et al. Does vertebral level of pedicle subtraction osteotomy correlate with degree of spinopelvic parameter correction? In: North American Spine Society 23rd Annual Meeting. Austin, September 10-13, 2008.

26. Schwab F, Bess S, Blondel B, et al. Combined Assessment of pelvic tilt, pelvic incidence/lumbar lordosis mismatch and sagittal vertical axis predicts disability in adult spinal deformity: a prospective analysis. Louisville (KY): Scoliosis Research Society; September 14-17, 2011.

27. Schwab F, Ungar B, Blondel B, et al. Scoliosis Research Society-Schwab adult spinal deformity classification: a validation study. Spine 2012;37:1077–82.

28. Schwab F, Lafage V, Shaffrey C, et al. Pre-operative pelvic parameters must be considered to achieve adequate sagittal balance after lumbar osteotomy. In: international meeting for advanced spinal techniques. Vienna. July 15-18, 2009.

29. Schwab F, Lafage V, Shaffrey C, et al. The SRS-Schwab Adult Spinal Deformity Classification: assessment and clinical correlations based on a prospective operative and non-operative cohort. Chicago: Scoliosis Research Society; September 5-8, 2012.

30. Smith J, Klineberg E, Schwab F, et al. Change in classification grade by the SRS-Schwab Adult Spinal Deformity (ASD) classification predicts impact on health related quality of life (HRQOL) measures: prospective analysis of operative and nonoperative treatment. Chicago: Scoliosis Research Society; September 5-8, 2012.

Coronal Realignment and Reduction Techniques and Complication Avoidance

Kai-Ming G. Fu, MD, PhD[a],*, Justin S. Smith, MD, PhD[b],
Christopher I. Shaffrey, MD[b], Christopher P. Ames, MD[c],
Shay Bess, MD[d]

KEYWORDS

- Scoliosis • Congenital deformity • Idiopathic scoliosis • Severe degenerative scoliosis

KEY POINTS

- Multiple reduction/realignment techniques have been described for treating coronal plane deformity.
- Rigid deformities may require anterior release or osteotomies before correction.
- Each deformity is unique and requires a tailored approach, often combining several techniques.
- Minimizing complications from spinal reconstructions requires adequate preoperative planning and attention to detail in the perioperative period.

Advances in technology, such as segmental pedicle screw instrumentation, have dramatically increased the number and effectiveness of realignment and reduction techniques for the treatment of coronal spinal deformity. Historically, distraction–compression was the primary technique used to correct coronal curvature.[1,2] However, employing this technique has deleterious effects on sagittal alignment, and it is rarely used as the sole maneuver to correct spinal deformity today. Other techniques, including cantilever bending, in situ bending, translation, derotation, direct vertebral rotation, and vertebral column resection have been described and are more commonly employed today.[3–5] Each patient's spinal deformity is unique; therefore spinal realignment must be individualized and employ a combination of techniques. The treatment of coronal deformity often requires substantial spinal reconstruction and involves significant risk of complications. Minimizing complications requires attention to detail in planning, positioning, and in perioperative management.

CORONAL CORRECTION CONCEPTS

The correction of spinal malalignment requires the application of appropriate forces counter to the direction of the deformity. All reduction strategies

Disclosures: Kai-Ming G. Fu is a consultant for Medtronic. Justin Smith is a consultant for Medtronic, Depuy, Biomet; Honoraria for teaching: Medtronic, Depuy, Biomet, Globus; research study group support: Depuy. Christopher Shaffrey: Biomet: consultant, patent; Medtronic: royalties, consultant; Depuy: honoraria; National Institutes of Health: research support; Department of Defense: research support; North American Clinical Trials Network: research support; AO: research support, fellowship support; Globuus: consultant; Nuvasive: consultant. Christopher Ames is a consultant: DePuy, Medtronic, Stryker; Employment: University of California San Francisco; Grants: Trans1; Patents, Fish & Richardson, Professional Corporation; Royalties: Aesculap, LAWX. Shay Bess is a consultant for Alphatec, Allosource, Depuy Spine, Medtronic; Royalties: Pioneer Spine; Research Support: Depuy Spine, Medtronic, Orthopedic Research and Education Foundation; Scientific Advisory Board: Allosource.
[a] Department of Neurosurgery, Weill Cornell Medical center, 525 East 68th Street, New York, NY 10065, USA;
[b] Department of Neurosurgery, University of Virginia, PO Box 800212, Charlottesville, VA 22908, USA;
[c] Department of Neurological Surgery, University of California, 505 Parnassus Avenue, Room 779 M, San Francisco, CA 94143-0112, USA; [d] Rocky Mountain Hospital for Children, 1719 E. 19th Avenue, Denver, CO 80218, USA
* Corresponding author.
E-mail address: kaimingfu@gmail.com

Neurosurg Clin N Am 24 (2013) 195–202
http://dx.doi.org/10.1016/j.nec.2012.12.011
1042-3680/13/$ – see front matter © 2013 Published by Elsevier Inc.

employ one or more of the following forces. Distraction of the vertebrae may be employed to address the concavity of the curve but also results in kyphosis in the sagittal plane. Compression is best applied over the convexity of the curve and results in increased lordosis in the sagittal plane. Other forces that can be applied in correction include the application of cantilever forces, translation or reducing the vertebra to a straight construct, tilting, and derotation or applying force in the axial plane to correct rotational deformity.[6–8]

The use of these forces requires a spine with some degree of flexibility. In certain cases, applying these forces will not result in adequate reduction due to the rigidity of the deformity. In other cases, previous operations may have led to arthrodesis of the spine in the deformed state. In these cases, the principles of rigid and revision surgery are applied. These include anterior releases designed to increase flexibility of a rigid curve, or osteotomies, including smith-petersen, pedicle subtraction, or vertebral column resection, which offer varying degrees of sagittal and coronal plane correction.[9,10]

PROCEDURES AND TECHNIQUES

Historically, scoliosis was treated with the principles of correction pioneered by Harrington.[2] **Fig. 1** demonstrates this technique. Distraction is applied to the concave side, and compression is applied over the convex side. Reduction is not segmental, but the technique can correct lateral and angular displacement. The technique does not correct rotational deformity and places high stress on the spine and instrumentation. Furthermore, the application of a straight rod reduced thoracic kyphosis and reduced lumbar lordosis, resulting in flat back deformity and sagittal spinopelvic malalignment. Subsequently, many patients required revision surgeries, which entailed complex osteotomy procedures to correct the iatrogenic sagittal plane deformity.[11] **Fig. 2** demonstrates such a case in which attempted coronal realignment resulted in thoracolumbar junction kyphosis, necessitating revision. Attention to detail in all planes is required to avoid long-term complications.

With the advent of segmental instrumentation, other techniques have been described to affect coronal reduction with less deleterious effects in the sagittal plane. First described by Luque,[12] translational reduction involves the placement of a contoured rod, during which each segment is brought toward the rod. **Fig. 3** demonstrates this technique. In general, the proximal and distal ends of the rod are provisionally placed. After this, each vertebral segment is reduced to the

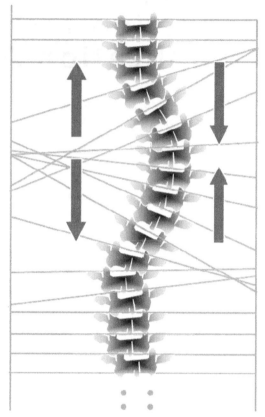

Fig. 1. Graphical demonstration of regional distraction compression technique as described by Harrington. Distraction is applied on the concave side, while compression is applied on the convex side. *Arrows* represent direction of correctional forces.

construct. This technique is useful in correcting lateral and rotational deformity. Proper contouring of the rod allows for the maintenance of physiologic lumbar lordosis and thoracic kyphosis. Translation, however, places high stress on the bone/implant interface, and there are limits to reduction before implants fail, either by loss of fixation (loosened screw), failure (instrumentation fracture), or failure to maintain correction.

In situ bending is another method for obtaining coronal correction. **Fig. 4** demonstrates this technique. In this method, the rod is shaped and fixed to the spine. The deformity is then corrected by bending the rod to the desired shape with in situ bending tools. This method provides for correction of lateral deformity. Again, this technique results in high stress on the instrumentation and bone. With titanium rods, multiple bends can lead to increased rod notching and structural weakening of the rod with associated risk of rod fracture.[13]

Segmental rod translation applies the techniques of translation in a segmental fashion. Again, the rod is contoured to the appropriate shape with

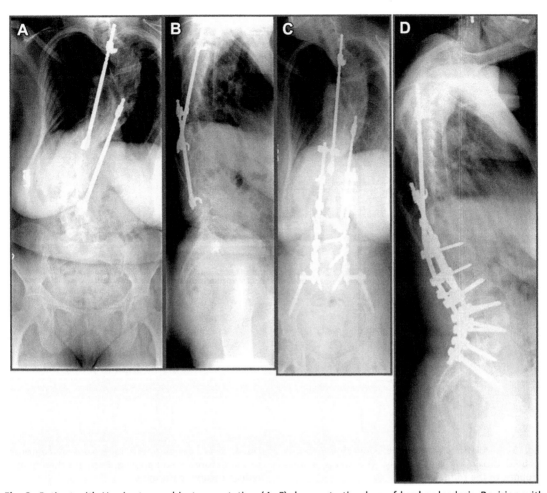

Fig. 2. Patient with Harrington rod instrumentation (*A, B*) demonstrating loss of lumbar lordosis. Revision with extension to pelvis was required (*C, D*) to restore sagittal alignment.

care taken to address the physiologic contours of the sagittal plane. As opposed to the translation techniques describe previously, the rod is secured at 1 end only. Each segment is brought to the rod, and the deformity is reduced at each segment, leading to a realigned spine (**Fig. 5**). A benefit of this approach is that less stress is applied to the instrumentation and bone, as the reduction is gradual and controlled. In addition, lateral and rotational components of deformity can be readily addressed.

Derotation has been advocated as another method for correcting deformity. Rod derotation was introduced theoretically to produce a 3-dimensional correction of deformity. **Fig. 6** demonstrates this technique. The rod is properly contoured to reflect the desired physiologic sagittal profile. including restoration of thoracic kyphosis and lumbar lordosis. According to derotation theory, this contour approximates the spinal deformity

rotated 90°. The rod is applied with the spine translated to the rod. The rod is then rotated in the axial plane to correct the coronal deformity while preserving or promoting a proper sagittal alignment. The benefit of this technique is that the procedure is simple and quick. One drawback is the high level of stress placed on the construct and bone interface. In addition, the amount of reported rotational correction varies, with some reports as low as 11°.[4,14] However, derotation has been demonstrated to be superior to Harrington techniques in curve correction and maintenance of correction.[15] A comparison of derotation with translation techniques among 70 adolescent idiopathic scoliosis patients demonstrated no significant difference between the procedures, with the exception of improved coronal thoracic curve reduction with the translation technique.[4] Direct vertebral derotation (DVD) has also been advocated as a method for potentially addressing thoracic rib hump and

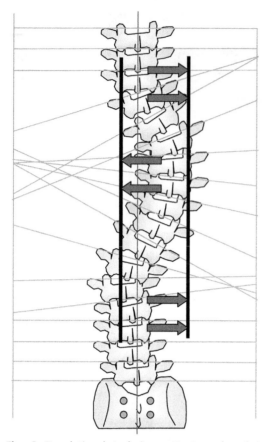

Fig. 3. Translational technique. Contoured rod is secured proximally and distally. The spine is then brought to the rod (*arrows*).

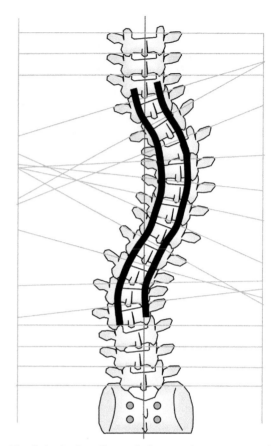

Fig. 4. In situ bending technique. Rods are contoured to the deformity and applied. Rods are then bent to reduce coronal deformity.

avoiding the need for a thoracoplasty. A recent report suggests that thoracic rib humps are addressed equally with and without DVD, but that DVD provides less correction in the thoracolumbar region.[16] DVD has been reported to have a deleterious effect on lumbar lordosis also. In patients undergoing DVD for adolescent idiopathic scoliosis, those treated with DVD demonstrated about a 12° loss of lumbar lordosis and an 8° loss of thoracic kyphosis.[17] Therefore, when employing this technique, care must be taken to avoid further flattening maneuvers.

A comparison of all these techniques demonstrates some benefits and drawbacks with each type of procedure. Segmental instrumentation has led to great improvements in techniques affording proper alignment in multiple planes. Each patient's deformity has individual characteristics, and the approach to each patient requires a customized plan for coronal realignment and reduction. **Fig. 7** demonstrates a combination technique for addressing coronal plane deformity. The technique requires distraction, compression,

and/or translation applied segment by segment. Reduction screws used at the apex may facilitate a controlled sequential reduction. A combination technique provides a comprehensive approach to the deformity addressing each segment in turn while building a construct with appropriate coronal and sagittal plane contours. In addition, individual segments may be derotated to address axial deformity. The combination technique places the bone and instrumentation under less stress, allowing for smaller rods and lower profile connectors.

The application of all of the previously described techniques is requisite on the flexibility of the spine. Rigid deformities may require additional procedures before attempted reduction. Osteotomies, including Smith-Petersen (facet osteotomies) or pedicle subtraction osteotomies, may used posteriorly to facilitate manipulation. Vertebral column resection provides the largest amount of correction in the sagittal and coronal planes. Anterior release can be performed before posterior coronal reduction procedures. Anterior release procedures reduce the stiffness of a curve and are usually

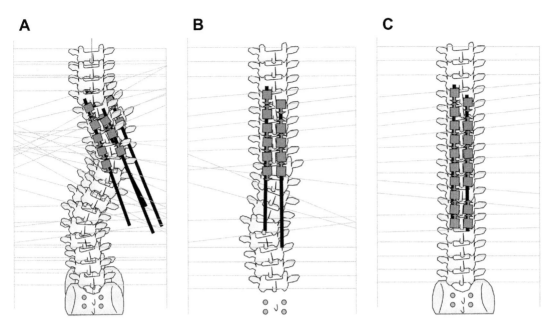

Fig. 5. Segmental rod translation. Contoured rods are applied (here proximally), and the spine is sequentially transferred to the rod segment by segment as shown progressively from panels A–C.

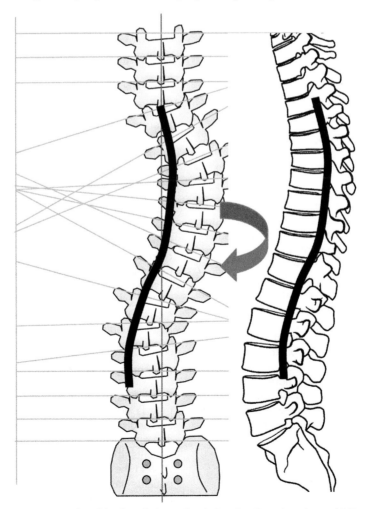

Fig. 6. Rod rotation. A contoured rod is placed along the deformity. Rotating the rod 90° reduces the coronal deformity while maintaining a proper sagittal alignment. *Arrows* represents direction of rotational correction.

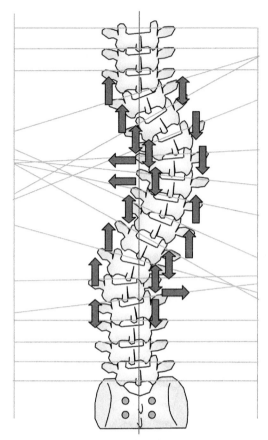

Fig. 7. Segmental correction. Each segment is translated, compressed, and distracted as indicated. *Arrows* represent segmental corrective maneuvers to be applied for correction.

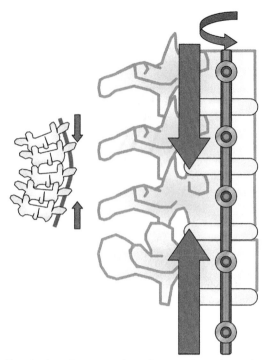

Fig. 8. Anterior correction. Compression along the convexity of the curve results in coronal plane reduction. *Arrows* represent direction of anterior reduction.

performed at areas of rigidity as determined by preoperative radiographs (lateral bending, bolster). The technique includes an anterior or anterolateral approach. For each segment, the disk is incised and removed. Structural interbody grafts may be placed. Such grafts may be contoured to aid in correction in both the sagittal and coronal planes. Anterior osteotomies can be performed for extremely rigid deformities.

Some deformities may be best approached with an anterior correction as demonstrated in **Fig. 8**. Anterior correction is effected with segmental distraction and compression, addressing lateral displacement. Derotation can be performed for correction of sagittal displacement. In situ bending is also used. However, effective translation is difficult to perform anteriorly.

DIAGNOSTIC CRITERIA

Coronal plane deformity encompasses a multitude of pathologies, ranging from neuromuscular to idiopathic to degenerative scoliosis. Affected patients range from infants to the elderly. Indications for intervention vary for each pathology; therefore, a complete discussion on the indications for treatment is beyond the context of this article. In general, adolescent idiopathic patients are considered for treatment if the major curve is greater than 45°. Imaging required for these patients includes long cassette scoliosis radiographs as well as others as needed to assess rigidity (bending, bolster). Older patients may require surgery for the sagittal plane deformity as much as a coronal deformity. Imaging generally includes advanced imaging studies (magnetic resonance imaging or computed tomography myelogram) to assess for spinal stenosis with resultant neurogenic claudication and or/radiculopathy. Patients often proceed with operative intervention for radicular pain or neurologic deficit.

COMPLICATIONS

Correction of thoracic and thoracolumbar deformity is not without potential complications. Depending on the size of the procedure, degree of correction, and age and comorbidities of the patients, the complication rates can be as high as 71% in the elderly.[18] Pediatric and younger adult patients have been reported to have complication rates much lower, in the 10% to 20% range.[18–20] Longer-term alignment complications can be minimized with proper preoperative planning.

Evaluating and addressing pelvic obliquity and leg length discrepancy are important in planning the extent of coronal correction. Fractional lumbral curves may need to be addressed to maintain coronal balance.

Other common complications are infections, dural tears, implant complications, and new neurologic deficits. Vancomycin powder and pulse irrigation have been used in longer cases.[21] Introperative guidance can be used to assess placement of instrumentation. Neurologic monitoring, including both motor-evoked potentials and somatosensory-evoked potentials should used intraoperatively and be monitored frequently during reduction techniques.[22–24] In the event of a new neurologic postoperative deficit, with appropriate intervention most deficits have been demonstrated to improve, most back to near baseline.[25]

Other common potential perioperative complications include postoperative anemia, deep vein thrombosis (DVT), and pulmonary embolus. Proper resuscitation should be performed to correct intraoperative blood loss. Care should be taken to perform mechanical DVT prophylaxis before induction through mobilization and discharge. Antibiotics can be given prophylactically while closed drainage systems are maintained in place. Immediate postoperative management in an intensive care unit setting may be indicated based upon duration and operative blood loss, or for frequent neurologic monitoring. Postoperative anemia is treated with transfusions as necessary. Long-term complications include adjacent level disease, proximal junction kyphosis, and pseudoarthrosis rates approaching 20%, necessitating longer-term postoperative patient follow-up.[26,27]

SUMMARY

Realignment of scoliosis in the coronal plane requires extensive spinal reconstruction. Various reduction techniques have been described. Each deformity is unique and requires a tailored approach to correction. Often, a combination of techniques must be employed. Preoperative planning is essential. Attention to detail is required in all aspects of the procedure, from positioning to postoperative mobilization. Despite these precautions, complications can occur, and a thorough discussion of risks and benefits should be held with the patient and family.

REFERENCES

1. Dickson JH. An eleven-year clinical investigation of Harrington instrumentation. A preliminary report on 578 cases. Clin Orthop Relat Res 1973;(93):113–30.

2. Harrington PR. Treatment of scoliosis. Correction and internal fixation by spine instrumentation. J Bone Joint Surg Am 1962;44:591–610.

3. Chang KW. Cantilever bending technique for treatment of large and rigid scoliosis. Spine (Phila Pa 1976) 2003;28(21):2452–8.

4. Delorme S, Labelle H, Aubin CE, et al. Intraoperative comparison of two instrumentation techniques for the correction of adolescent idiopathic scoliosis. Rod rotation and translation. Spine (Phila Pa 1976) 1999;24(19):2011–7 [discussion: 2018].

5. Lenke LG, O'Leary PT, Bridwell KH, et al. Posterior vertebral column resection for severe pediatric deformity: minimum two-year follow-up of thirty-five consecutive patients. Spine (Phila Pa 1976) 2009; 34(20):2213–21.

6. Dabney KW, Salzman SK, Wakabayashi T, et al. Experimental scoliosis in the rat. II. Biomechanical analysis of the forces during Harrington distraction. Spine (Phila Pa 1976) 1988;13(5):472–7.

7. Ghista DN, Viviani GR, Subbaraj K, et al. Biomechanical basis of optimal scoliosis surgical correction. J Biomech 1988;21(2):77–88.

8. Viviani GR, Ghista DN, Lozada PJ, et al. Biomechanical analysis and simulation of scoliosis surgical correction. Clin Orthop Relat Res 1986;(208):40–7.

9. Auerbach JD, Lenke LG, Bridwell KH, et al. Major complications and comparison between 3-column osteotomy techniques in 105 consecutive spinal deformity procedures. Spine (Phila Pa 1976) 2012; 37(14):1198–210.

10. Cho KJ, Bridwell KH, Lenke LG, et al. Comparison of Smith-Petersen versus pedicle subtraction osteotomy for the correction of fixed sagittal imbalance. Spine (Phila Pa 1976) 2005;30(18):2030–7 [discussion: 2038].

11. Connolly PJ, Von Schroeder HP, Johnson GE, et al. Adolescent idiopathic scoliosis. Long-term effect of instrumentation extending to the lumbar spine. J Bone Joint Surg Am 1995;77(8):1210–6.

12. Luque ER. Segmental spinal instrumentation for correction of scoliosis. Clin Orthop Relat Res 1982;(163):192–8.

13. Smith JS, Shaffrey CI, Ames CP, et al. Assessment of symptomatic rod fracture following posterior instrumented fusion for adult spinal deformity. Neurosurgery 2012. [Epub ahead of print].

14. Cheng I, Hay D, Iezza A, et al. Biomechanical analysis of derotation of the thoracic spine using pedicle screws. Spine (Phila Pa 1976) 2010;35(10):1039–43.

15. Helenius I, Remes V, Yrjönen T, et al. Harrington and Cotrel-Dubousset instrumentation in adolescent idiopathic scoliosis. Long-term functional and radiographic outcomes. J Bone Joint Surg Am 2003; 85(12):2303–9.

16. Hwang SW, Dubaz OM, Ames R, et al. The impact of direct vertebral body derotation on the lumbar

prominence in Lenke Type 5C curves. J Neurosurg Spine 2012;17(4):308–13.

17. Mladenov KV, Vaeterlein C, Stuecker R. Selective posterior thoracic fusion by means of direct vertebral derotation in adolescent idiopathic scoliosis: effects on the sagittal alignment. Eur Spine J 2011; 20(7):1114–7.

18. Smith JS, Shaffrey CI, Glassman SD, et al. Risk–benefit assessment of surgery for adult scoliosis: an analysis based on patient age. Spine (Phila Pa 1976) 2011;36(10):817–24.

19. Reames DL, Smith JS, Fu KM, et al. Complications in the surgical treatment of 19,360 cases of pediatric scoliosis: a review of the scoliosis research society morbidity and mortality database. Spine (Phila Pa 1976) 2011;36(18):1484–91.

20. Sansur CA, Smith JS, Coe JD, et al. Scoliosis research society morbidity and mortality of adult scoliosis surgery. Spine (Phila Pa 1976) 2011;36(9):E593–7.

21. Sweet FA, Roh M, Sliva C. Intrawound application of vancomycin for prophylaxis in instrumented thoracolumbar fusions: efficacy, drug levels, and patient outcomes. Spine (Phila Pa 1976) 2011;36(24):2084–8.

22. Flynn JM, Sakai DS. Improving safety in spinal deformity surgery: advances in navigation and neurologic monitoring. Eur Spine J 2012. [Epub ahead of print].

23. Emerson RG. NIOM for spinal deformity surgery: there's more than one way to skin a cat. J Clin Neurophysiol 2012;29(2):149–50.

24. Malhotra NR, Shaffrey CI. Intraoperative electrophysiological monitoring in spine surgery. Spine (Phila Pa 1976) 2010;35(25):2167–79.

25. Hamilton DK, Smith JS, Sansur CA, et al. Rates of new neurological deficit associated with spine surgery based on 108,419 procedures: a report of the scoliosis research society morbidity and mortality committee. Spine (Phila Pa 1976) 2011; 36(15):1218–28.

26. Kim YJ, Bridwell KH, Lenke LG, et al. Pseudarthrosis in adult spinal deformity following multisegmental instrumentation and arthrodesis. J Bone Joint Surg Am 2006;88(4):721–8.

27. Kim YJ, Bridwell KH, Lenke LG, et al. Pseudarthrosis in primary fusions for adult idiopathic scoliosis: incidence, risk factors, and outcome analysis. Spine (Phila Pa 1976) 2005;30(4):468–74.

Spinal Osteotomies for Rigid Deformities

Munish C. Gupta, MD[a], Khalid Kebaish, MD[b],
Benjamin Blondel, MD[c], Eric Klineberg, MD[a,*]

KEYWORDS

- Rigid spinal deformities • Wide posterior release • Smith-Petersen • Osteotomy • Ponte osteotomy
- Pedicle subtraction osteotomy • Vertebral column resection

KEY POINTS

- Rigid deformities of the spine pose a significant challenge to the even the most experienced spine surgeon.
- The definition of a rigid deformity is one that does not correct more than 50% on bending or traction radiographs.
- There are many surgical options for the treatment of rigid spinal deformity.
- Understanding the character of the curve can help surgeons choose the most appropriate surgical corrective.

INTRODUCTION: NATURE OF THE PROBLEM

Rigid deformities of the spine pose a challenge to the most experienced spine surgeons. Rigid deformities can be encountered in primary or revision spinal procedures. Rigid deformity denotes a deformity that does not correct more than 50% on bending or traction radiographs. The deformity can be large or small, but rigid (eg, a flat lumbar spine that has been previously operated on from anteriorly and posteriorly). The other scenario is a sharp angular deformity that is rigid and causes cord compression. Usually, the deformity is not only rigid but also severe in the coronal plane, sagittal plane, or both. The definition of an osteotomy is cutting of bone. A rigid spine that is almost ankylosed often requires a thorough release or an osteotomy. The choice is to either accept the deformity or use osteotomies to make the spine flexible enough to be corrected to a balanced coronal and sagittal plane.

PREOPERATIVE PLANNING

The type of release or osteotomy chosen depends on the type of deformity, location of the deformity, presence of spinal cord compression, and previous surgical procedures that have already been performed on the spine.

There are rigid deformities that are round and smooth and others that are sharp and angular. Large round and smooth deformities are more amenable to a release at multiple segments to give a correction that is smooth and harmonious over several levels. This strategy avoids correction at the middle of the round smooth curve, creating 2 semicircles with a kink in the middle. Sharp angular deformities can be in the coronal as well as the sagittal plane. Sharp angular deformities are more amenable to a resection procedure regardless whether the resection is performed via an anterior or a posterior approach. Large sharp angular deformities are the easiest to

[a] Department of Orthopaedic Surgery, University of California, Davis, 4860 Y Street, Suite 3800, Sacramento, CA 95817, USA; [b] Department of Orthopaedic Surgery, Johns Hopkins University, 601 North Caroline Street, Suite 5223, Baltimore, MD 21287–0882, USA; [c] Department of Orthopaedic Surgery, NYU Hospital for Joint Diseases, 306 East 15th Street, Suite 1F, New York, NY 10003, USA
* Corresponding author.
E-mail address: eric.klineberg@ucdmc.ucdavis.edu

Neurosurg Clin N Am 24 (2013) 203–211
http://dx.doi.org/10.1016/j.nec.2012.12.001
1042-3680/13/$ – see front matter © 2013 Elsevier Inc. All rights reserved.

approach from a posterior-only approach than from an anterior and posterior approach. It is difficult to reach the posterior part of the vertebral body and the canal through the anterior approach in such cases.

The location of the deformity also determines the approach, which might be more facile and less morbid. For example, a high thoracic deformity is more difficult to approach anteriorly than posteriorly. The thoracic, thoracolumbar, and lumbar spine can easily be approached anteriorly. The anterior approach is useful in performing a release in a rigid smooth curve, which can be scoliotic or kyphotic. Multiple disk spaces can be released by removing the annulus and disk in almost its entirety. In addition, support of the anterior column can be addressed by providing strut grafting for either disk space or vertebral body deficiencies. The anterior approach has recently been used less, because of more powerful instrumentation systems and techniques such as preoperative traction and intraoperative temporary distraction.

Previous surgery may limit the options for correcting a deformity. Previous multiple decompressions may limit the amount of posterior elements for obtaining a solid arthrodesis. An anterior arthrodesis may be helpful in ensuring a successful fusion. Previous fusion from the posterior approach only can still be approached anteriorly for either enhancing the ability to fuse or trying to achieve correction with a release or resection procedure. A previously fused spine that has had a previous anterior approach cannot be easily approached from the same side and certainly not from the opposite side, endangering the vascular supply to the spinal cord. In these cases, a posterior-only approach is the most useful in achieving correction using a pedicle subtraction osteotomy (PSO) or a vertebral column resection (VCR).

Spinal cord or cauda equina compression in the presence of a rigid deformity necessitates decompression in addition to the spinal realignment procedure. If the compression is posterior-only, the approach for deformity correction is seldom influenced. But if the compression is anterior or circumferential, then a formal anterior approach, posterolateral approach such as a costotransversectomy or a posterior VCR, enters the decision making for choosing the surgical procedure.

The available hospital facilities and resources also influence the procedure that is chosen. An advanced anesthesia team with neuromonitoring and an intensive care unit with ventilators are mandatory in the care of these complex patients. The surgeon's experience and comfort level are also paramount in deciding the nature of the procedure.

PREPARATION AND PATIENT POSITIONING

The patient is usually placed in a right lateral decubitus position for a thoracic, thoracolumbar, and lumbar left-sided anterior approach. The table can be flexed to open the interval between the pelvis and the ribs in the flank. An axillary roll is always placed in the axilla of the right shoulder. A pillow is placed below the right knee and between the legs. The patient can be held with the help of a beanbag or tape. The left arm is placed in a 90/90 position, with the help of a universal arm holder. It is important to pad all the pressure points. The draping for the preparation includes a midline-to-midline drape at the umbilicus and the posterior spinous processes.

Posterior positioning is usually performed on a 4-poster frame either on a regular operating table or a Jackson frame. It is important to place bolsters underneath the thighs to gain hip extension, which helps achieve better lumbar lordosis. All the pressure points should be well padded, especially when a 4-poster similar to a Relton-Hall frame is used, to prevent pressure damage to the chest and anterior iliac crest area. Reflexing the bed can assist with closure of a PSO. A regular operating table or adjustable Jackson frame can be used.

After positioning, the patient is prepared with an alcohol scrub followed by a ChloraPrep solution (care fusion corporation, San Diego, CA). The perioperative prophylactic antibiotics used are vancomycin and cefazolin. The flora of every hospital have different sensitivities. The sensitivities of a particular hospital have to be assessed to decide which antibiotics should be used for prophylaxis. Use of fibrinolytics such as tranexamic acid and aminocaproic acid have been shown to decrease operative blood loss in spine surgery.[1] A Cochrane review[2] showed safety and efficacy of antifibrinolytics in pediatric patients with idiopathic scoliosis.

SURGICAL APPROACH
Wide Posterior Release

Shufflebarger and Clark described wide posterior release.[3] They first described wide posterior release in patients with idiopathic scoliosis in whom partial resection of the spinous process, ligamentum flavum, facet capsule, and facet joint is performed. The release helped correction in both coronal and sagittal planes of the lumbar deformity. This release was then applied in a situation in which the adult degenerative lumbar spine was usually flat and rigid. A 3-stage sequential same-day procedure using a posterior, anterior, and then posterior approach was described. The first approach included placement of pedicle screws in the lumbar spine, followed by wide posterior release. An anterior release was then performed by diskectomies and placement of mesh cages in the disk space for disk height restoration. The posterior part of the spine was again approached to achieve the final correction by shortening the posterior column and realigning the spine in both the coronal and sagittal planes (**Fig. 1**).

Wide posterior release involves removing the interspinous ligament and inferior and superior portion of the spinous process to expose the interlaminar space, ligamentum flavum and facet capsule and a partial removal of the facet joint. A distracter is used to distract the posterior elements between the spinous processes or the lamina to help visualize the resection of the ligamentum flavum as well as the facet capsule through to the foramen. Partial facet joint resection is enough to release the level so that the facet joint can be separated with a simple distracter rather than a Ponte osteotomy. While performing the Ponte osteotomy, a large part of the superior and inferior facet is resected, creating a large gap that is closed for a posterior shortening procedure. Wide posterior release is commonly performed to disengage all the soft tissues between segments to correct deformity in the coronal and sagittal

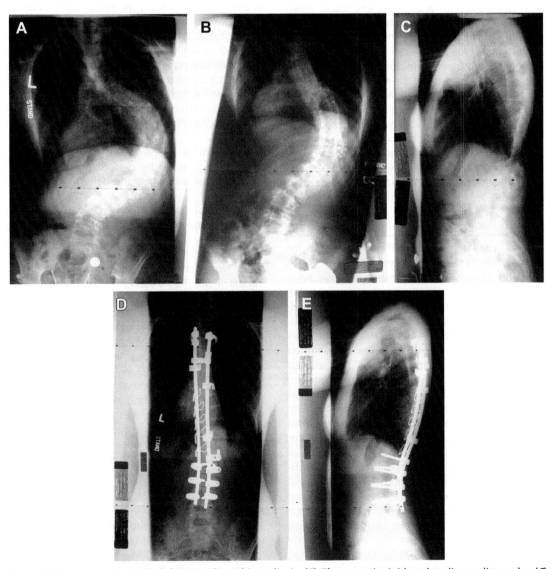

Fig. 1. (A) Large round rigid adolescent idiopathic scoliosis. (B) The curve is rigid on bending radiographs. (C) Preoperative lateral radiographs. (D) Postoperative correction obtained by anterior release, wide posterior release, and spinal instrumentation. (E) Postoperative lateral radiograph.

planes. This release can facilitate correction in rigid curves, especially in combination with segment instrumentation, when in previous years, an anterior release may have been performed.

Smith-Petersen Osteotomy

Smith-Petersen osteotomies (SPOs) were first described in 1945[4] for correcting sagittal plane deformities in the already fused spine either surgically or with an ankylosing condition such as ankylosing spondylitis. From Smith-Petersen's first reports, the technique improved with modifications such as foraminotomies and addition of rigid internal fixation.[5] The osteotomy relies on a mobile disk space for correction. The spinous process, lamina, and facet joints are resected. The foramen is fully exposed and the soft tissue is removed to prevent impingement of the nerve root when the osteotomy is closed. If the disk is ankylosed, the osteotomy produces a fracture through the disk space or the end plate of the vertebral body. The separation that can occur anteriorly has been reported with rare devastating injury to the large vessels, such as a tear of the aorta, which was deadly.[6] The term SPO has been used loosely to describe any posterior release. The major difference between the SPO and wide posterior release or Ponte osteotomy is that the SPO was described for already fused spines.

Ponte Osteotomy

Alberto Ponte described the Ponte osteotomy for treatment of Scheuermann kyphosis.[7] The vertebral end plates in Scheuermann disease have growth plates that are abnormal and weak. The disk material goes through these weak end plates, giving rise to the classic picture on magnetic resonance imaging (MRI) of a Schmorl node. Scheuermann disease with kyphosis results in elongated posterior elements compared with the anterior column consisting of the abnormal vertebral bodies and disks. The Ponte osteotomy involved removal of the inferior part of the spinous process, lamina, and facet joints. The superior and the inferior facets are resected in their entirety. After removal, the kyphosis is corrected with posterior column shortening. The main maneuver is a cantilever moment and compression across the apex of the kyphosis. Ponte described this procedure for Scheuermann disease and kyphosis in mostly the thoracic spine. The main difference between the Ponte osteotomy and the wide posterior release is the amount of facet resection. In the Ponte osteotomy, the entire superior and inferior facet is removed. The main difference between the SPO and the Ponte osteotomy is that the

SPO was described for treatment of already fused spines.

Pedicle Subtraction Osteotomy

Fixed sagittal imbalance or fixed kyphotic deformities have been treated with SPO and PSO. Osteotomies such as SPO as well as PSO have been described and used for more than 5 decades.[4,5,8,9] PSOs have been used mainly to correct the sagittal plane, but, in addition, has been used recently to correct coronal plane deformities as well. PSO is performed from a posterior-only approach, avoiding anterior release in many cases. Pedicle subtraction has been mostly used in revision surgeries in the past but this technique is often used in primary as well as revision deformity corrections.[10,11]

The limitation of the Smith-Petersen technique is the lengthening of the anterior column, which may lead to stretching of the cauda equina and possible vascular complications, such as aortic rupture.[6] Thomasen[8] in 1985 described a 3-column posterior wedge osteotomy in 11 patients with ankylosing spondylitis. The anterior column did not lengthen as in SPO.[4] No complications such as stretching of the cauda equina or vascular complications were noted by performing the posterior compression or wedging through the L2 vertebral body.

Several clinical studies have attempted to document the efficacy of both SPO and PSO. Van Royen[9] reported on 856 patients with ankylosing spondylitis who underwent lumbar osteotomies. No difference was reported between SPO versus PSO for treating fixed sagittal plane deformity.

Recently, Cho and colleagues[10] assessed the clinical and radiographic outcomes between PSO and SPO in a total of 71 patients. Although there was greater blood loss with the PSO group compared with the SPO, no significant difference was noted in the clinical outcome measures. However, when more than 3 levels of osteotomies were compared, there was a statistically significant difference with correction of the sagittal and coronal planes of PSO versus SPO.[10] PSO is an excellent tool for the orthopedic spine surgeon to tackle the difficulty of fixed sagittal plan deformities.

Indications

The indications for a PSO keep widening. Pedicle subtraction was and still is used for treating a fixed sagittal deformity. PSO has been used to treat not only the iatrogenic flatback but also sagittal plane deformities that have other causes in combination with coronal deformities. The simplest example is degenerative scoliosis with significant loss of lumbar lordosis. Using wide releases and, if needed, a PSO can help correct these deformities from a posterior-only approach. We have primarily used PSO in patients who are undergoing revision surgery with fixed sagittal plane deformities. This technique has been used less frequently in revision surgeries of a combined coronal and sagittal plane deformity.

Preoperative planning

Long films for posteroanterior and lateral radiographs are mandatory. Supine anteroposterior and lateral radiographs are helpful. Supine radiographs help define the flexibility of the deformity in the sagittal and coronal planes. The amount of correction necessary can be reevaluated if the spine corrects significantly in the supine position. The rigid parts of the spine and the more flexible or compensatory parts of the spine can be identified in this manner. Bending radiographs also are performed in a supine position to gain the help of removing gravity and access any flexibility of the coronal deformities. In addition, a lateral radiograph while the patient is in supine hyperextension over a bolster is helpful in assessing the flexibility of the focal kyphotic segment of the spine. The hyperextension radiograph frequently reveals areas of nonunion in a patient with a previous attempt at arthrodesis, such as air in the disk space or angular correction between erect and supine radiographs. The preoperative planning includes measuring all the sagittal and coronal parameters. The sagittal parameters have to include the sagittal vertical axis, thoracic kyphosis, lumbar lordosis, pelvic incidence, pelvic tilt, and sacral slope. The analysis of these parameters helps determine the amount of correction needed in order to achieve sagittal balance.

Having MRI as well as computed tomography (CT) scans preoperatively allows the surgeon to be prepared for the complexity of revision surgery. Arachnoiditis can be found after spinal surgery with clumping of the cauda equina. The presence of arachnoiditis may be a prognostic indicator of subtotal improvement in lower extremity symptoms after decompression and should be discussed with the patient preoperatively. Stenosis, whether central or foraminal, can be defined properly and decompressed during surgery before performing the PSO. CT is helpful in outlining the bony landmarks and elucidating the extent of the fusion mass. The CT scan can be used for planning the placement of the spinal instrumentation such as pedicle screws. A CT scan after a myelogram is a useful tool in cases, for example, in which a patient who has claustrophobia cannot have MRI because of a pacemaker. In revision cases, it is essential to define the neural elements and the canal.

Surgical Technique

Patient positioning

PSO requires the patient to be in the prone position with bony prominences well padded and the abdomen free during surgery. The abdomen hanging free helps increase venous drainage away from the epidural plexus. The procedure lends itself to large blood loss because of the cancellous bone of the vertebral body as well as the disrupted epidural vessels during the procedure. A bed that reflexes is useful not only in the initial accommodation or positioning of the patient with kyphotic deformity but closing the wedge osteotomy in a controlled manner using the bed can be a useful technique. Using temporary rods and a bed that reflexes helps guide the closure safely and effectively.

Operative technique

First, adequate exposure is performed exposing all the previous instrumentation. Then, new pedicle screws are placed before performing PSO. Once instrumentation is in place, we proceed with laminectomy and removal of the posterior elements. The decompression laminectomy is performed from pedicles above and below the proposed pedicle resection. The nerve roots above and below are followed all the way out to the paraspinal muscles. Attention is then turned to removal of the pedicles. It is helpful to keep the medial part of the pedicle intact initially to protect the neural elements. The medial part of the pedicle acts as a nerve root retractor while the pedicles are removed and the resection of the body is performed.

The transverse process is removed. The lateral portion of the vertebral body is dissected with a Cobb elevator and a malleable retractor is placed on the lateral portion of the vertebral body. The pedicle is then cannulated as if a pedicle screw was being placed. Once adequate exposure of the lateral wall has been achieved, Leksell rongeurs are used to remove the lateral wall of the vertebral body to the level of the anterior cortex. The vertebral body is decancelled through the partially resected pedicles and lateral wall of the body by serially using larger curettes.

The next step requires resecting the posterior wall of the vertebral body. Often, it is necessary to use reversed angled curettes to thin the cortex enough to create a controlled fracture. Care must be taken to protect the anterior aspect of the dura and the posterior aspect of the vertebral body. Bipolar cautery can be used to coagulate the epidural vessels before removal of the posterior wall of the vertebral body. Hemostasis is critical at this junction, using topical hemostatic agents such as Gelfoam, bone wax, and thrombin-soaked Cottonoids (particularly if there is bleeding form the epidural vessels). Remnants of the posterior cortex are then removed.

The next step involves closing the osteotomy in a controlled manner. Using a bed that has ability to reflex can assist. If a bed that reflexes is not available, hyperextension of the patient's chest and pelvis also aids in closing the osteotomy. In preoperative planning, we decide to correct for coronal plane deformities by adjusting the asymmetric closure of the osteotomy. Short rods to control our correction in a gradual manner are placed and tightened once the PSO is complete. The short rods help to stop the osteotomy from shifting and provide additional stability to the highest stress region around the pedicle subtraction site (**Figs. 2 and 3**).

VCR

VCR was performed first in cases of hemivertebrae resection. The resection was performed via an anterior approach followed by posterior resection of the posterior elements.[12] VCR was also described in treatment of rigid deformities with removal of the vertebral bodies from the anterior approach. Gelfoam was left on the dura and loose bone graft anteriorly. The posterior elements were then resected before achieving any correction.[13–15] Suk[16] recently described using the posterior-only approach for performing a VCR. Posterior VCR (PVCR) is being performed with more frequency than ever before.

Indications

The indications of VCR or PVCR are severe rigid deformities that are not amenable to correction with an anterior and posterior release alone. Disk space release is not adequate in achieving correction, and more shortening is needed for correction. Thus, a vertebral body has to be removed anteriorly and from the corresponding posterior elements to gain correction, to avoid residual deformity. Severe rigid scoliosis with a previous fusion posteriorly can be treated with an anterior and posterior VCR. However, there are circumstances in which the anterior approach is not possible (eg, in a patient with previous anterior and posterior fusion). In such cases, PVCR is a viable option. A severe sharp angular kyphosis is also easier to treat with PVCR, because it is difficult to reach the canal at the apex with an anterior approach (**Fig. 4**).

Preoperative planning

Preoperative planning includes a thorough medical workup to evaluate the cardiac and pulmonary status. Patients with severe curves can have associated pulmonary restrictive disease from the scoliosis as well as obstructive disease, which

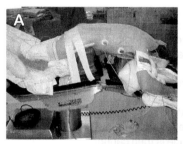
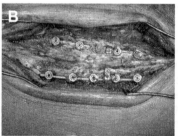
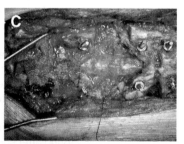
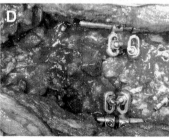
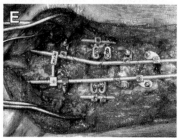

Fig. 2. (*A*) Positioning for PSO. (*B*) An example of an exposure of previous instrumentation and fusion. (*C*) After removal and reinstrumentation, wide decompression is performed from pedicle to pedicle, delineating 4 nerve roots. (*D*) After correction using the help of the operating room table and short rods. Notice the redundancy of the dural sac. (*E*) The longitudinal members are placed without disturbing the correction already obtained and secured with the short rods.

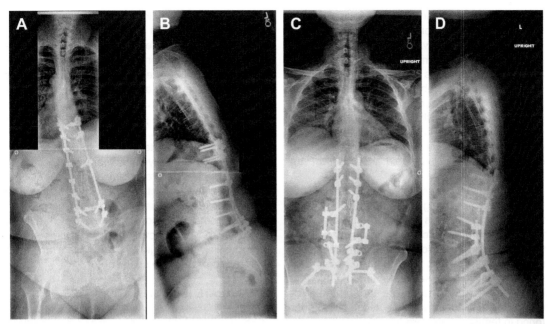

Fig. 3. (*A*) A rigid fusion after anterior and posterior fusion with instrumentation in coronal imbalance. (*B*) The patient has a severe positive sagittal imbalance after instrumentation and fusion. (*C*) Coronal balance obtained after PSO and extension to the pelvis. (*D*) Sagittal balance has markedly improved after PSO and extension to the pelvis.

is treatable. Beside the normal radiographs, as described for PSO, the use of additional studies such as MRI and CT can further delineate the anatomy and help in planning the resection and instrumentation. It is also possible to make a three-dimensional (3D) model in resin before the surgery. These models are helpful not only in operative planning of the resection but also in

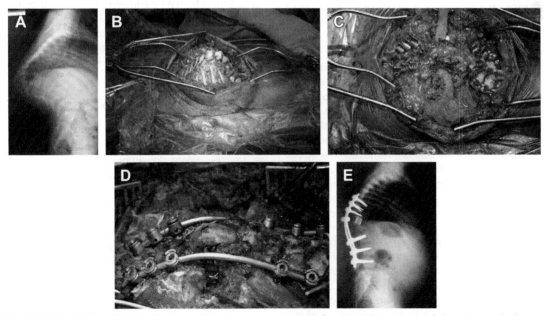

Fig. 4. (*A*) Posttuberculosis kyphosis resulting in a severe rigid deformity. (*B*) Exposure of the spine and rib cage for posterior VCR. (*C*) Ribs have been removed. Nerve roots had to be ligated. Anterior exposure has been performed, and vital structures protected with a sponge. (*D*) Correction of the kyphosis after resection and shortening. A cage has been placed anteriorly. (*E*) Correction of the kyphosis after PVCR kyphosis; improved but not perfect.

placing instrumentation. The models also help define the patient's congenital anomalies, which would be difficult to visualize from a CT scan. Anterior vertebral anomalies are sometimes not at the same level as posterior elements. For example, a hemivertebra at T4 in the thoracic spine may have redundant hemilamina of the posterior elements at the T5 level. The mismatch can occur anywhere in the spine. The 3D model not only makes it easy to visualize the anomalies clearly but also helps avoid resection of the unplanned levels.

Neuromonitoring is essential in performing these cases. Neuromonitoring is an early warning system that points out if there is a problem with spinal cord function. The warning can lead to adjustments to the correction and also to spinal cord perfusion parameters to prevent a devastating spinal cord injury. There are large savings in terms of the time if several wake-up tests are performed. The wake-up test is not as accurate as the neuromonitoring in testing spinal cord function.

Patient positioning

Positioning is lateral decubitus for an anterior approach if a VCR is being performed for the anterior portion of the resection, then prone for the posterior approach and resection. PVCR, which is all posterior, requires a regular operating table with a 4-poster frame or Jackson table. The table does not require a reflex function, as in PSO, because the correction is obtained from resection and sequential rod contouring.

Operative technique

PVCR is the most challenging osteotomy. The dissection of the spine requires not only a thorough posterior approach but also an anterior approach exposing the vertebral bodies that are to be removed. After the exposure is complete, the transverse process and ribs have to be removed. The more lateral the ribs are removed, the easier it is to reach the front of the spine safely. Usually, the ribs that are removed are above and below the vertebral body that is to be removed. For example, if a T4 vertebra has to be removed, the T4 rib is articulated with the T3 and T4 vertebrae or a high-speed burr. After the body has been mostly removed except the posterior cortex, temporary rods are used to stabilize the construct. The posterior cortex is then removed by using either a Kerrison or a reverse-angle curette.

The size of the cage to be put in place of the vertebral body is determined. The cage is then placed with local bone and allograft. The deformity is then corrected using compression, distraction, and in situ contouring. The rods are replaced sequentially as the correction is dialed into the rods. The spinal cord is assessed manually each time a correction maneuver is completed to ensure that there is no compression of the spinal cord or the nerve roots. After the final correction, the radiographs as well as the neuromonitoring are checked for transcranial motor-evoked potentials and somatosensory potentials from the upper and lower extremities. If there are any changes in neuromonitoring, a Stagnara wake-up test is performed. The hemodynamic parameters can be adjusted to ensure proper spinal cord perfusion.

After all the correction is achieved, the spinal cord is assessed to see if it is vulnerable by lying supine from the muscle and fascia. If the spinal cord is above the level of the instrumentation, a cross-link or a cage can be placed on top of the rod to protect the spinal cord.

IMMEDIATE POSTOPERATIVE CARE

Postoperative care usually requires admission to the intensive care unit. The patient may require blood products and ventilator support, as well as intravenous analgesia. If there were any neuromonitoring changes during surgery, the mean blood pressure should be kept higher than 80. Sometimes a dopamine drip is used to increase the blood pressure artificially for spinal cord perfusion. There have been reports of spinal cord compromise in the next few days after surgery as a result of lack of adequate perfusion of the spinal cord.

Mobilization of the patient is important to prevent deep venous thrombosis and pneumonia. An orthosis is seldom required for mobilization because of the pedicle screw segmental instrumentation.

REHABILITATION AND RECOVERY

The rehabilitation required is not different from other long segment spinal construct. The patient is usually asked to ambulate daily for 20 to 30 minutes. The precautions are: no driving for 6 weeks, no tub baths for 6 weeks, no repetitive bending and stooping, and refraining from lifting more than 13.6 kg (30 pounds). Children usually fare better than adults. Elderly patients usually require a transitional stay at a skilled nursing facility for 2 weeks before they can go home. After 4 to 6 weeks, children can go back to school. Adults feel better after about 3 months and feel much better about 1 year postoperatively.

COMPLICATIONS

PSOs have a significant complication rate of 35%, as reported by Auerbach and colleagues.[18] The

PSO complication rate was 38% and VCR, 22%.[13,16]

Transient neurologic deficit has been reported to range from 11.1 to 9.2% and major permanent neurologic deficit from 5.7 to 2.8%.[16,17] The VCR neurologic injury rate was 5.6%. Suk reported a neurologic deficit rate of 17%. There were only 2 complete cord deficits.

SUMMARY

Rigid deformities of the spine pose a challenge in achieving correction. The type of deformity, location of the deformity, presence of cord compression, hospital facilities, and surgeon experience help determine the approach used to correct that particular deformity. PSO and VCR should be used only when other simpler approaches are not possible.

REFERENCES

1. Baldus CR, Bridwell KH, Lenke LG, et al. Can we safely reduce blood loss during lumbar pedicle subtraction osteotomy procedures using tranexamic acid or aprotinin? A comparative study with controls. Spine (Phila Pa 1976) 2010;35(2):235–9.

2. Tzortzopoulou A, Cepeda MS, Schumann R, et al. Antifibrinolytic agents for reducing blood loss in scoliosis surgery in children. Cochrane Database Syst Rev 2008;(3):CD006883.

3. Shufflebarger HL, Clark CE. Effect of wide posterior release on correction in adolescent idiopathic scoliosis. J Pediatr Orthop B 1998;7(2):117–23.

4. Smith-Petersen MN, Larson CB, Aufranc OE. Osteotomy of the spine for correction of flexion deformity in rheumatoid arthritis. J Bone Joint Surg Am 1945;27:1–11.

5. Briggs H, Keats S, Schlesinger PT. Wedge osteotomy of the spine with bilateral, intervertebral foraminotomy: correction of flexion deformity in five cases of ankylosing arthritis of spine. J Bone Joint Surg Am 1947;29:1075–82.

6. Weatherley C, JaVray D, Terry A. Vascular complications associated with osteotomy in ankylosing spondylitis: a report of two cases. Spine 1988;13:43–6.

7. Geck MJ, Macagno A, Ponte A, et al. The Ponte procedure: posterior only treatment of Scheuermann's kyphosis using segmental posterior short-ening and pedicle screw instrumentation. J Spinal Disord Tech 2007;20(8):586–93.

8. Thomasen E. Vertebral osteotomy for correction of kyphosis in ankylosing spondylitis. Clin Orthop 1985;194:142–52.

9. Van Royen BJ, De Gast A. Lumbar osteotomy for correction of thoracolumbar kyphotic deformity in ankylosing spondylitis. A structured review of three methods of treatment. Ann Rheum Dis 1999;58:399–406.

10. Cho KJ, Bridwell KH, Lenke LG, et al. Comparison of Smith-Petersen versus pedicle subtraction osteotomy for the correction of fixed sagittal imbalance. Spine (Phila Pa 1976) 2005;30(18):2030–7 [discussion: 2038].

11. Colomina MJ, Bagó J, Fuentes I. Efficacy and safety of prophylactic large dose of tranexamic acid in spine surgery: a prospective, randomized, double-blind, placebo-controlled study. Spine (Phila Pa 1976) 2009;34(16):1740–1 [author reply: 141]. Spine 2008;33:2577–80.

12. Leatherman K, Dickson R. Two stage corrective surgery for congenital deformities of the spine. J Bone Joint Surg Br 1979;61-B(3):324–8.

13. Lenke LG, Sides BA, Koester LA, et al. Vertebral column resection for the treatment of severe spinal deformity. Clin Orthop Relat Res 2010;468(3):687–99.

14. Bradford D, Tribus C. Vertebral column resection for the treatment of rigid coronal decompensation. Spine 1997;22(14):1590–9.

15. Lenke LG, O'Leary PT, Bridwell KH, et al. Posterior vertebral column resection for severe pediatric deformity: minimum two-year follow-up of thirty-five consecutive patients. Spine (Phila Pa 1976) 2009;34(20):2213–21.

16. Suk SI, Chung ER, Kim JH, et al. Posterior vertebral column resection for severe rigid scoliosis. Spine 2005;30(14):1682–7.

17. Buchowski JM, Bridwell KH, Lenke LG, et al. Neurologic complications of lumbar pedicle subtraction osteotomy: a 10-year assessment. Spine (Phila Pa 1976) 2007;32(20):2245–52.

18. Auerbach JD, Lenke LG, Bridwell KH, et al. Major complications and comparison between 3-column osteotomy techniques in 105 consecutive spinal deformity procedures. Spine (Phila Pa 1976) 2012;37(14):1198–210.

Proximal Junctional Kyphosis and Proximal Junctional Failure

Robert A. Hart, MD[a],*, Ian McCarthy, PhD[b],
Christopher P. Ames, MD[c], Christopher I. Shaffrey, MD[d],
David Kojo Hamilton, MD[a], Richard Hostin, MD[b]

KEYWORDS

• Proximal junctional failure • Proximal junctional kyphosis • Complications • Spine deformity

KEY POINTS

• Proximal junctional failure should be distinguished from proximal junctional kyphosis, which is a recurrent deformity with limited clinical impact.
• Proximal junctional failure is a significant complication following adult spinal deformity surgery with potential for neurologic injury and increased need for surgical revision.
• Risk factors for proximal junctional failure include age, severity of sagittal plane deformity, and extent of operative sagittal plane realignment.
• Techniques for avoiding proximal junctional failure will likely require multiple refinements in perioperative and surgical strategies.

BACKGROUND AND DEFINITIONS

Proximal junctional kyphosis (PJK) is a recognized complication for patients undergoing posterior segmental instrumented fusion for spinal deformity.[1–5] However, descriptions of criteria for defining PJK, its incidence and clinical impact, and the basis for its development vary in the literature. Measured radiographically with a sagittal view, PJK has traditionally been defined by a 10° or greater increase in kyphosis at the proximal junction as measured by the Cobb angle from the caudal endplate of the uppermost instrumented vertebrae (UIV) to the cephalad endplate of the vertebrae 2 segments cranial to the UIV. This was the measurement used by Glattes and colleagues[1] and proved reliable in a study by Sacramento-Dominguez and colleagues[6] testing the reproducibility of different methods of measuring PJK.

Several investigators have reported that PJK according to the definition mentioned earlier does not generate significant clinical or quality-of-life issues.[1,4] In general, PJK is often well tolerated and does not lead to revision surgery in most cases.[7] Yagi and colleagues[8] reported that 4 of 32 PJK patients underwent additional surgery because of local pain but found no significant differences in Scoliosis Research Society (SRS) or Oswestry Disability Index (ODI) scores at final follow-up. Kim and colleagues[7] found no significant differences in clinical outcomes with SRS scores except in the self-image domain when PJK was greater than 20°. Similarly, no differences in clinical outcomes were found among PJK patients in the studies of Glattes and colleagues[1] and Hyun and Rhim.[9] Collectively, these reports support the idea that PJK defined radiographically amounts really to recurrent deformity, which is both infrequently associated with revision surgery and has a limited impact on clinical outcomes (**Fig. 1**).

a Department of Orthopaedic Surgery, Oregon Health and Science University, 3181 SW Sam Jackson Park Road, Portland, OR 97239, USA; b Department of Orthopaedic Surgery, Baylor Scoliosis Center, 478 Alliance Building, Suite 800, Plano, TX 75093, USA; c Department of Neurosurgery, Spine Tumor Surgery, Spinal Deformity Surgery, UCSF Medical, 505 Parnassus Avenue, Room M779, San Francisco, CA 94143-0112, USA; d Neurological and Orthopaedic Surgery, University of Virginia, P.O. Box 800386, Charlottesville, VA 22908-0386, USA
* Corresponding author.
E-mail address: hartro@ohsu.edu

Neurosurg Clin N Am 24 (2013) 213–218
http://dx.doi.org/10.1016/j.nec.2013.01.001
1042-3680/13/$ – see front matter © 2013 Elsevier Inc. All rights reserved.

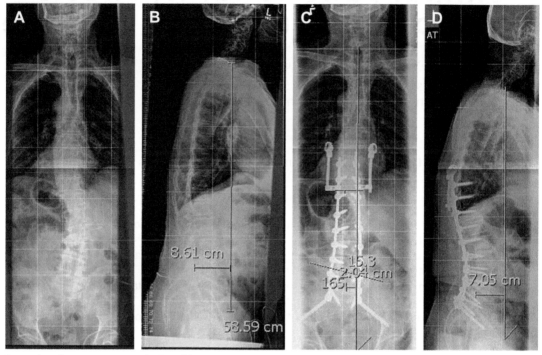

Fig. 1. (A, B) Posteroanterior (PA) and lateral full length views of a 77-year-old man with a history of 3 lumbar laminectomies, with persistent complaints of sciatica, low back pain, and sagittal imbalance. Preoperative lumbar lordosis is 43°, thoracic kyphosis is 27°, and junctional kyphosis (T8–T10) is 2°. Pelvic incidence measures 44°. (C, D) PA and lateral full length views following posterior instrumented fusion from T10-pelvis. Prophyllactic stabilization of T9 rib without fusion has been performed. Anterior diskectomy and fusion from L2-S1 was performed as a separate stage 6 weeks postoperatively. Postoperative lumbar lordosis is 53° (PI-LL = −9°), thoracic kyphosis has increased to 44°, and junctional kyphosis (T8–T10) has increased to 17°, meeting the definition of PJK. Patient was asymptomatic at the junction of his construct and was delighted with his clinical outcome.

Despite these relatively benign reports, other investigators have recognized that there is a subset of patients with a more severe version of PJK, which does seem to increase need for revision surgery and even carries a risk of neurologic deficit in addition to increased deformity and pain. This phenomenon has been variously termed "topping-off syndrome," proximal junctional acute collapse, or fractures of the vertebrae at the top of long pedicle screw constructs.[2,10–14] More recently, the term proximal junctional failure (PJF) has been proposed to distinguish between junctional kyphosis because of structural failure and more common, but less severe, PJK.[15–17]

The definition and classification of PJF is ongoing. *Hart* and colleagues[12] (2008) offered a definition of proximal junctional acute collapse as a failure of greater severity based on the clinical impact of the fracture. Similarly, Watanabe and colleagues[2] described a group of patients with fractures above pedicle screw constructs, which resulted in greater clinical effect but did not offer a clear definition of the phenomenon, and did not describe cases that resulted more from soft tissue

failure than from fracture. Finally, although Yagi and colleagues[8] provided a classification of PJK, their description included less severe cases with deformity as opposed to mechanical failure, and ultimately concluded that PJK has limited clinical impact.

Increasingly, the phenomenon of PJF has been distinguished from PJK in that it includes not only an increase in kyphosis but also structural failure of either the UIV or the vertebra immediately proximal to the fusion construct (UIV +1).[15–17] Structural failure is considered a vertebral body fracture, disruption of the posterior osseo-ligamentous complex, or both. Unlike traditionally defined PJK, PJF has been clearly shown to be associated with higher morbidity including increased pain, spinal instability, risk of neurologic injury, and need for revision surgery.[15–17] PJF is thus defined as a change of more than 10° of kyphosis between the UIV and the vertebra 2 levels above the UIV (UIV +2), along with one or more of the following: fracture of the vertebral body of UIV or UIV +1, posterior osseo-ligamentous disruption, or pull-out of instrumentation at the UIV (**Fig. 2**).

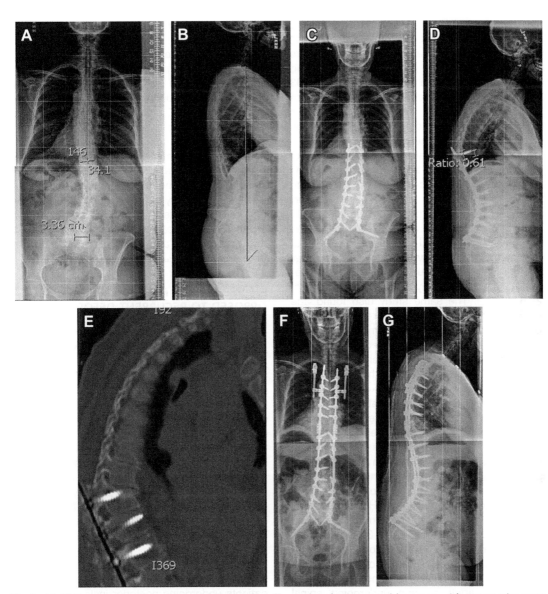

Fig. 2. (*A, B*) Posteroanterior and lateral full length radiographs of a 61-year-old woman with progressive symptoms of spinal stenosis and scoliosis. There was no history of prior surgery, and bone density was normal. Preoperative lumbar lordosis is 68°, thoracic kyphosis is 65°, and junctional kyphosis (T8–T10) is 11°. Pelvic incidence measures 75°. (*C–E*) Six week postoperatively from T10-pelvis instrumented fusion with transforaminal lumbar interbody fusion at L4/5 and L5/S1, she demonstrated a fracture of T10 vertebral body with disruption of the posterior tension band, although nondisplaced. She was symptomatic with significant axial pain and was quite bothered by the junctional kyphosis. Immediate postoperative radiographs had shown lumbar lordosis of 79° (PI-LL = −4°), thoracic kyphosis of 71°, and junctional kyphosis of 16°. Thus her immediate postoperative films did not display PJK despite early reciprocal increase in thoracic kyphosis and good matching of lumbar lordosis to pelvic incidence. (*F, G*) At 3 months postoperatively she underwent extension of the fusion to T4 with a Smith-Petersen osteotomy at T9–10 and prophylactic rib fixation at T3 without fusion. Early postoperative results from her revision surgery have been encouraging.

PREVALENCE AND RISK FACTORS FOR PJK AND PJF

With respect to the prevalence of PJK and PJF, it is important to assess the timing of occurrence

of these events. Kim and colleagues[7] found that the development of PJK was most frequent in the first 8 weeks after surgery, representing 59% of total kyphosis progression; however, it was also noted that after 2 years, the progression was also substantial with 41% of total progression. In a study on adolescent idiopathic scoliosis (AIS) correction and PJK with average age of 14.3 years and an average 11.6 levels fused, Kim and colleagues[5] reported a prevalence of 50/193 (26%). PJK did not progress significantly from 2 to 7.3 years average final follow-up period. It thus appears that the most dramatic progression of PJK occurs early in the postoperative period.

Several studies have analyzed the incidence of PJK after instrumented spinal fusion operations for adolescent idiopathic scoliosis, Scheuermann kyphosis,[4,14,18–22] and adult spinal deformity[1,7,9,23–25] as well as risk factors for the complication. With respect to adult patients, Kim and colleagues[7] investigated prevalence of PJK at a minimum 5-year follow-up following segmental posterior instrumented fusion of 5 or more vertebrae in 161 adults. They found a prevalence of 62/161 (39%). The same study also found age over 55 years to be a significant risk factor for development of PJK as well as a combined anterior/posterior fusion versus an isolated posterior approach. As described earlier, patients in this study had no significant differences in their clinical outcomes as measured by SRS-22 except in the self-image domain when PJK was greater than 20°.[7]

Glattes and colleagues[1] reported a lower PJK prevalence of 21/81 (26%) in their study, which retrospectively examined 81 adults with a minimum of 6 levels fused posteriorly with an average follow-up of 5.3 years. Again there were no differences in SRS-24 outcome scores and also no identifiable risk factors for the complication. Hyun and Rhim[9] investigated the clinical outcomes of pedicle subtraction osteotomy and found 3 of 13 patients (23%) with PJK on a 3-year follow-up although again no effects of PJK on clinical outcome scores were found. Mendoza-Lattes and colleagues[24] analyzed 54 adult patients undergoing spinal deformity surgery with an average follow-up of 26.8 months in a retrospective case-control study. They found a PJK prevalence of 19/54 (35%), with risks for PJK including a smaller difference in magnitude between lumbar lordosis and thoracic kyphosis (measured as LL-TK) at baseline and early postoperatively. In a retrospective case series of 157 adult scoliosis patients undergoing long fusion (>5 vertebrae) by Yagi and colleagues,[8] the PJK prevalence was 32/157 (20%), with an average follow-up of 4.3 years. These investigators also reported no differences in SRS and ODI outcomes scores, although 4 patients did undergo additional surgery due to local pain. They reported fusion to the sacrum and posterior fusion with segmental instrumentation risk factors for PJK and felt that the incidence of PJK could be minimized with normal sagittal global realignment postoperatively.[8]

The common theme among these studies suggesting limited clinical impact of PJK is that they combine PJF with PJK patients and typically do not have a PJF cohort of sufficient size to make stronger statistical statements. Although several of the investigators have commented on the more significant impact on patients of PJF, the data of single-center studies have not allowed a more detailed analysis of PJF as a distinct entity. Despite the commonality of increased proximal kyphosis shared by both PJK and PJF, it appears that PJF represents a separate phenomenon with a substantial clinical impact in patients suffering this complication and thus deserves separation from analyses of PJK.

PJF VERSUS PJK: MECHANICAL FAILURE AS OPPOSED TO RECURRENT DEFORMITY

The underlying pathology of PJF appears to be an acute event rather than a progressive deformity. Some cases of PJK may develop from similar structural issues. For example, Hollenbeck and colleagues[20] focused on adolescent patients and postulated that PJK was due to posterior ligament disruption and muscular support. Rhee and colleagues[22] also support this claim in a study focusing on adolescents, which found an increased incidence of PJK with posterior instrumentation compared with an anterior approach. They hypothesized that PJK is at least partially a result of damage to the posterior tension band from surgery, deformity correction forces applied during surgery, and a resulting compensation for reduced kyphosis in the thoracic region.

Denis and colleagues[18] expands on the idea of soft tissue injury during surgery in their study of patients undergoing posterior instrumentation for Scheuermann kyphosis. In 67 patients with an average age of 37 years and a PJK prevalence of 20/67 (30%), they reported that 3/20 were attributable to ligamentum flavum damage and an additional 2 were due to a combination of ligamentum flavum trauma and failure to incorporate the proximal end vertebrae. Helgeson and colleagues[19] draw a similar conclusion in their study examining PJK after AIS corrective surgery comparing pedicle screw only (n = 37), hook-only (n = 51), hybrid (n = 177), and pedicle screws with hooks at the UIV (n = 18) in a sample of 283 adolescent patients. A significant increase in PJK was found with the screw-only patients compared with both the hybrid and hook-only groups.[19] It thus seems that some juvenile PJK may result from structural injury and that the stronger correction forces applied with pedicle screw constructs may also increase the impact on adjacent segments. Given this, the overlap in definition and description is perhaps not surprising.

With respect to adult patients, Watanabe and colleagues[2] also studied the effects of segmental pedicle screw constructs on the incidence of proximal vertebral fracture in 10 adult spinal deformity patients. It was conjectured that the vertebral body fractures were at least in part because of the mechanical stress generated by pedicle screw instrumentation at the proximal junction, especially with inclusion of the sacrum.[2] Yagi and colleagues[8] also found that fusion to the sacrum and segmental posterior instrumentation were risk factors for PJK in their adult study. Both of these reports support the idea that correction force, and possibly surgical dissection, contribute to PJK and PJF in adults as well as adolescents.

Several preoperative risk factors have consistently emerged among adult deformity patients. These include age and preoperative sagittal malaignment.[1,2,7–10,15,16] Hart and colleagues[16] reported a multicenter comparison of adult deformity patients experiencing PFJ with a large prospective cohort of non-PJF patients. Age-matched and procedure-matched control groups were developed. Besides age, they found that several measures of preoperative sagittal imbalance correlated strongly with development of PJF, including increased sagittal vertical alignment (SVA), increased mismatch of pelvic incidence with lumbar lordosis (LL-PI), and increased thoracic kyphosis.

Concordant with the preoperative sagittal malalignment of patients at highest risk for PJF is the demonstration that patients undergoing greater sagittal realignments are also at higher risk of PJF.[2,8,15,16] In this regard, the analysis by Hart and colleagues[16] showed that adult patients experiencing PJF underwent a greater number of pedicle subtraction osteotomies, and had greater corrections of SVA, greater increases in lumbar lordosis, and greater reduction in the difference between pelvic incidence and lumbar lordosis (LL-PI). This is consistent with the findings of prior investigators.[2,8]

Most importantly from a clinical perspective is increasing evidence that patients with PJF do suffer a worsened clinical course than patients without this complication. Hostin and colleagues[15] reported a retrospective consecutive case review of 1218 adult deformity surgeries, with 68 cases of PJF identified (5.6%). Twenty-eight of the 68 patients underwent revision surgery within 6 months of the index operation. Patients undergoing revision surgery were identified with PJF on average of 9 weeks after index, in comparison to 13 weeks for patients who did not undergo revision, again demonstrating the impact of mechanical failure as opposed to recurrent deformity.[15] The results of the cohort comparison by Hart and colleagues[16] further validated the concept that PJF results in a higher rate of revision surgery in the early postoperative course after adult deformity reconstruction.

Given the frequent need for extension of instrumentation proximal to junctional failures, the occurrence of PJF has clear clinical significance. From a clinical standpoint, revisions subject the patient to additional risks of perioperative and postoperative complications and hospitals and payers to greater economic costs. Given the expected increase in frequency of surgical reconstruction for patients with adult spinal deformity, efforts at defining and ultimately preventing PJF appear warranted.

SUMMARY

Although several studies have reported incidence and risk factors for PJK, understanding of risk factors and means of prevention of PJF remains incomplete. Most patients experiencing PJF develop the complication in the early postoperative period, resulting from a combination of reciprocal kyphosis in the unfused portions of the spine, increased loads in the mobile segments adjacent to the fusion, and surgical trauma to soft tissues at the proximal junction. PJF appears to be increasing in incidence, due perhaps both to increasing numbers of older patients undergoing extended spinal reconstruction, as well as changes in surgical techniques producing more substantial spinal realignment and greater construct stiffness. Although some patients with PJF may be successfully followed without intervention, there is a consistent relationship between development of PJF and a need for early revision surgery. Further efforts to define this complication, and more importantly to reduce its incidence, remain an important goal for adult spinal deformity surgeons.

REFERENCES

1. Glattes RC, Bridwell KH, Lenke LG, et al. Proximal junctional kyphosis in adult spinal deformity following long instrumented posterior spinal fusion: incidence, outcomes, and risk factor analysis. Spine (Phila Pa 1976) 2005;30(14):1643–9.
2. Watanabe K, Lenke LG, Bridwell KH, et al. Proximal junctional vertebral fracture in adults after spinal

deformity surgery using pedicle screw constructs: analysis of morphological features. Spine (Phila Pa 1976) 2010;35(2):138–45.

3. Nowakowski A. Some aspects of spine biomechanics and their clinical implications in idiopathic scoliosis. Chir Narzadow Ruchu Ortop Pol 2004; 69(5):349–54.

4. Lee GA, Betz RR, Clements DH 3rd, et al. Proximal kyphosis after posterior spinal fusion in patients with idiopathic scoliosis. Spine (Phila Pa 1976) 1999;24(8):795–9.

5. Kim YJ, Lenke LG, Bridwell KH, et al. Proximal junctional kyphosis in adolescent idiopathic scoliosis after 3 different types of posterior segmental spinal instrumentation and fusions: incidence and risk factor analysis of 410 cases. Spine (Phila Pa 1976) 2007;32(24):2731–8.

6. Sacramento-Dominguez C, Vayas-Diez R, Coll-Mesa L, et al. Reproducibility measuring the angle of proximal junctional kyphosis using the first or the second vertebra above the upper instrumented vertebrae in patients surgically treated for scoliosis. Spine (Phila Pa 1976) 2009;34(25):2787–91.

7. Kim YJ, Bridwell KH, Lenke LG, et al. Proximal junctional kyphosis in adult spinal deformity after segmental posterior spinal instrumentation and fusion: minimum five year follow-up. Spine (Phila Pa 1976) 2008;33(20):2179–84.

8. Yagi M, Akilah KB, Oheneba B. Incidence, risk factors and classification of proximal junctional kyphosis: surgical outcomes review of adult idiopathic scoliosis. Spine (Phila Pa 1976) 2010; 36(1):9.

9. Hyun SJ, Rhim SC. Clinical outcomes and complications after pedicle subtraction osteotomy for fixed sagittal imbalance patients: a long-term follow-up data. J Korean Neurosurg Soc 2010;47(2):95–101.

10. Lewis SJ, Abbas H, Chua S, et al. Upper instrumented vertebra (UIV) fractures in long lumbar fusions-What are the associated risk factors? Spine (Phila Pa 1976) 2012;37(16):1407–14.

11. Venu V, Vertinsky AT, Malifair D, et al. Plain radiograph assessment of spinal hardware. Semin Musculoskelet Radiol 2011;15(2):151–62.

12. Hart RA, Prendergast MA, Roberts WG, et al. Proximal junctional acute collapse cranial to multi-level lumbar fusion: a cost analysis of prophylactic vertebral augmentation. Spine J 2008;8(6):875–81.

13. Bridwell KH, Baldus C, Berven S, et al. Changes in radiographic and clinical outcomes with primary treatment adult spinal deformity surgeries from two years to three-to five- years follow-up. Spine (Phila Pa 1976) 2010;35(20):1849–54.

14. Hart RA, Prendergast M. Spine surgery for lumbar degenerative disease in the elderly and osteoporotic patient. Marsh JL, editor. AAOS instructional course lectures. vol. 56. Rosemont (IL): 2007. p. 257–72.

15. Hostin R, McCarthy I, O'Brien M, et al; International Spine Study Group. Incidence, mode, and location of acute proximal junctional failures following surgical treatment for adult spinal deformity. Spine (Phila Pa 1976) 2012. [Epub ahead of print].

16. Hart R, Hostin R, McCarthy I, et al; International Spine Study Group. Age, sagittal deformity and operative correction are risk factors for proximal junctional failure following adult spinal deformity surgery. AAOS. Spine, in press.

17. Hart R, Hostin R, McCarthy I, et al; International Spine Study Group. Development and validation of a classification system for proximal junctional failure, SRS Published Abstracts, 2012.

18. Denis F, Sun EC, Winter RB. Incidence and risk factors for proximal and distal junctional kyphosis following surgical treatment for Scheuermann kyphosis: minimum five-year follow-up. Spine (Phila Pa 1976) 2009;34(20):E729–34.

19. Helgeson MD, et al. Evaluation of proximal junctional kyphosis in adolescent idiopathic scoliosis following pedicle screw, hook, or hybrid instrumentation. Spine (Phila Pa 1976) 2010;35(2):177–81.

20. Hollenbeck SM, et al. The prevalence of increased proximal junctional flexion following posterior instrumentation and arthrodesis for adolescent idiopathic scoliosis. Spine (Phila Pa 1976) 2008;33(15):1675–81.

21. Lonner BS, et al. Operative management of Scheuermann's kyphosis in 78 patients: radiographic outcomes, complications, and technique. Spine (Phila Pa 1976) 2007;32(24):2644–52.

22. Rhee JM, et al. Sagittal plane analysis of adolescent idiopathic scoliosis: the effect of anterior versus posterior instrumentation. Spine (Phila Pa 1976) 2002;27(21):2350–6.

23. Kwon BK, et al. Progressive junctional kyphosis at the caudal end of lumbar instrumented fusion: etiology, predictors, and treatment. Spine (Phila Pa 1976) 2006;31(17):1943–51.

24. Mendoza-Lattes S, et al. Proximal junctional kyphosis in adult reconstructive spine surgery results from incomplete restoration of the lumbar lordosis relative to the magnitude of the thoracic kyphosis. Iowa Orthop J 2011;31:199–206.

25. O'Leary PT, Bridwell KH, Lenke LG, et al. Risk factors and outcomes for catastrophic failures at the top of long pedicle screw constructs: a matched cohort analysis performed at a single center. Spine (Phila Pa 1976) 2009;34(20):2134–9.

Treatment Algorithms and Protocol Practice in High-Risk Spine Surgery

Patrick A. Sugrue, MD[a],*, Ryan J. Halpin, MD[b],
Tyler R. Koski, MD[a]

KEYWORDS

- Evidence-based medicine • High-risk spine protocol • Spine surgery • Spinal deformity

KEY POINTS

- Protocol-based care has been shown to improve outcomes in many care pathways.
- Increasing understanding of surgical goals in spinal deformity surgery as well as improved techniques used to achieve such goals has led to improved outcomes.
- As more patients are considered for surgical intervention, the medical comorbidities and potential complications require thorough and appropriate workup.

INTRODUCTION

The treatment of complex spinal deformity is becoming increasingly more common as the population ages. Pain and difficulty with balance are the leading complaints of elderly (age >60 years) patients undergoing complex spinal reconstruction.[1–3] The focus of treatment for such abnormality is centered on the spinal deformity, but one must pay close attention to the overall medical condition and relevant comorbidities that may complicate the operative course. With improvements in surgical technique and anesthetic management, the surgical ability to tackle complex deformity is increasing, but enthusiasm must be tempered by the medical challenges and the patient's ability to tolerate surgery. Glassman and colleagues[4] have categorized a series of complications as either major or minor. This study reported a 10% rate of major complications in patients undergoing major adult spinal reconstruction, whereas more recent studies have shown a 34.3% rate of major complication including a 19.3% rate of perioperative complications and an 18.7% rate of long-term complications.[5] The risk factors for perioperative complications were advanced age, medical comorbidities, and obesity; however, the only factors that were found to negatively affect patient outcomes as demonstrated on the Scoliosis Research Society questionnaire and the Oswestry Disability Index (ODI) were those found at follow-up, such as presence of a 3-column osteotomy or progressive loss of sagittal correction.[5] In the setting of spinal deformity, the surgeon's goal is to apply various surgical techniques to restore sagittal alignment and safely decompress neurologic structures. The clinical importance and significant patient impact of restoring sagittal alignment has been demonstrated in the literature[6–9]; however, the magnitude of the operation that would be

Disclosures: P.A.S., R.J.H: None. T.R.K: Consultant: Medtronic, Nuvasive, Globus; Research Funding: Medtronic, NIAMS.

[a] Department of Neurological Surgery, Northwestern University Feinberg School of Medicine, 676 North Saint Clair, Suite 2210, Chicago, IL 60611, USA; [b] Division of Neurosurgery, Olympia Orthopaedics Associates, 3901 Capital Mall Drive Southwest, Olympia, WA 98502, USA
* Corresponding author.
E-mail address: p-sugrue@fsm.northwestern.edu

required to correct a complex deformity must be one that the patient can tolerate medically.

As much as 68% of the population older than 60 years has been shown to have some form of spinal deformity, and limitation in activity and overall disability are the most powerful factors driving individuals to surgery.[10] The overall complication rate in adult revision spinal surgery has been reported to be as high as 40%, and the factors associated with the highest rate of complication include patient age, medical comorbidities, and extension of fusion to the sacrum.[3,4,11–15] Because of the lack of physiologic reserve and multiple medical comorbidities, the complication rate can be even higher in the elderly population.[2,3] Despite the higher rate of complications, Drazin and colleagues[2] have demonstrated that elderly patients benefit from deformity correction. In fact they demonstrated, for patients with a mean age of 74.2 years, a mean reduction in ODI of 24.1 and a mean reduction in visual analog scale of 5.2.[2]

USE OF PREOPERATIVE PROTOCOL

In efforts to optimize outcomes and minimize complications, protocol-based care plans have been initiated in many disciplines. Specifically, protocol-based care has been shown to successfully decrease the number of days on mechanical ventilation,[16–21] reduce the incidence of thromboembolism,[22] improve mortality from sepsis,[23,24] reduce the costs of hospitalization,[24] and reduce

the incidence of drug-resistant bacterial infections.[25] Furthermore, Awissi and colleagues[26] have also shown that some protocol-based therapies can reduce overall cost. The purpose of the protocol-based interventions is to use evidence-based methods to comprehensively target specific medical issues before surgical intervention takes place. The Northwestern high-risk spine protocol[27] begins in the outpatient setting before any surgical intervention. The surgeon first determines the goals of surgery, and within that context a complete medical evaluation is initiated to determine how each of the patient's comorbidities can be optimized within the specific context of the planned surgical intervention. The protocol is designed for patients who will require more than 6 hours of surgery time, and for whom the surgeon plans more than 6 fusion levels or plans a staged procedure. The protocol is also initiated in the setting of specific medical comorbidities such as coronary artery disease, congestive heart failure, cirrhosis, dementia, emphysema, renal insufficiency, cerebrovascular disease, pulmonary hypertension, and age older than 80 years. The protocol can also be initiated in any instance whereby the clinical judgment of surgeon, internist, and/or anesthesiologist determines that the patient should be on the protocol (**Figs. 1** and **2**).[27]

The use of protocol-based therapies is designed to provide a comprehensive evaluation that can be discussed among all the care teams, including the surgeon, internist/hospitalist, anesthesiologist,

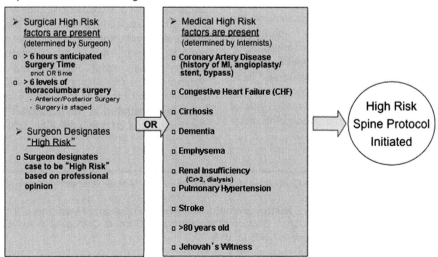

High Risk Spine – Patient Criteria

A patient is determined "High Risk" when:

➤ Surgical High Risk factors are present (determined by Surgeon)
□ > 6 hours anticipated Surgery Time anot OR time
□ > 6 levels of thoracolumbar surgery
  · Anterior/Posterior Surgery
  · Surgery is staged

➤ Surgeon Designates "High Risk"
□ Surgeon designates case to be "High Risk" based on professional opinion

OR

➤ Medical High Risk factors are present (determined by Internists)
□ Coronary Artery Disease (history of MI, angioplasty/ stent, bypass)
□ Congestive Heart Failure (CHF)
□ Cirrhosis
□ Dementia
□ Emphysema
□ Renal Insufficiency (Cr>2, dialysis)
□ Pulmonary Hypertension
□ Stroke
□ >80 years old
□ Jehovah's Witness

High Risk Spine Protocol Initiated

Fig. 1. Initiation of the high-risk spine protocol is based on the complexity of planned surgical intervention, patient-specific medical comorbidities, and clinical judgment.

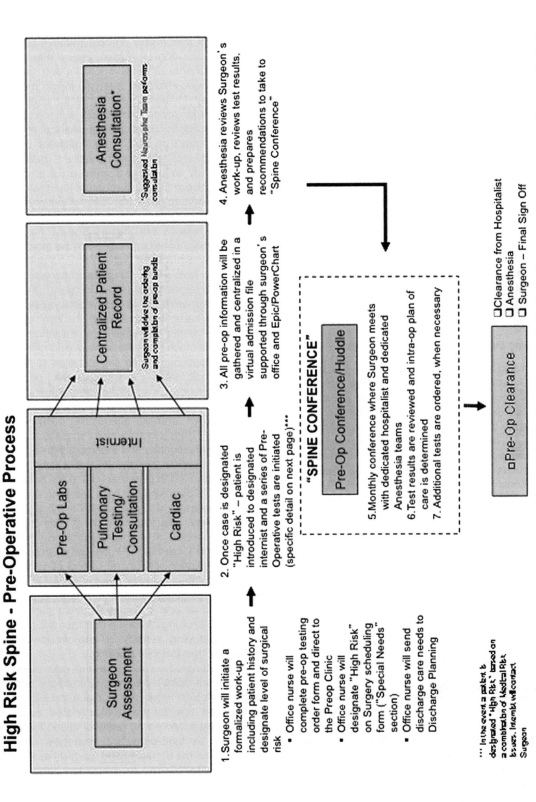

Fig. 2. The preoperative evaluation of a patient scheduled to undergo high-risk spine surgery begins in the clinic setting and continues through evaluation by the internist/hospitalist, anesthesiologist, and critical care team, to create a comprehensive evaluation and medical optimization.

and critical care physician, so as to fully understand the risk profile for the patient within the context of the patient's specific medical history and the planned surgical intervention. With this information the surgeon can have a detailed discussion with the patient addressing a true patient-specific risk profile for the planned procedure. With this in mind, a key element of the protocol is communication between the various teams involved. Each member of the high-risk team provides a unique skill set. By using the established protocol, each team member can better understand and appreciate the importance or goal of each intervention specific to the patient. Likewise, the importance of communication between the team members cannot be overemphasized as the patient transitions from the clinic, to the operating room, to the intensive care unit.

In the Northwestern high-risk spine protocol, areas specifically addressed include the patient's cardiac, pulmonary, hepatic, renal, nutritional (including bone quality), and psychosocial status.[27]

Cardiac Evaluation

According to the American College of Cardiology and American Heart Association, the following conditions have been identified as increasing the risk of perioperative cardiac complications: unstable coronary syndromes, decompensated heart failure, significant arrhythmias, or severe valvular disease. The presence of any one of these conditions may require the delay or cancellation of any nonemergent surgical intervention. Patients with a history of ischemic heart disease, history of compensated or prior heart failure, history of stroke, diabetes mellitus, renal insufficiency, or poor exercise tolerance from smoking or limited activity due to pain may also require additional workup, including a stress test or consultation with a cardiologist.[28] Often these patients will benefit from the use of a β-blocker with a goal heart rate of 55 to 65 beats/min, which has been shown to lead to a 90% reduction in cardiac events at 30 days postoperatively as well as a reduction in 1- and 2-year mortality rates.[29]

Pulmonary Evaluation

Pulmonary complications in the postoperative setting include pneumonia, pleural effusions, respiratory failure, with prolonged mechanical ventilation, bronchospasm, atelectasis, and exacerbations of chronic lung disease, and can be just as common as cardiac complications.[3,30] Presence of decreased breath sounds, dullness to percussion, wheezes, rhonchi, or prolonged expiratory phase

in the preoperative evaluation predict an increased risk of pulmonary complications postoperatively.[30,31] Furthermore, 64% of patients will have some form of abnormality on postoperative chest radiograph, including atelectasis, pleural effusion, infiltrate, or lobar collapse, and patients with radiographic changes also tend to have a longer mean length of stay[3,14] The use of a ventilator-weaning protocol by Blackwood and colleagues[32] demonstrated a reduction in duration on mechanical ventilation and length of stay in the intensive care unit. Poor exercise tolerance/capacity is defined by the inability to perform 2 minutes of supine bicycle exercise sufficient to raise the heart rate to 99 beats/min, and predicts 79% of pulmonary complications in patients undergoing surgical intervention.[33] In patients with cough, dyspnea, or exercise intolerance, consideration should be given to evaluation by a pulmonary specialist, and pulmonary function tests (PFTs) should be obtained.[34] In children undergoing scoliosis surgery, PFTs decreased by as much as 60% postoperatively, reaching a nadir approximately 3 days after surgery.[35] Patients undergoing a transthoracic approach are much more likely to develop pulmonary complications,[36,37] so the decision to use a transthoracic versus a posterior-only based approach must be considered in the preoperative discussion.

Patients with chronic obstructive pulmonary disease (COPD) are at increased risk for pleural effusion and/or pneumonia, and treatment with bronchodilators, physical therapy, antibiotics, smoking cessation, and corticosteroids can help reduce this risk.[34,38–40] Smoking has been shown to significantly increase the risk of pulmonary complications postoperatively. The relative risk of pulmonary complication rates in smokers compared with nonsmokers is 1.4 to 4.3.[27,34] Patients with an acute COPD exacerbation are at increased risk of complications and should consider delaying surgery.[40] In patients undergoing coronary artery bypass surgery, Warner and colleagues[41] have demonstrated that smoking cessation less than 8 weeks before undergoing surgery is associated with a higher risk than is active smoking.

In the setting of surgery involving high blood loss, such as spinal deformity correction, high blood-transfusion requirements place the patient at increased risk for transfusion-related acute lung injury (ALI). Moreover, protocol-based therapies such as lung-protective strategies have helped reduce the morbidity and mortality associated with ALI.[42,43] Acute respiratory distress syndrome (ARDS) and other forms of ALI are associated with critically ill patients and potential complications following spinal surgery.[44–46]

Hepatic Evaluation

Patients with chronic liver disease are at risk for increased morbidity and mortality following surgical procedures[47] whereby the most common complications are secondary to acute or chronic liver failure leading to severe coagulopathy, encephalopathy, ARDS, acute renal failure, and sepsis.[48] As part of the comprehensive preoperative assessment, the use of the Model for End-Stage Liver Disease (MELD) can be a useful predictor of mortality in patients with liver disease. Northup and colleagues[49] reported a direct correlation between MELD scores and postoperative mortality, demonstrating that a MELD score of less than 10 predicts a low likelihood of complication whereas a score greater than 20 suggests a high risk of complication. Furthermore, patients with acute viral or alcoholic hepatitis, fulminant hepatic failure, severe chronic hepatitis, Child-Pugh class C cirrhosis, severe coagulopathy, or severe extrahepatic complications such as hypoxia, cardiomyopathy, or acute renal failure should not undergo elective surgery.[27]

Renal Evaluation

Patients with chronic renal failure or dialysis-dependent end-stage renal disease (ESRD) are at risk for osteoporosis, electrolyte imbalances, and anemia, which can each complicate the intraoperative and postoperative course. In particular, patients at risk for osteoporosis are also at risk for pseudarthrosis, which may influence the planned surgical intervention biomechanically when considering fusion levels, circumferential procedures, type and material of instrumentation used, or the use of osteobiologics.[50–52] The most common abnormality found in patients with ESRD is hyperkalemia, so electrolyte levels should be monitored closely in conjunction with overall fluid balance.[53,54] Patients with ESRD should be dialyzed within 24 hours after surgery.[53]

Nutrition Evaluation

Risk factors for poor nutrition status include age older than 60 years, diabetes, osteomyelitis, and spinal cord injury.[29,55] The metabolic demands on a patient following major spinal reconstruction are likely much higher than their baseline metabolic needs, therefore nutritional status before surgery can greatly affect outcome. Preoperative albumin level, prealbumin level, and total lymphocyte counts can be useful for estimating nutritional reserves, as nutritional stores following major reconstructive surgery can take 6 to 12 weeks to return to baseline.[56] The use of hyepralimentation

with total parenteral nutrition during the perioperative period, particularly in the setting of staged procedures, can be used to augment nutritional stores.[57]

Aggressive glucose control is associated with improved outcomes, as diabetes or poor glucose control has been shown to increase the risk of infection and pneumonia as well as the length of stay in hospital and the intensive care unit.[27,29,55,58–61] The use of protocol-driven therapies in the intensive care unit has shown that using an intensive glucose control protocol designed to maintain serum glucose levels at 110 mg/dL reduced in-hospital mortality by 34%, bloodstream infections by 46%, acute renal failure by 41%, and the rate of red blood cell transfusions by 50%.[62] Hemmila and colleagues[63] have also demonstrated a reduced incidence of pneumonia and urinary tract infection in burn patients with intensive glucose control.

Osteoporosis, as defined by a bone mineral density more than 2.5 standard deviations below peak bone mineral density, measured using dual-energy radiograph absorptiometry, can lead to increased rates of proximal junctional kyphosis, pseudarthrosis, and distal screw loosening.[64] Risk factors for osteoporotic fractures include Caucasian race, age older than 50 years, postmenopausal status, active smoking, history of any fracture sustained after age 40 years, or history of fractures of the hip, spine, or wrist in a first-degree relative.[65] In addition to nutritional supplementation with calcium and vitamin D, antiresorptive agents such as bisphosphonates, calcitonin, estrogens, and estrogen-receptor modulators have been used to treat osteoporosis, but animal studies have shown varying effects on the amount of fusion mass and radiographic evidence of fusion.[66–69] More recently, teriparatide has been introduced as an alternative to the antiosteoclastic activity of bisphosphonates. Nakamura and colleagues[70] have shown that once-weekly injections of teriparatide reduced the incidence of new vertebral fractures in patients with known osteoporosis and prior fractures: 3.1% in the teriparatide cohort compared with 14.5% in the placebo cohort. Furthermore, Ohtori and colleagues[71] demonstrated an increased fusion rate and decreased time to radiographic fusion in osteoporotic women with degenerative spondylolisthesis undergoing decompression and instrumented posterolateral fusion with teriparatide compared with bisphosphonate. Transient exposure to parathyroid hormone has been shown to improve bone formation by altering the activities of osteoblasts, osteoclasts, and osteocytes.[72] Potential side effects include hypercalcemia and hypercalciuria, and studies in animals have shown only some increase in sarcoma formation.[72]

Thromboembolism

Rates of deep venous thrombosis (DVT) after spine surgery have been reported widely in the literature, ranging from 0.3% to 31%.[73–84] Owing to concerns for postoperative hematoma formation and potential severe neurologic decline, the use of chemical DVT prophylaxis among spine surgeons varies widely. However, the use of DVT prophylaxis protocols in specialties such as orthopedics, general surgery, and plastic surgery has been shown to reduce the incidence of DVT and pulmonary embolism.[22,85,86] The application of such a protocol must take into consideration the preoperative risk factors of the specific patient and must include the intraoperative findings. A podium presentation from the Scoliosis Research Society Annual Meeting reviewed 445 high-risk patients who were given prophylactic low molecular weight heparin on average postoperative day 4 (42% within 72 hours) without sequelae.[87] The use of prophylactic inferior vena cava filters has also been shown to reduce the risk of pulmonary embolism in particularly high-risk patients.[78,88–90]

USE OF INTRAOPERATIVE PROTOCOL

Once the preoperative risk stratification and medical optimization is complete, the patient is finally brought to the operating room for the planned surgical intervention. A key component of maximizing the benefits of the high-risk spine protocol is communication. Both the surgical and anesthetic teams must be well versed in the medical history and preoperative evaluation of the patient, and both are encouraged to discuss the goals and risks of each intervention throughout the case. Likewise, verbal communication between the surgical, anesthetic, and neuromonitoring teams occurs at least on an hourly basis and more frequently during times of higher-risk interventions such as performing osteotomies. Any change in the patient's condition is communicated immediately to all parties.

A worksheet/checklist is maintained throughout the procedure as part of the anesthetic record. Laboratory values including complete blood count, prothrombin time, partial thromboplastin time, international normalized ratio, fibrinogen,

High Risk Spine - Post-Operative Care Communication

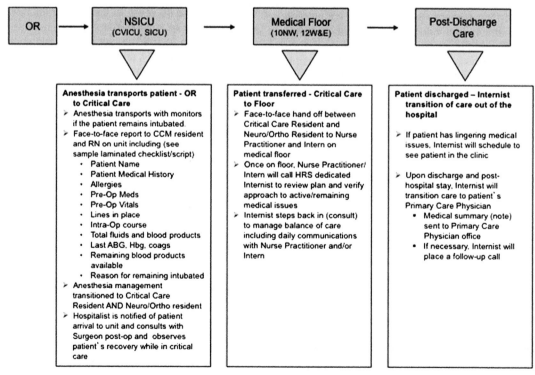

Fig. 3. A crucial element of executing the high-risk spine protocol is the use of effective and open communication as the patient advances from the clinic, to the operating room (OR), to the intensive care unit. ABG, arterial blood gas; CCM, critical care medicine; coags, coagulation studies; CVICU, cardiovascular intensive care unit; Hbg, hemoglobin; HRS, high-risk spine; NSICU, neuro-spine intensive care unit; RN, registered nurse; SICU, surgical intensive care unit.

High Risk Spine - Post-Operative Care Guidelines

- Complications identified Intraop or during pre-op assessment may require specific care

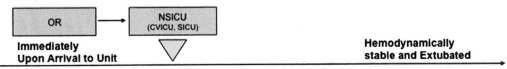

- Stabilize Hemodynamics
  Ensure euvolemia
  Maintain Hgb > 9.5 until hemodynamically stable with minimal drain output
  Maintain preoperative blood pressure unless otherwise specified
- Correct Hypothermia to > 96°F
  Fluid warmers
  Forced Air Warmers
- Correct acidosis
  Resuscitate volume status
  Transfuse RBCs as necessary
  Optimize Ventilator Settings for goal eucapnia. Consider the use of PEEP.
- Correct coagulopathy
  See Blood/Fluid Management Protocol
- Order and Review initial postoperative labs and ECG
  ABG, CBC, basic Chem, Coags with fibrinogen, Lactic Acid, Troponin
- Oder and Review postoperative Chest Xray
  ETT position and central line placement
- Electrolyte Replacement per CCM service
- Sedation per CCM service
- Wean Mechanical Ventilation and Extubate per Weaning Protocol
  Assess the patient for appropriateness for extubation (positive leak, hemodynamic stability, normal acid base status) at least every 4 hours for the first 24 hours postop
  Ensure adequate sedation and analgesia while intubated with RASS goal of -2 to 0 when not undergoing Spontaneous Breathing Trial (SBT). Re-sedate if the patient does not meet extubation criteria after 30min of SBT
  Maintain analgesia with IV opioids titrated to RR 10-20 during spontaneous breathing trial and extubation

Fig. 4. On arrival to the intensive care unit, intraoperative events are discussed with establishment of immediate specific plans for resuscitation and recovery. CBC, complete blood count; ECG, electrocardiogram; ETT, endotracheal tube; IV, intravenous; PEEP, positive end-expiratory pressure; RASS, Regional Anesthesia Surveillance System; RBCs, red blood cells; RR, respiratory rate.

High Risk Spine – Post-Operative Protocol Guidelines

Blood /Fluid Management

High Risk Spine Cryo Guidelines*
➢ORDER cryo to be thawed at fibrinogen <200
➢ADMINISTER cryo when fibrinogen <150

High Risk Spine Platelet Guidelines*
➢ORDER platelets when <150,000
➢ADMINISTER platelets when <100,000

IF patient is oozing **AND**
- Fibrinogen is normal
- Platelet count is corrected (>100,000)
➢ORDER and ADMINISTER Desmopressin (DDAVP, Sanofi-Aventis) – dose 0.3 µ g/kg placed in 50 ml saline, infused intravenously over 20 minutes

IF patient is still oozing after DDAVP **AND**
- INR > 2
➢ORDER and ADMINISTER recombinant factor VIIa (NovoSeven, NovoNordisk, Princeton, NJ) – dose 20 µg/kg for a 80 kg patient injected directly intravenously over 2-5 minutes
  [Pharmacy can obtain dose form 2.4 mg vial and keep the remainder should the patient require a second dose]

❖**Fresh frozen plasma is generally not indicated**

* Algorithms outlined above have been developed
specifically for designated High Risk Spine Procedures

Fig. 5. Coagulation parameters and transfusion thresholds are established based on the high-risk spine protocol. INR, international normalized ratio.

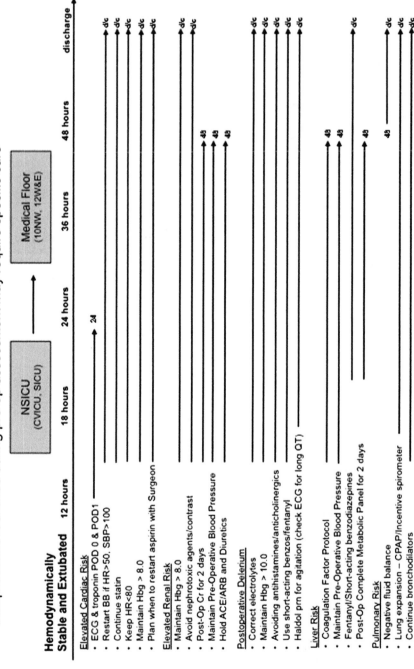

Fig. 6. Patient-specific laboratory values and clinical parameters tailored to the specific patient comorbidities are followed immediately postoperatively throughout the patient's hospital course. ACE, angiotensin-converting enzyme inhibitor; ARB, angiotensin receptor blocker; BB, β-blocker; CPAP, continuous positive airway pressure; Cr, creatinine; HR, heart rate; POD, postoperative day; SBP, systolic blood pressure.

and ionized calcium are initially followed every 2 hours, and after 6 hours they are checked and reported hourly. The transfusion protocol as presented by Halpin and colleagues[27] uses packed red blood cells, cryoprecipitate, platelets, desmopressin, and activated factor VII, but does not use fresh frozen plasma because of the excessive volume associated with it.

The use of antifibrinolytics has become increasingly common in spinal deformity operations. Aprotinin, ε-aminocaproic acid, and tranexamic acid have all been used in various studies. A meta-analysis by Gill and colleagues[91] determined that all 3 agents are effective at reducing blood loss and transfusion requirements in patients undergoing spine surgery, and that both ε-aminocaproic acid and tranexamic acid do so without increasing the risk of a thromboembolic event. Elwatidy and colleagues[92] confirmed the efficacy and safety of tranexamic acid in a randomized, double-blind, placebo-controlled trial of 64 adult patients undergoing high-blood-loss spinal procedures, and Yagi and colleagues[93] likewise demonstrated a reduction in blood loss and blood-transfusion requirements in 106 adolescents undergoing posterior spinal fusion. The use of antifibrinolytics during high-risk spine surgery has become part of the standard protocol for many institutions, and can help reduce complications associated with significant blood loss/anemia and transfusion-related reactions.

USE OF POSTOPERATIVE PROTOCOL

Following the completion of the procedure, the patient is transported to the neuro-spine intensive care unit (NSICU), and a face-to-face report from the anesthesia team is given to the critical care team along with the surgical team (**Figs. 3** and **4**). The intraoperative checklist is reviewed and a new set of laboratory values is established. Postoperative resuscitation and subsequent transfusion is performed according to the high-risk spine protocol and is tailored to the needs of that specific patient (**Figs. 5** and **6**). Specifically, in the setting of active hemorrhage or high subfascial drain output the coagulation profile is determined, which may necessitate transfusion of blood product clotting factor. Once the patient is fully resuscitated, the use of restrictive transfusion strategies is typically implemented[94,95] and the ventilator-weaning protocol is initiated. At this time the hospitalist who evaluated the patient preoperatively then engages again in helping to manage the patient's ongoing medical issues until the time of discharge. At the time of discharge a summary letter is sent to the patient's primary care physician for established follow-up.

SUMMARY

The use of early goal-directed evidence-based therapies has led to improved outcomes and has helped to minimize complications.[23,24] The Institute for Healthcare Improvement in the Surviving Sepsis Campaign advocates for widespread adoption of the bundle protocol with a program of "education, practice improvement, and performance measurement" in the treatment of sepsis.[23,96] Likewise, the application of protocol-based care in the treatment of complex spinal pathology in an aging and medically complex patient population helps to unify and direct the various medical and surgical subspecialists toward one overall patient goal. In this context, the protocol provides a comprehensive evaluation of the patient that also helps the transition of care from the outpatient setting through surgery and until the time of discharge, with multiple transitions of care among health care providers. The goal of this or any protocol-based therapy is to improve outcomes through improved communication and collaboration between health care providers when caring for these medically and surgically complex patients.

REFERENCES

1. Bess S, Boachie-Adjei O, Burton D, et al. Pain and disability determine treatment modality for older patients with adult scoliosis, while deformity guides treatment for younger patients. Spine (Phila Pa 1976) 2009;34:2186–90.
2. Drazin D, Shirzadi A, Rosner J, et al. Complications and outcomes after spinal deformity surgery in the elderly: review of the existing literature and future directions. Neurosurg Focus 2011;31:E3.
3. Baron EM, Albert TJ. Medical complications of surgical treatment of adult spinal deformity and how to avoid them. Spine (Phila Pa 1976) 2006;31: S106–18.
4. Glassman SD, Hamill CL, Bridwell KH, et al. The impact of perioperative complications on clinical outcome in adult deformity surgery. Spine (Phila Pa 1976) 2007; 32:2764–70.
5. Cho SK, Bridwell KH, Lenke LG, et al. Major complications in revision adult deformity surgery: risk factors and clinical outcomes with two- to seven-year follow-up. Spine (Phila Pa 1976) 2012; 37:489–500.
6. Glassman SD, Berven S, Bridwell K, et al. Correlation of radiographic parameters and clinical symptoms in adult scoliosis. Spine (Phila Pa 1976) 2005; 30:682–8.
7. Glassman SD, Bridwell K, Dimar JR, et al. The impact of positive sagittal balance in adult spinal deformity. Spine (Phila Pa 1976) 2005;30:2024–9.

8. Mac-Thiong JM, Transfeldt EE, Mehbod AA, et al. Can C7 plumbline and gravity line predict health related quality of life in adult scoliosis? Spine (Phila Pa 1976) 2009;34:E519–27.

9. Schwab F, Patel A, Ungar B, et al. Adult spinal deformity-postoperative standing imbalance: how much can you tolerate? An overview of key parameters in assessing alignment and planning corrective surgery. Spine (Phila Pa 1976) 2010;35:2224–31.

10. Pekmezci M, Berven SH, Hu SS, et al. The factors that play a role in the decision-making process of adult deformity patients. Spine (Phila Pa 1976) 2009;34:813–7.

11. Bradford DS, Tay BK, Hu SS. Adult scoliosis: surgical indications, operative management, complications, and outcomes. Spine (Phila Pa 1976) 1999;24:2617–29.

12. Emami A, Deviren V, Berven S, et al. Outcome and complications of long fusions to the sacrum in adult spine deformity: Luque-Galveston, combined iliac and sacral screws, and sacral fixation. Spine (Phila Pa 1976) 2002;27:776–86.

13. Faciszewski T, Winter RB, Lonstein JE, et al. The surgical and medical perioperative complications of anterior spinal fusion surgery in the thoracic and lumbar spine in adults. A review of 1223 procedures. Spine (Phila Pa 1976) 1995;20:1592–9.

14. Jules-Elysee K, Urban MK, Urquhart BL, et al. Pulmonary complications in anterior-posterior thoracic lumbar fusions. Spine J 2004;4:312–6.

15. McDonnell MF, Glassman SD, Dimar JR 2nd, et al. Perioperative complications of anterior procedures on the spine. J Bone Joint Surg Am 1996;78:839–47.

16. Clifford C, Spencer A. An evaluation of the impact of a tracheostomy weaning protocol on extubation time. Nurs Crit Care 2009;14:131–8.

17. Crocker C. Nurse led weaning from ventilatory and respiratory support. Intensive Crit Care Nurs 2002;18:272–9.

18. Horst HM, Mouro D, Hall-Jenssens RA, et al. Decrease in ventilation time with a standardized weaning process. Arch Surg 1998;133:483–8 [discussion: 8–9].

19. Kollef MH, Shapiro SD, Silver P, et al. A randomized, controlled trial of protocol-directed versus physician-directed weaning from mechanical ventilation. Crit Care Med 1997;25:567–74.

20. Robinson BR, Mueller EW, Henson K, et al. An analgesia-delirium-sedation protocol for critically ill trauma patients reduces ventilator days and hospital length of stay. J Trauma 2008;65:517–26.

21. Saura P, Blanch L, Mestre J, et al. Clinical consequences of the implementation of a weaning protocol. Intensive Care Med 1996;22:1052–6.

22. Gonzalez Della Valle A, Serota A, Go G, et al. Venous thromboembolism is rare with a multimodal prophylaxis protocol after total hip arthroplasty. Clin Orthop Relat Res 2006;444:146–53.

23. Talmor D, Greenberg D, Howell MD, et al. The costs and cost-effectiveness of an integrated sepsis treatment protocol. Crit Care Med 2008;36:1168–74.

24. Shorr AF, Micek ST, Jackson WL Jr, et al. Economic implications of an evidence-based sepsis protocol: can we improve outcomes and lower costs? Crit Care Med 2007;35:1257–62.

25. Bennett KM, Scarborough JE, Sharpe M, et al. Implementation of antibiotic rotation protocol improves antibiotic susceptibility profile in a surgical intensive care unit. J Trauma 2007;63:307–11.

26. Awissi DK, Begin C, Moisan J, et al. I-SAVE Study: impact of sedation, analgesia, and delirium protocols evaluated in the intensive care unit: an economic evaluation (January). Ann Pharmacother 2012;46:21–8.

27. Halpin RJ, Sugrue PA, Gould RW, et al. Standardizing care for high-risk patients in spine surgery: the Northwestern high-risk spine protocol. Spine (Phila Pa 1976) 2010;35:2232–8.

28. Fleisher LA, Beckman JA, Brown KA, et al. ACC/AHA 2007 guidelines on perioperative cardiovascular evaluation and care for noncardiac surgery: a report of the American College of Cardiology/American Heart Association Task Force on Practice Guidelines (Writing Committee to Revise the 2002 Guidelines on Perioperative Cardiovascular Evaluation for Noncardiac Surgery): developed in collaboration with the American Society of Echocardiography, American Society of Nuclear Cardiology, Heart Rhythm Society, Society of Cardiovascular Anesthesiologists, Society for Cardiovascular Angiography and Interventions, Society for Vascular Medicine and Biology, and Society for Vascular Surgery. Circulation 2007;116:e418–99.

29. Hu SS, Berven SH. Preparing the adult deformity patient for spinal surgery. Spine (Phila Pa 1976) 2006;31:S126–31.

30. Lawrence VA, Dhanda R, Hilsenbeck SG, et al. Risk of pulmonary complications after elective abdominal surgery. Chest 1996;110:744–50.

31. Kocabas A, Kara K, Ozgur G, et al. Value of preoperative spirometry to predict postoperative pulmonary complications. Respir Med 1996;90:25–33.

32. Blackwood B, Alderdice F, Burns KE, et al. Protocolized versus non-protocolized weaning for reducing the duration of mechanical ventilation in critically ill adult patients. Cochrane Database Syst Rev 2010;(5):CD006904.

33. Williams-Russo P, Charlson ME, MacKenzie CR, et al. Predicting postoperative pulmonary complications. Is it a real problem? Arch Intern Med 1992;152:1209–13.

34. Smetana GW. Preoperative pulmonary evaluation. N Engl J Med 1999;340:937–44.

35. Yuan N, Fraire JA, Margetis MM, et al. The effect of scoliosis surgery on lung function in the immediate

postoperative period. Spine (Phila Pa 1976) 2005; 30:2182–5.

36. Rawlins BA, Winter RB, Lonstein JE, et al. Reconstructive spine surgery in pediatric patients with major loss in vital capacity. J Pediatr Orthop 1996; 16:284–92.

37. Zhang JG, Wang W, Qiu GX, et al. The role of preoperative pulmonary function tests in the surgical treatment of scoliosis. Spine (Phila Pa 1976) 2005;30: 218–21.

38. Stein M, Cassara EL. Preoperative pulmonary evaluation and therapy for surgery patients. JAMA 1970; 211:787–90.

39. Stein M, Koota GM, Simon M, et al. Pulmonary evaluation of surgical patients. JAMA 1962;181:765–70.

40. Tarhan S, Moffitt EA, Sessler AD, et al. Risk of anesthesia and surgery in patients with chronic bronchitis and chronic obstructive pulmonary disease. Surgery 1973;74:720–6.

41. Warner MA, Offord KP, Warner ME, et al. Role of preoperative cessation of smoking and other factors in postoperative pulmonary complications: a blinded prospective study of coronary artery bypass patients. Mayo Clin Proc 1989;64:609–16.

42. Brower RG, Ware LB, Berthiaume Y, et al. Treatment of ARDS. Chest 2001;120:1347–67.

43. Ware LB, Matthay MA. The acute respiratory distress syndrome. N Engl J Med 2000;342:1334–49.

44. Naunheim KS, Barnett MG, Crandall DG, et al. Anterior exposure of the thoracic spine. Ann Thorac Surg 1994;57:1436–9.

45. Urban MK, Beckman J, Gordon M, et al. The efficacy of antifibrinolytics in the reduction of blood loss during complex adult reconstructive spine surgery. Spine (Phila Pa 1976) 2001;26:1152–6.

46. Urban MK, Urquhart B, Boachie-Adjei O. Evidence of lung injury during reconstructive surgery for adult spinal deformities with pulmonary artery pressure monitoring. Spine (Phila Pa 1976) 2001;26:387–90.

47. Rice HE, O'Keefe GE, Helton WS, et al. Morbid prognostic features in patients with chronic liver failure undergoing nonhepatic surgery. Arch Surg 1997; 132:880–4 [discussion: 4–5].

48. Wiklund RA. Preoperative preparation of patients with advanced liver disease. Crit Care Med 2004; 32:S106–15.

49. Northup PG, Wanamaker RC, Lee VD, et al. Model for End-Stage Liver Disease (MELD) predicts nontransplant surgical mortality in patients with cirrhosis. Ann Surg 2005;242:244–51.

50. Burval DJ, McLain RF, Milks R, et al. Primary pedicle screw augmentation in osteoporotic lumbar vertebrae: biomechanical analysis of pedicle fixation strength. Spine (Phila Pa 1976) 2007;32:1077–83.

51. Glassman SD, Alegre GM. Adult spinal deformity in the osteoporotic spine: options and pitfalls. Instr Course Lect 2003;52:579–88.

52. Sawakami K, Yamazaki A, Ishikawa S, et al. Polymethylmethacrylate augmentation of pedicle screws increases the initial fixation in osteoporotic spine patients. J Spinal Disord Tech 2012;25:E28–35.

53. Han IH, Kim KS, Park HC, et al. Spinal surgery in patients with end-stage renal disease undergoing hemodialysis therapy. Spine (Phila Pa 1976) 2009;34:1990–4.

54. Pinson CW, Schuman ES, Gross GF, et al. Surgery in long-term dialysis patients. Experience with more than 300 cases. Am J Surg 1986;151:567–71.

55. Klein JD, Hey LA, Yu CS, et al. Perioperative nutrition and postoperative complications in patients undergoing spinal surgery. Spine (Phila Pa 1976) 1996; 21:2676–82.

56. Lenke LG, Bridwell KH, Blanke K, et al. Prospective analysis of nutritional status normalization after spinal reconstructive surgery. Spine (Phila Pa 1976) 1995; 20:1359–67.

57. Lapp MA, Bridwell KH, Lenke LG, et al. Prospective randomization of parenteral hyperalimentation for long fusions with spinal deformity: its effect on complications and recovery from postoperative malnutrition. Spine (Phila Pa 1976) 2001;26:809–17 [discussion: 17].

58. Browne JA, Cook C, Pietrobon R, et al. Diabetes and early postoperative outcomes following lumbar fusion. Spine (Phila Pa 1976) 2007;32:2214–9.

59. Fang A, Hu SS, Endres N, et al. Risk factors for infection after spinal surgery. Spine (Phila Pa 1976) 2005;30:1460–5.

60. Glassman SD, Alegre G, Carreon L, et al. Perioperative complications of lumbar instrumentation and fusion in patients with diabetes mellitus. Spine J 2003;3:496–501.

61. Simpson JM, Silveri CP, Balderston RA, et al. The results of operations on the lumbar spine in patients who have diabetes mellitus. J Bone Joint Surg Am 1993;75:1823–9.

62. van den Berghe G, Wouters P, Weekers F, et al. Intensive insulin therapy in the critically ill patients. N Engl J Med 2001;345:1359–67.

63. Hemmila MR, Taddonio MA, Arbabi S, et al. Intensive insulin therapy is associated with reduced infectious complications in burn patients. Surgery 2008;144:629–35 [discussion: 35–7].

64. DeWald CJ, Stanley T. Instrumentation-related complications of multilevel fusions for adult spinal deformity patients over age 65: surgical considerations and treatment options in patients with poor bone quality. Spine (Phila Pa 1976) 2006;31:S144–51.

65. Cummings SR, Nevitt MC, Browner WS, et al. Risk factors for hip fracture in white women. Study of Osteoporotic Fractures Research Group. N Engl J Med 1995;332:767–73.

66. Lehman RA Jr, Kuklo TR, Freedman BA, et al. The effect of alendronate sodium on spinal fusion: a rabbit model. Spine J 2004;4:36–43.

67. Xue Q, Li H, Zou X, et al. The influence of alendronate treatment and bone graft volume on posterior lateral spine fusion in a porcine model. Spine (Phila Pa 1976) 2005;30:1116–21.

68. Huang RC, Khan SN, Sandhu HS, et al. Alendronate inhibits spine fusion in a rat model. Spine (Phila Pa 1976) 2005;30:2516–22.

69. Babat LB, McLain R, Milks R, et al. The effects of the antiresorptive agents calcitonin and pamidronate on spine fusion in a rabbit model. Spine J 2005;5:542–7.

70. Nakamura T, Sugimoto T, Nakano T, et al. Randomized Teriparatide [human parathyroid hormone (PTH) 1-34] Once-Weekly Efficacy Research (TOWER) trial for examining the reduction in new vertebral fractures in subjects with primary osteoporosis and high fracture risk. J Clin Endocrinol Metab 2012;97: 3097–106.

71. Ohtori S, Inoue G, Orita S, et al. Teriparatide accelerates lumbar posterolateral fusion in women with postmenopausal osteoporosis: prospective study. Spine (Phila Pa 1976) 2012;37:E1464–8.

72. Deal C. Future therapeutic targets in osteoporosis. Curr Opin Rheumatol 2009;21:380–5.

73. Catre MG. Anticoagulation in spinal surgery. A critical review of the literature. Can J Surg 1997;40: 413–9.

74. Ferree BA, Stern PJ, Jolson RS, et al. Deep venous thrombosis after spinal surgery. Spine (Phila Pa 1976) 1993;18:315–9.

75. Cheng JS, Arnold PM, Anderson PA, et al. Anticoagulation risk in spine surgery. Spine (Phila Pa 1976) 2010;35:S117–24.

76. Ferree BA, Wright AM. Deep venous thrombosis following posterior lumbar spinal surgery. Spine (Phila Pa 1976) 1993;18:1079–82.

77. Glotzbecker MP, Bono CM, Wood KB, et al. Thromboembolic disease in spinal surgery: a systematic review. Spine (Phila Pa 1976) 2009;34:291–303.

78. Leon L, Rodriguez H, Tawk RG, et al. The prophylactic use of inferior vena cava filters in patients undergoing high-risk spinal surgery. Ann Vasc Surg 2005;19:442–7.

79. Oda T, Fuji T, Kato Y, et al. Deep venous thrombosis after posterior spinal surgery. Spine (Phila Pa 1976) 2000;25:2962–7.

80. Rokito SE, Schwartz MC, Neuwirth MG. Deep vein thrombosis after major reconstructive spinal surgery. Spine (Phila Pa 1976) 1996;21:853–8 [discussion: 859].

81. Smith MD, Bressler EL, Lonstein JE, et al. Deep venous thrombosis and pulmonary embolism after major reconstructive operations on the spine. A prospective analysis of three hundred and seventeen patients. J Bone Joint Surg Am 1994;76:980–5.

82. West JL 3rd, Anderson LD. Incidence of deep vein thrombosis in major adult spinal surgery. Spine (Phila Pa 1976) 1992;17:S254–7.

83. Dearborn JT, Hu SS, Tribus CB, et al. Thromboembolic complications after major thoracolumbar spine surgery. Spine (Phila Pa 1976) 1999;24:1471–6.

84. Piasecki DP, Poynton AR, Mintz DN, et al. Thromboembolic disease after combined anterior/posterior reconstruction for adult spinal deformity: a prospective cohort study using magnetic resonance venography. Spine (Phila Pa 1976) 2008;33:668–72.

85. Pannucci CJ, Dreszer G, Wachtman CF, et al. Postoperative enoxaparin prevents symptomatic venous thromboembolism in high-risk plastic surgery patients. Plast Reconstr Surg 2011;128:1093–103.

86. Pannucci CJ, Jaber RM, Zumsteg JM, et al. Changing practice: implementation of a venous thromboembolism prophylaxis protocol at an academic medical center. Plast Reconstr Surg 2011;128:1085–92.

87. Koski TR, Halpin RJ, Vaz K, et al. Risks of chemoprophylaxis for venous thromboembolism following spinal fusions: a retrospective review of 351 consecutive patients. Scoliosis Research Society Annual Meeting. Kyoto, September 21-24, 2010.

88. Dazley JM, Wain R, Vellinga RM, et al. Prophylactic inferior vena cava filters prevent pulmonary embolisms in high-risk patients undergoing major spinal surgery. J Spinal Disord Tech 2012;25:190–5.

89. Ozturk C, Ganiyusufoglu K, Alanay A, et al. Efficacy of prophylactic placement of inferior vena cava filter in patients undergoing spinal surgery. Spine (Phila Pa 1976) 2010;35:1893–6.

90. Rosner MK, Kuklo TR, Tawk R, et al. Prophylactic placement of an inferior vena cava filter in high-risk patients undergoing spinal reconstruction. Neurosurg Focus 2004;17:E6.

91. Gill JB, Chin Y, Levin A, et al. The use of antifibrinolytic agents in spine surgery. A meta-analysis. J Bone Joint Surg Am 2008;90:2399–407.

92. Elwatidy S, Jamjoom Z, Elgamal E, et al. Efficacy and safety of prophylactic large dose of tranexamic acid in spine surgery: a prospective, randomized, double-blind, placebo-controlled study. Spine (Phila Pa 1976) 2008;33:2577–80.

93. Yagi M, Hasegawa J, Nagoshi N, et al. Does the intraoperative tranexamic acid decrease operative blood loss during posterior spinal fusion for treatment of adolescent idiopathic scoliosis? Spine (Phila Pa 1976) 2012;37:E1336–42.

94. Carson JL, Carless PA, Hebert PC. Transfusion thresholds and other strategies for guiding allogeneic red blood cell transfusion. Cochrane Database Syst Rev 2012;(4):CD002042.

95. Carson JL, Grossman BJ, Kleinman S, et al. Red blood cell transfusion: a clinical practice guideline from the AABB*. Ann Intern Med 2012;157:49–58.

96. Dellinger RP, Carlet JM, Masur H, et al. Surviving Sepsis Campaign guidelines for management of severe sepsis and septic shock. Crit Care Med 2004;32:858–73.

The Role of Minimally Invasive Techniques in the Treatment of Adult Spinal Deformity

Praveen V. Mummaneni, MD[a], Tsung-Hsi Tu, MD[a,b,c],*,
John E. Ziewacz, MD, MPH[a], Olaolu C. Akinbo, MBBS[a],
Vedat Deviren, MD[d], Gregory M. Mundis, MD[e]

KEYWORDS

- Adult spinal deformity • Minimally invasive surgery • Scoliosis

KEY POINTS

- Minimally invasive techniques are feasible options for the treatment of certain subtypes of adult degenerative spinal deformity.
- Careful patient selection for minimally invasive deformity surgery is critical to achieve the best surgical outcome.
- An algorithm is provided to help guide spinal surgeons on the use of minimally invasive techniques for the treatment of patients with degenerative spinal deformity.

INTRODUCTION

Adult degenerative scoliosis is becoming more prevalent in the rapidly growing elderly population. This disease represents a process of degenerative changes of the disks and facets that leads to progressive deformity in both the coronal and sagittal plane. The coronal Cobb angles range from mild (10°–20°) to moderate (20°–40°), with the apex of the curve most frequently located between L2 and L4. The loss of lumbar lordosis (LL) is common and can cause significant sagittal imbalance, which is predictive of a poor quality of life in this patient group.[1] The surgical treatment of adult spinal deformity aims to reduce pain, arrest progression of the deformity, restore sagittal and coronal balance, improve neurologic function, and improve cosmesis.

There are substantial surgical risks for patients with adult degenerative deformity, especially because of their increased age and frequently associated medical comorbidities. Long-segment reconstruction is associated with prolonged operative times under general anesthesia and significant blood loss. The reported complication rates of adult deformity surgery are as high as 41.2%[2] and the rates are even higher in the population older than 75 years,[3] and in the revision setting. A recent multi-center study from the International Spine Study Group[4,5] reviewed a total of 953 adult patients with spinal deformity with minimum 2-year follow-up to identify patients with major perioperative complications. Ninety-nine major complications were observed in 72 patients (7.6%). The most common complications were excessive blood loss (EBL) (>4 L), deep wound infection requiring reexploration of the wound, and pulmonary embolism.

To decrease surgical morbidity and complications, minimally invasive surgery (MIS) approaches

[a] Department of Neurosurgery, University of California, San Francisco, 505 Parnassus Avenue, Room M-780, San Francisco, CA 94143-0332, USA; [b] Department of Neurosurgery, Neurological Institute, Taipei Veterans General Hospital, 201 Sec. 2, Shipai Road, Taipei 112, Taiwan; [c] School of Medicine, National Yang-Ming University, 155, Sec. 2, Linong Street, Taipei 112, Taiwan; [d] Department of Orthopaedic Surgery, University of California, San Francisco, 500 Parnassus MU 320 West, San Francisco, CA 94143, USA; [e] San Diego Center for Spinal Disorder, 4130 La Jolla Village Drive, Suite 300La Jolla, La Jolla, CA 92037, USA
* Corresponding author. 505 Parnassus Avenue, Room M-780, San Francisco, CA 94143-0332.
E-mail address: thtu0001@gmail.com

Neurosurg Clin N Am 24 (2013) 231–248
http://dx.doi.org/10.1016/j.nec.2012.12.004
1042-3680/13/$ – see front matter © 2013 Elsevier Inc. All rights reserved.

for the treatment of adult spinal deformity have been proposed. However, not every adult patient with deformity can be managed with MIS. Proper patient selection is the key to successfully treating adult patients with deformity using MIS techniques.

The Rationale of MIS to Treat Adult Degenerative Spinal Deformity

Before using various MIS techniques to treat degenerative scoliosis, several questions need to be clarified. First, can MIS achieve adequate decompression?[6] Second, can instrumentation be placed appropriately with MIS? Third, can solid fusion be established? Fourth, can global coronal and sagittal balance be restored? Recent publications have shed some light on these issues.

Kelleher and colleagues[7] reported a single-surgeon 75-patient consecutive series of minimally invasive bilateral decompression via a unilateral approach at 1 (n = 48) or 2 (n = 27) levels for focal lumbar spinal stenosis. The patients were divided into 4 groups: (A) stenosis with no deformity (n = 22); (B) stenosis with spondylolisthesis only (n = 25); (C) stenosis with scoliosis (n = 16); and (D) stenosis combined with spondylolisthesis and scoliosis (n = 12). The average ages were 68 years and the mean follow-up was 31.8 months. The Oswestry Disability Index (ODI) score improved from 49.1 preoperatively to 23.9 postoperatively. Significant improvement in the ODI score was observed in all 4 subgroups, without intergroup differences. The overall revision surgery rate during a mean 42.8-month postoperative period was 10% and included revision surgery (n = 2) or addition of instrumented fusion (n = 6). The revision rate in the subgroups was (A) 0%; (B) 4%; (C) 25%; and (D) 25%, respectively; and the mean number of months to surgical revision was (B) 25.4, (C) 26.1, and (D) 27.8, respectively. The revision rate was significantly higher in patients with scoliosis than those without. There were 12 patients who had a lateral listhesis (average 13.9%, range, 6%–21%). Six of the 8 revised patients had a lateral listhesis (3 in C and 3 in D, all had >10% listhesis).

Yamada and colleagues[8] reported the outcomes of 46 patients who had microscopic lumbar foraminotomy for degenerative lumbar foraminal stenosis (DLFS). The duration of follow-up was more than 1 year in these patients. Degenerative lumbar scoliosis (DLS) was noted in 26 of the patients, whereas 20 patients were in the non-DLS group. Overall, the Japanese Orthopaedic Association (JOA) scores improved from 13.8 to 21.9 postoperatively. The leg pain was reduced in 44 patients (95.7%) immediately after surgery but recurred in 9 patients (19.6%). The leg pain

recurred in 8 (30.8%) of the patients with DLS compared with 1 (5%) of the non-DLS group (P = .027). Also, the outcome was good or excellent for 46% of the patients with DLS compared with 80% of the non-DLS group (P = .029). Amongst the patients with DLS in whom the difference between standing and supine Cobb angle was less than 3°, 70% had good or excellent outcome and there was no recurrence of leg pain. This result was better than in the patients with DLS with Cobb angle difference of 3° or more; 50% of these patients had recurrent radiculopathy, and only 32% had good or excellent outcomes. Patients with recurrent radiculopathy had significantly higher preoperative Cobb angles than those without recurrence (17.8 ± 3.2 vs 13.8 ± 4.1; P = .007).

Anand and colleagues[9] reported 28 patients treated with 3 or more levels of minimally invasive lateral transpsoas interbody fusion (LIF) and percutaneous pedicle screw (PPS) fixation, with a mean age of 67.7 years and mean follow-up time of 22 months. Mean intraoperative blood loss was of 500 mL for both stages, and the operative times were a mean of 500 minutes. The visual analogue scale (VAS), treatment intensity scale, 36-Item Short Form Health Survey, and ODI scores at 1 year were statistically better than preoperative values. The mean coronal Cobb angles were 22° preoperatively and 7.5° postoperatively, but the investigators did not report results of sagittal balance correction. All patients had a solid fusion assessed by plain radiographs at 1 year. However, complications were noted in 23 patients, mostly transient dysesthesia (17/23) related to the LIF approach. The investigators also reported 2 transient quadriceps palsies, 1 retrocapsular renal hematoma, and 1 cerebellar hemorrhage in this cohort.

Tormenti and colleagues[10] reported their retrospective review of 8 cases performed with a combined anterior LIF and open posterior fixation and compared this cohort with 4 cases who underwent posterior-only open surgery. The mean preoperative and postoperative coronal Cobb angles were 39° and 13°, respectively, in the LIF group versus 19° and 11°, respectively, in the posterior-approach-only group. One case of cecal perforation during the anterior approach was reported in this series. The investigators also reported 6 cases of sensory lower extremity dysesthesias as well as 2 cases of lower extremity motor dysfunction after the lateral approach. In most cases, these neurologic issues resolved over several months. The investigators also reported 1 case of infection and meningitis, 1 case of ileus, 1 case of pleural effusion, and 1 patient who had a pulmonary embolus after surgery.

There were no pseudarthrosis or instrumentation failures. The investigators did not report sagittal balance parameters.

Dakwar and colleagues[11] retrospectively reviewed 25 adult patients with degenerative deformity who underwent anterior reconstruction with LIF for 3 or more levels with a mean follow-up of 11 months. The mean intraoperative blood loss was 53 mL per level, with a mean length of stay of 6.2 days. VAS scores and ODI scores improved significantly postoperatively. Complications included 3 cases of transient postoperative anterior thigh numbness, 1 case of rhabdomyolysis requiring temporary hemodialysis, 1 case of implant failure, and 1 case of asymptomatic subsidence. One-third of their cases failed to restore sagittal balance. Reported perioperative complications included 1 patient with rhabdomyolysis requiring temporary hemodialysis, 1 patient with implant subsidence, and 1 patient with hardware failure. In addition, 3 patients (12%) experienced transient postoperative anterior thigh numbness in the distribution of the anterior femoral cutaneous nerve after the LIF procedure.

Wang and Mummaneni[12] retrospectively reviewed 23 patients with thoracolumbar deformity treated with minimally invasive approaches. The mean age was 64.4 years, with a mean follow-up of 13.4 months. The mean blood loss was 477 mL. The coronal Cobb angles improved from 31.4° preoperatively to 11.5° postoperatively. The LL improved from 37.4° preoperatively to 47.5° postoperatively. All of the 16 patients achieved solid fusion at the levels of interbody fusion. Of the 7 cases without use of interbody fusion at every level, 2 patients had pseudarthrosis. Seven patients developed thigh dysesthesia or numbness on the side of the LIF. All of these cases recovered except for 1 patient who had thigh numbness and quadriceps weakness that persisted. Other complications included 1 patient with postoperative atrial fibrillation, 1 case of pneumothorax requiring a chest tube, 1 cerebrospinal fluid (CSF) leak, and 1 patient who needed reoperation for S1 screw pull-out.

Isaacs and colleagues[13] performed a prospective nonrandomized observational study of 107 adult patients with deformity with mean age of 68.4 years who were treated with LIF alone (24.3%) or LIF with either open or percutaneous posterior fixation (75.7%). The mean operative time was 177.9 minutes. A total of 62.5% of patients had a recorded EBL of less than 100 mL and only 8.4% had greater than 300 mL EBL. The overall complication rate was 24.3%. These investigators found that the patients undergoing MIS-only procedures (LIF stand alone or with percutaneous pedicle screws) had significantly lower complications (9% had 1 or more major complications) than those undergoing combined MIS LIF procedures with posterior open pedicle screw fixation procedures (20.7% had 1 or more major complications). The most common major surgical complications were posterior wound infections (3 patients who had open posterior surgery) and postoperative motor deficits (7 cases of persistent motor weakness or having 2 grades decrease in motor strength after LIF procedures). The investigators did not report the preoperative and postoperative sagittal balance parameters as well as fusion status.

Scheufler and colleagues[14,15] reviewed 30 prospectively collected adult patients with degenerative deformity who were treated with mini-open transforaminal lumbar interbody fusion (TLIF) and computed tomography (CT)-guided PPS with an average of 19 months' follow-up. The mean age was 73.2 years. In the 30 patients, a total of 179 segments were fused, among which 134 segments had a TLIF. Mean LL and coronal Cobb angles correction were 44.8° ± 10.7° and 31.7° ± 13.7°, respectively. Mean LL increased from 8.8° ± 8.9° to −36° ± 6.9°, and sagittal vertical axis was reduced from 31.6 ± 15.2 to 8 ± 8.4 mm. Solid fusion was confirmed with CT scan in 90% of the instrumented segments at 18 months. The rate of major and minor complications was 23.4% and 59.9%, respectively. The fusion was not extended to the pelvis, and 2 patients developed symptomatic lumbosacral pseudarthrosis, mandating extension of fusion to the pelvis.

Acosta and colleagues[16] retrospectively evaluated the changes in the coronal and sagittal plane after LIF for the treatment of degenerative lumbar disease in 36 patients. Of this cohort, only 8 patients had degenerative scoliosis; the mean regional lumbar coronal Cobb angles improved significantly from 21.4° preoperatively to 9.7° postoperatively. The mean global coronal alignment was 19.1 mm preoperatively and 12.5 mm postoperatively (P<.05). In the sagittal plane, the mean segmental Cobb angle measured −5.3° preoperatively and −8.2° postoperatively (P<.0001). The mean preoperative and postoperative regional LL was 42.1° and 46.2°, respectively (P>.05). The mean global sagittal alignment was 41.5 mm preoperatively and 42.4 mm postoperatively (P = .7). The postoperative ODI and VAS scores improved significantly. However, the fusion status was not reported.

Mundis and colleagues[17] performed a literature review on minimally invasive lateral approaches for interbody fusion to treat degenerative spinal deformity. Both patient-centered outcomes and objective radiographic parameters showed significant improvement in most studies. The complications rates varied between studies, but the major complications were low. Thigh dysesthesia was the most commonly reported complication associated with LIF but was transient in most cases. The investigators concluded that the minimally invasive lateral approach was an effective surgical strategy for adult degenerative deformity.

Berjano and Larmatina[18] also reviewed the current literature for minimally invasive lateral approaches in the treatment of adult deformity, and they proposed a classification of adult lumbar deformity to guide formulation of a surgical strategy for LIF use.

From these published articles, it can be surmised that (1) decompression can be achieved with minimally invasive approaches for a subset of adult deformity cases (because the ODI and VAS are regarded as the surrogates for extent of decompression)[6]; (2) instrumentation can be safely placed with minimally invasive approaches; (3) LIF is effective in treating the coronal deformity (however, restoring the sagittal plane remains an issue); (4) pseudarthrosis is problematic in cases with posterolateral MIS fusion without interbody support; (5) the complication profile of LIF remains to be determined on a large scale, with temporary sensory deficits and transient leg weakness being most common. Because these deficits are approach-related and mostly transient, the question remains whether these temporary neurological changes should be considered as approach related temporary morbidity or as complications.

PATIENT EVALUATION
Physical Examination

A detailed neurologic examination, including muscle power, reflexes, sensory testing, and gait testing, is necessary for patients with spinal deformity. Any degree of shoulder or pelvic asymmetry as well as pelvic obliquity and leg length discrepancy are evaluated and noted. The patients are assessed for any local tenderness in the facets, trochanters, or sacroiliac joints. The range of motion in hip and knee joints is evaluated to identify any contracture.

Radiographic Studies

Patients with adult deformity usually seek medical attention because of radicular leg or back pain, rather than the magnitude of the deformity itself.[19] It is important to identify whether the nature of the pain is radicular, axial, or combined. For pure radicular pain, it is important to confirm that the pain is congruent with the foraminal stenosis on imaging. It is also important to clarify if the stenosis is central, paracentral (lateral recess), foraminal, or extraforaminal. Axial back pain often originates from advanced disk or facet degeneration, worsening subluxation or listhesis (instability), or

muscle fatigue from deformity (sagittal or coronal imbalance). It is important to evaluate the dynamic flexion and extension radiographs to identify any instability. The sagittal and coronal balance is assessed on 91.44-cm (36-in) radiographs taken with patients in the standing position with their hips and knees fully extended. This positioning is particularly important in minimally invasive versus open approach planning because it helps the surgeon decide whether an osteotomy is needed for fixed sagittal imbalance to restore the sagittal vertebral axis (SVA) to within 5 cm. Spinopelvic parameters (LL, pelvic incidence [PI], pelvic tilt, and sacral slope) should be assessed for appropriate preoperative planning. The PI and pelvic tilt should be measured. The pelvic tilt is a compensatory parameter that can be altered by patients in an attempt to realign their SVA, but there is a limit to this compensation. The PI, on the other hand, is a fixed parameter that cannot be varied. The surgeon should pay close attention to the parameters of the spinopelvic region, including mismatch of the LL to the PI. Ideally, LL should match the PI ± 10°. This strategy is important in planning any degree of balance correction necessary to alleviate the patient's symptoms, because sagittal balance correction has been associated with improved clinical outcomes in patients undergoing scoliosis surgery.[20–22]

Magnetic resonance imaging (MRI) is essential in evaluating the location and severity of neural element compression, the degree of disk degeneration, and also any anatomic variations that may hinder certain approaches. Special attention must be paid to the location of the psoas, particularly at L4 to L5 if an LIF is to be used. When the psoas lies more anterior, consideration should be given to an alternate approach. An anterior location of the psoas relative to the vertebral body indicates a narrower corridor for retractor placement and interbody work, because the neural elements similarly lie more anteriorly. It is also important to appreciate the location of the vasculature (iliac vessels, vena cava, and aorta) and their relationship to a rotated lumbar spine.[23] Identification of the position of other retroperitoneal structures is important, including the descending colon on the left side and the kidneys.

CT can be used as a valuable adjunctive tool in evaluating bony anatomy and the three-dimensional anatomy of the spinal deformity, especially in more severe cases. The information gained can also be used to plan the proper diameter and length of the pedicle screws. In patients who have cardiac pacemakers or other MRI-incompatible metal implants, a CT myelogram is the study of choice to evaluate both bony and neural/soft tissue anatomy.

To further elucidate the pain generators, provocative testing such as facet and nerve root blocks can be of value to the deformity surgeon.

MINIMALLY INVASIVE FIXATION/FUSION TECHNIQUES
LIF

The LIF technique begins with preoperative evaluation of the lumbar spine on MRI and CT, when available. Special note is taken regarding the position of the psoas and the location of the great vessels, as well as their bifurcation. Contraindications for this approach include previous retroperitoneal dissection, unfavorable anatomy (including anterior position of the psoas on axial MRI at L4–5), the radiographic appearance of adherent vasculature, previous pyogenic kidney infection or retroperitoneal infection. The decision regarding the side of the approach is dependent on the curve type. Our preference is to approach the spine on the concavity; however, the convex approach may be technically less challenging because the spine rotates toward the convexity in some cases of scoliosis. When approaching the convex side, the release is performed directly over the apex of the curve, and it is possible to perform 3 to 4 levels of LIF through a single skin incision.

The patient is positioned in the lateral position after the appropriate neuromonitoring leads are placed. An axillary roll is used and the peroneal nerve is supported on the down side. The hips and knees are flexed as much as possible to place the psoas under as little tension as possible. The patient is then secured to the operating table with tape and a gentle flexion of the operating table is performed; however, care is taken not to overbreak the table to avoid excess tension on the psoas.

Positioning is confirmed with fluoroscopy in both the anteroposterior (AP) and lateral planes. Because the spine is scoliotic, only 1 vertebra can be perfectly fluoroscopically aligned and imaged at a time, and it is therefore recommended to start imaging the caudal vertebrae. The procedure cannot be initiated until the fluoroscopic views are orthogonal in the AP and lateral plane.

The approach to the spine is a retroperitoneal transpsoas approach. Access can be obtained through 1 or 2 skin incisions. The first incision is located directly over the disk space and the second a finger length posterior to the first and is used as a direct access point to the retroperitoneal space. Using the first incision, dissection is carried bluntly through the abdominal musculature until the fascia is reached. If a second incision is used, the initial dilator is then placed through the first incision and guided to the retroperitoneum via the second incision. The psoas is easily palpable as well as the transverse process, confirming the position in the retroperitoneum. Then, using biplanar fluoroscopy and directional electromyographic (EMG) testing on the initial dilator, the dilator is placed through the psoas onto the disk space and secured with a guidewire. Sequential dilation is performed followed by placement of the retractor, which is secured to the operating table. Then AP and lateral images are used to confirm position of the working corridor.

Next, an 8-step process for disk preparation is performed. First, a knife is used to make an annulotomy, a pituitary rongeur is used to remove the disk material, and next a Cobb elevator is used to dissect the cartilage off both end plates and to gently release the contralateral annulus. The pituitary rongeur is again used to remove excess disk; however, one should not devote too much time to this step to improve efficiency. A 16-mm-long box cutter is then used to further open up the disk space and remove excess disk. Care should be taken to avoid placement of the box cutter too anteriorly to avoid inadvertent removal of the anterior longitudinal ligament. Lateral fluoroscopy is used to ensure the location of the passage of the box cutter. Next, trials are used to pick the appropriate height and width of the interbody cages. The investigators prefer to use cages long enough to slightly overlie the lateral aspects of the vertebral bodies to avoid complications such as subsidence and to allow for the most load-sharing environment. While the cage is being prepared (filled with allograft or other fusion substance) on the back table, the endplates are prepared with stirrup curettes to ensure a good bleeding bony endplate surface exists for bony ingrowth. The implant is then placed into the disk space under fluoroscopic guidance.

Neuromonitoring, specifically directional EMG testing, is integral to the safety of this procedure. It is vital to have a clear neurologic path through the psoas muscle to access the spine using directional EMG to identify the nerves at risk at each level being worked on. During the remainder of the procedure, free running EMG allows identification of any abnormal activity. Long retractor times are not favorable because the static/rigid retraction of these peripheral nerves within the psoas muscle can result in paresthesias and neuropraxia.

Posterior Mini-Open TLIF and Mini-Open Pedicle Screw Fixation

The pelvic rim obstructs the lateral access to the L5/S1 disk space. Mini-open TLIF is an option to achieve a solid interbody fusion for this level.

Table 1
Summary of Prior MIS Deformity Surgery Publications

Reference	Patients/Procedures	Outcomes				Complications	Remarks
Acosta et al 2011[16]	36 patients with lumbar degenerative disease; LIF + posterior percutaneous screw	Fusion rate: N/A				N/A	No report fusion rates; Mean f/u: not reported
		Clinical	Pre	Post	P<.05		
		VAS	7.7	2.9			
		ODI	43	21			
		Coronal plane correction					
		Segmental Cobb	4.5°	1.5°	P<.0001		
		Regional lumbar Cobb	7.6°	3.6°	P<.0001		
		Sagittal plane correction					
		Segmental Cobb	5.3°	8.2°	P>.05		
		Regional lumbar lordosis	42.1°	46.2°	P = .7		
		Global sagittal alignment (mm)	41.5	42.4			
Anand et al 2010[9]	28 adult scoliosis patients/(LIF ± AxiaLIF) plus post percutaneous screw (LIF > 3 levels)	Fusion 1 y: 100%				23 complications:	Fusion is determined by static radiograph and CT in 21 patients; Mean f/u: 22 mo
		Surgical data				Transient dysarthria 17	
		EBL Anterior procedures: 241 mL				Quadriceps palsy 2	
		Posterior procedures: 231 mL				Retrocapsular renal hematoma 1	
		Operating room times Anterior 232 min				Cerebellar hemorrhage 1	
		Posterior 248 min				Screw prominence 1	
		Cobb angles Preoperative 22.3°			P<.05	Asymptomatic proximal screw fracture 1	
		Postoperative 7.47°			P<.05		
		Clinical	Preoperative	Postoperative			
		VAS	7.05	3.03			
		TIS	53.5	25.88			
		SF-36	55.73	61.50			
		ODI	39.13	7.00			

Dakwar et al 2010[11]	25 adult patients with degenerative deformity	Fusion rate: 100% for those with f/u >6 mo (n = 20) EBL: 53 mL/level OP time: 108 min/level			Rhabdomyolysis	1	Fusion is determined by CT and flexion/extension radiograph
	LIF only	2	Clinical	Preoperative	Postoperative	P: N/A	Subsidence	11	Mean f/u: 11 mo
	LIF + LP	15	VAS	8.1	2.4		Hardware failure	1	
	LIF + PSF	7					Thigh numbness (transient)	3	
	LIF + PSF + LP	1	ODI	53.6	29.9				
Isaacs et al 2010[13]	107 adult patients with degenerative deformity	Fusion rate: N/A EBL: <100 mL in 62.5% >300 mL in 8.4% OP times: 177.9 min per surgery (57.9 min per interbody fusion level) Patients with entirely minimally invasive procedures had significantly lower incidence of having any complication than patients with open posterior instrumentation (19.2% vs 37.9%) (P = .0450).					13 (12.1%) patients experienced 14 major complications Of 36 patients (33.6%) with some evidence of weakness after surgery, 29 had isolated proximal hip weakness (25 patients are transient weakness) 7 cases had weakness last longer than 6 mo or was decreased by 2 grades at any time point		Focused on complications within 6 wk postoperatively
	XLIF stand alone	20							
	XLIF + LF	6							
	XLIF with open PSF	29							
	XLIF with MIS PSF	52							
Kelleher et al 2010[7]	75 consecutive patients who underwent MIS decompression for focal lumbar spinal stenosis		ODI	Pre	Post	P<.05	The revision rate for patient with scoliosis (C + D) was significant (P = .0035) compared with those without (A + B) Six of the 8 revised patients had a preoperative lateral (rotatory) listhesis (3 in C and 3 in D)		Mean postoperative f/u: 31.8 mo
	(A) Stenosis with no deformity (n = 22)		A	48%	18.7%				
	(B) Stenosis with spondylolisthesis only (n = 25;		B	48%	24.6%				
	(C) Stenosis with scoliosis (n = 16;		C	50.7%	31.5%				
	(D) Stenosis combined with spondylolisthesis and scoliosis (n = 12)		D	53%	22%				
			Revision rates (overall: 10%) (A) 0%; (B) 4%; (C) 25%;(D) 25%;						

(continued on next page)

Table 1
(continued)

Reference	Patients/ Procedures	Outcomes			Complications	Remarks
			Preoperative	12 mo postoperative		
Scheufler et al 2010[14,15]	30 patients with degenerative lumbar kyphoscoliosis Mini-open TLIF and CT-guided PPS (179 segments were fused, among which 134 segment had a TLIF)	Fusion rates: 90% for instrumented segment by CT criteria				Mean f-u was 19.6 mo
		Clinical			P<.05	
		VAS	7.5	2.63	Major complication rates: 23.4% Minor complication rates: 59.9%	
		SF12V2PCS	20.2	34.6		
		ODI	57.2	24.8		
		Coronal plane correction				
		Cobb angles	42°	10.3°		
		Coronal balance (mm)	n/a	3.7		
		Sagittal plane correction				
		LL	8.8 ± 8.9°	−36 ± 6.9°		
		SVA (mm)	31.6 ± 15.2	8 ± 8.4		
Tormenti et al 2010[10]	8 patients XLIF + open PSF 4 patients TLIF/ PLIF + open PSF	Fusion rate: N/A				Mean f-u: ~11 mo
			Preoperative	Postoperative		
		XLIF + PSF			P<.001	
		Cobb angles	38.5°	10.0°	XLIF + PSF	
		AVT (cm)	3.6	1.8	Motor radiculopathy 2	
		Lumbar Lordosis	47.3°	40.4°	Thigh paresthesia 6	
		VAS	8.8	3.5	Cecal perforation 1	
		PLIF/TLIF + PSF			Pleural effusion 2	
		Cobb angles	19°	11°	Pulmonary embolism 1	
		AVT (cm)	2.2	1.1	Durotomy 1	
					PLIF/TLIF + PSF:	
					Clostridium difficile colitis 1	
		LL	30°	37.7°	Durotomy 1	
		VAS	9.5	4	Junctional kyphosis 1	

Study	Population / Technique	Results	Complications	Follow-up
Wang and Mummaneni 2010[12]	23 patients with thoracolumbar deformity Mini-open LIF + PPS	Fusion rate: 91.3% Mean 3.7 intersegmental levels/patient EBL: 477 mL OP times: 401 min Preoperative Postoperative Cobb angles 31.4° 10.3° LL 34.7° 47.5° VAS leg pain 4.35 1.57 VAS axial back pain 7.30 3.35	Postoperative thigh numbness 1 CSF leak 1 Large blood loss 1 Screw pull-out 1 Pneumothorax 1 New-onset atrial fibrillation 1	Mean f-u: 13.4 mo
Yamada et al 2011[8]	46 patients with DLFS were treated with microscopic lumbar foraminotomy Group 1: Cobb angle ≥10° n = 26 Group 2: Cobb angle <10° n = 20	Clinical Pre Post JOA 13.8 21.9 JOA score improvement ratio: Group 1 < group 2 P = .027 Preoperative Cobb angle and Cobb angle difference between supine and standing position are significantly higher in patients with recurrent leg pain than those without P = .007 Subgroup analysis of group 1: Cobb angle difference <3°: P = .006 No recurrence; 70% showed good or excellent results Cobb angle difference ≥3°: 50% patients had recurrence; 23% had good or excellent results	Recurrent leg pain: group 1 (30.8%) vs group 2 (5%) P = .029	Mean f-u: 21.9 mo

Abbreviations: AVT, apical vertebral translation; DLFS, degenerative lumbar foraminal stenosis; f-u, follow-up; JOA, Japanese Orthopaedic Association; LIF, Lateral Interbody Fusion; LL, Lumbar Lordosis; LP, lateral plate; N/A, not applicable; ODI, Oswestry Disability Index; PSF, pedicle screw fixation; SF-12V2 PCS, 12-Item Short Form Health Survey Version 2 physical component summary; SF-36, 36-Item Short Form Health Survey; SVA, sagittal vertical axis; TIS, Treatment intensity scale; TLIF, transforaminal lumbar interbody fusion; VAS, Visual Analogue Scale; XLIF, extreme lateral interbody fusion.

The patient is positioned prone on a Jackson table in reverse Trendelenburg position to help provide better visualization of the L5/S1 disk space.

For 1 or 2 level cases, the Wiltse plane incision location is identified by AP fluoroscopy to identify the lateral aspect of the pedicles and marked on the skin. For 3 or more levels, a midline skin incision and then a paramedian fascial incision are used. The fascial incisions are made at the outside margins of the pedicles (3–4 cm laterally to midline). After the skin and fasciae are incised, the Wiltse plane between multifidus and longissimus muscles is developed bluntly and serially enlarged with sequential dilators. The expandable tubular retractor is inserted. The optimal position and angle of the retractor are confirmed by lateral fluoroscopy.

The lateral facet complex, the transverse process, and pars interarticularis are identified and exposed with Bovie electrocautery and dissecting curettes. The pedicle screw entry point is located at the junction of midpoint of transverse process with the lateral aspect of the superior articulating facet in the mini-open technique. After decorticating the entry point with a high-speed drill, a gear shift is used to navigate through the cancellous bone of the pedicle into the vertebral body. A pedicle marker is placed into the hole. The marker provides an anatomic visual cue during the facetectomy and diskectomy. The same procedure is repeated for the remaining planned pedicle instrumentation levels. The pedicle screws are placed after completion of the diskectomy, end plate preparation, and insertion of the interbody cage.

Facetectomy and foraminotomy are performed with a drill and chisel to expose the disk space. The diskectomy and end plate preparation are performed efficiently with end plate shaver, pituitary rongeurs, and curettes. It is critical to remove the cartilaginous end plate without violating the bony end plate, to prevent cage subsidence. Next, an appropriately sized cage is selected based on interbody dilators used during serial dilation of the disk space. Autograft is packed into the disk space before cage insertion using a bone funnel. Next, the interbody cage is packed with autograft and implanted into the disk space.

Decompression of the neural elements is performed after cage insertion. The expandable retractor may need to be realigned medially onto the ipsilateral hemilamina to perform decompression. The contralateral decompression can be achieved by aligning the retractor even more medially to visualize and thin the contralateral lamina (so called ipsicontra decompression). The ligamentum flavum can be removed after all the drill work is finished to decrease the risk of dural tear.

The appropriate-sized pedicle screw is inserted into the formerly prepared bony entry points. EMG stimulation on the pedicle screw can help verify the integrity of the cortical bone around the pedicle. The bone graft is placed in between the transverse process before the rods are secured to the pedicle screw heads.[24,25]

Percutaneous Pedicle Screw Fixation

The pedicle screws may be inserted percutaneously on the contralateral side of the TLIF approach or to supplementally fixate a lateral interbody fusion. The true AP fluoroscopic view of each particular vertebral body intended for fixation is critical for accurate screw insertion. A true AP image can be identified by the single radiopaque shadow of the upper end plate, and the properly aligned image can be confirmed by the centrally located spinous process between the pedicles. With the true AP image, the trajectory to reach the pedicle can be achieved by placing a Jamshidi needle over the skin and adjusting the position to be in line with the centers of the bilateral pedicles of interest. Skin incisions are marked 1 cm lateral to the AP superimposed position of the pedicle to allow for a lateral to medial screw trajectory. After the skin and fasciae are incised, the tract to the transverse process can be developed using index finger blunt dissection. A Jamshidi needle is inserted and docked at the base of the transverse process, as mentioned earlier. An AP view is obtained, and the needle is adjusted to position its tip over the lateral border of the pedicle (3 o'clock for left pedicle/9 o'clock for right). After confirming the ideal entry point, the needle is tapped a few millimeters into the pedicle after making a 2-cm mark on the shaft. The shaft of the needle must be aligned parallel to the end plate on AP view. The Jamshidi needle is tapped gently under fluoroscopy to advance 2 cm in depth. The tip of the needle is now at the junction of the pedicle with the vertebral body. A true AP view is obtained to confirm that the tip of the needle is not medial to the medial shadow of the pedicle. The obturator is removed and a blunt-tipped guidewire is introduced through the needle into the cancellous bone. The Jamshidi needle shaft is removed with special attention to hold the guidewire in place. The pedicle is then tapped with a cannulated tap and the cannulated pedicle screw is inserted over the guidewire. Lateral fluoroscopy is taken to ensure proper trajectory for tapping and screw placement.[24,26] Care is taken to prevent K-wire migration through the ventral vertebral body during tapping and screw placement.

ALGORITHM FOR MINIMALLY INVASIVE APPROACHES TO TREATMENT OF ADULT DEGENERATIVE SPINAL DEFORMITY

The main goals for the treatment of adult degenerative spinal deformity are neural element decompression, establishing or maintaining sagittal and coronal global balance, and arthrodesis. Operative interventions require evaluation of the unique needs and goals of each patient. Several classification schemes as well as levels of treatment have been proposed for adult spinal deformity. In 2010, Silva and Lenke[6] published a treatment-level guide to adult degenerative deformity management. In this scheme, the patients who need treatment are classified into 6 treatment levels, based on clinical and radiographic findings. Of the 6 Lenke-Silva

treatment levels, treatment levels I to IV could be appropriately treated with current minimally invasive techniques based on published data (**Table 1**).[9,11,12] We have modified the Lenke-Silva paradigm to create an algorithm for the minimally invasive treatment of spinal deformity, which we have termed the MiSLAT (Mummaneni, M. Wang, Silva, Lenke, Amin, Tu) algorithm (**Fig. 1**).[24]

MiSLAT Treatment Level I

Patients with level 1 disease present with symptoms of neurogenic claudication or radiculopathy caused by central, lateral recess or foraminal stenosis. These patients (**Fig. 2**) have minimal back pain and symptoms with regard to their deformity. Radiographically and clinically, there is no sagittal

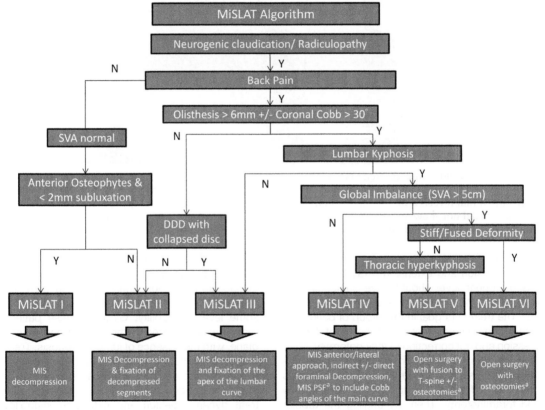

Fig. 1. MiSLAT algorithm for MIS treatment of adult degenerative deformity. MiSLAT I = decompression only; MiSLAT II = decompression and limited pedicle screw fixation of a portion of the coronal curve with posterolateral bone graft or TLIF; MiSLAT III = decompression and pedicle screw fixation of the apex of the lumbar curve with posterolateral bone graft or TLIF/extreme lateral interbody fusion (XLIF)/direct lateral interbody fusion (DLIF); MiSLAT IV = decompression and pedicle screw fixation of the lumbar spine with TLIF/XLIF/DLIF to include Cobb angles of the main curve[a]; MiSLAT V = decompression and pedicle screw fixation and fusion extending into thoracic region for thoracic hyperkyphosis ± osteotomies[a]; MiSLAT VI = correction of thoracolumbar scoliosis with 3-column or multiple-facet osteotomies and multisegmental pedicle fixation and fusion[a]. [a]Iliac screw insertion is suggested for constructs extending longer than L2 to S1. (*Adapted from* Mummaneni PV, Wang MY, Silva FE, et al. Minimally invasive evaluation and treatment for adult degenerative deformity–using the MiSLAT algorithm. In Scoliosis Research Society E-Textbook. Available at: http://etext.srs.org/book/. Accessed August 13, 2012; with permission.)

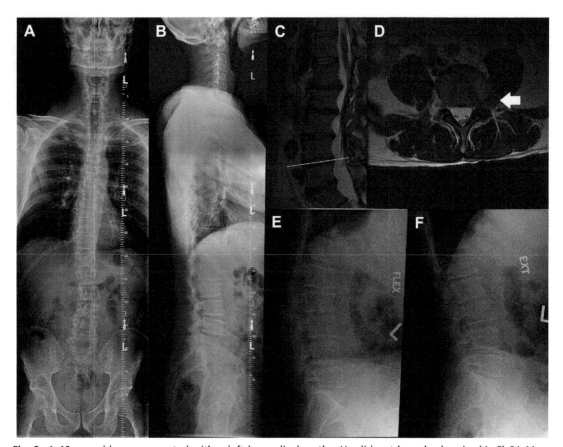

Fig. 2. A 46-year-old man presented with a left leg radiculopathy. He did not have back pain. (*A, B*) 91.44-cm (36-in) radiographs show mild thoracolumbar scoliosis and maintained sagittal balance. (*C, D*) Sagittal and axial T2-weighted MRI reveals a far lateral disk herniation (*arrow*) at the left L4/5 level. (*E, F*) Flexion and extension radiographs did not show any instability. This patient had a minimally invasive far lateral diskectomy without instrumentation (MiSLAT I treatment).

or coronal imbalance. There is no dynamic instability on flexion and extension X-rays. Patients in this treatment level should have subluxation of less than 2 mm, and the curve should be less than 30°. The treatment goal in this group of patients is central canal, lateral recess, and nerve root decompression and not correction of their deformity. Minimally invasive techniques are well suited to this type of decompression. Typically, a tubular retractor is used to perform an ipsilateral hemilaminotomy and foraminotomy. Then, by angling the tubular retractor medially, an undercutting contralateral decompression is also possible (ipsicontra decompression). This type of ipsicontra decompression may be performed at 1 or 2 contiguous levels through 1 small incision. The midline spinous processes and interspinous ligaments are spared.

MiSLAT Treatment Level II

Patients with level II disease (**Fig. 3**) complain of similar neurologic issues as those in level I;

however, they have a greater back pain component. Radiographically, there is more than 2 mm of subluxation, Cobb angles are less than 30°, and anterior osteophytes are present, indicating some level of stability. Globally, these patients remain well balanced in the sagittal and coronal plane, with the absence of lumbar kyphosis. Treatment involves decompression of the spine at one or two levels and concomitant focal instrumentation at the area of decompression is recommended to treat dynamic flexion and extension instability. We treat these patients with a minimally invasive decompression and limited instrumented fusion. It is important to understand the context of the limited fusion in light of the given deformity. Ideally, the fusion results in parallel end plates in the coronal plane and restoration of normal lordosis within the segment(s) fused. Fusion can be achieved through MIS or mini-open TLIF or LIF followed by percutaneous pedicle fixation and minimally invasive decompression with tubular retractors, as described earlier. The surgeon may

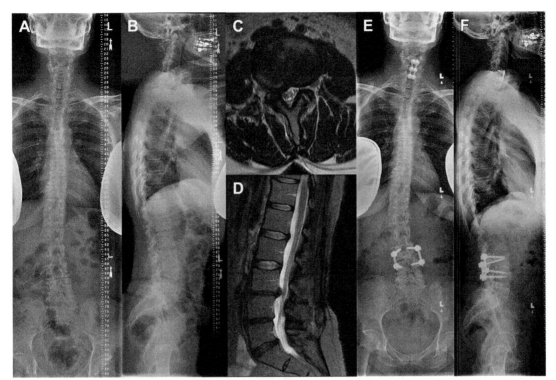

Fig. 3. A 52-year-old woman with radicular right leg pain and back pain. (*A, B*) 91.44-cm (36-in) preoperative radiographs showed a mild lumbar scoliosis (Cobb angle of 16°) and maintained sagittal balance (SVA = 2.0 cm). (*C, D*) T2-weighted axial and sagittal MRI shows a right herniated disk causing lateral recess stenosis at the L3 to 4 level. (*E, F*) Postoperative 91.44-cm (36-in) radiographs after a minimally invasive L3 to 4 TLIF (MiSLAT II treatment).

choose the TLIF or LIF depending on the patient's anatomy (ie, the position of the iliac crest precludes some L4–5 surgeries and L5–S1 cannot be accessed via LIF).

MiSLAT Treatment Level III

Patients with level III disease have a more dominant back pain component to their chief complaint in addition to their neurologic issues. Radiographically, they have more than 2 mm of subluxation/olisthesis, lack anterior bridging osteophytes, and present with Cobb angles greater than 30°. As with level II disease, decompression and fusion are necessary; however, these curve patterns and extent of the deformity usually require fusion beyond the levels involved for the decompression, and typically require fusion of the apex of the lumbar deformity. Minimally invasive techniques are well suited because they achieve the same goals as the open approaches. As with level I, decompression can be achieved at multiple levels through expandable tubular retractors, and, as with treatment level II, instrumentation can be performed via percutaneous or mini-open techniques, and interbody grafting achieved posteriorly via

tubular retractors or LIF. In addition, minimally invasive LIF may allow for indirect foraminal decompression by distracting the interbody space and recreating foraminal height.

MiSLAT Treatment Level IV

Patients with level IV disease have claudication-radicular pain, back pain, lumbar hypolordosis/kyphosis and lack anterior osteophytes. The goal of the operative intervention includes decompression, instrumentation, interbody fusion, and correction of the lumbar flat back. Radiographs of these patients show segmental instability and loss of LL, but no significant global imbalance (SVA <5 cm) (**Fig. 4**). As already delineated, decompression, instrumentation, and interbody graft placement and arthrodesis can all be achieved with minimally invasive techniques. Lordotic interbody grafts are placed from the lateral approach before posterior segmental mini-open or percutaneous pedicle screw instrumentation. The lordotic interbody cages not only serve in kyphoscoliosis correction and derotation but also place the pedicles at a more physiologic angle, making the landmarks for percutaneous pedicle

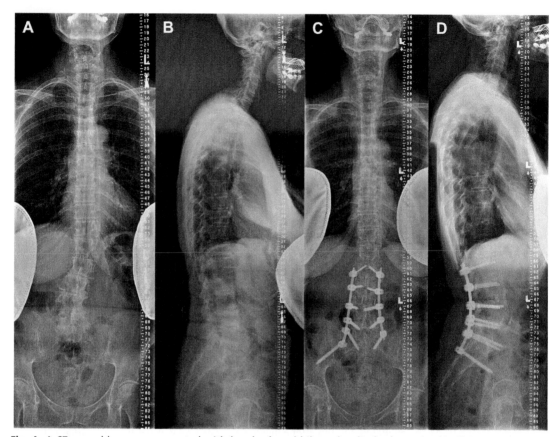

Fig. 4. A 67-year-old woman presented with low back and bilateral radicular leg pain. (*A, B*) Her preoperative 91.44-cm (36-in) radiographs revealed L2 to 3 lateral listhesis, an SVA of 4.3 cm, and a lumbar lordosis of 27°. (*C, D*) Postoperative 91.44-cm (36-in) radiographs after an L2 to L5 LIF and an L2 to the sacrum posterior MIS spinal fusion with a right iliac screw fixation (MiSLAT IV treatment).

screw fixation easier to identify. Particular attention is paid to restoring normal segmental lordosis in the lower levels of correction, particularly at L4 to L5 and L5to S1 (via TLIF or mini-anterior lumbar interbody fusion), because two-thirds of LL comes from these 2 segments. Also, it is important to match the LL to the patient's individual PI ± 10°.[21,27,28] MiSLAT IV treatment involves fixation of the entire spinal deformity, with special attention given to the lumbosacral fractional curve, because it needs to be included in the fusion construct. If the fusion extends to the sacrum, it may also be necessary to place iliac instrumentation long fusions (L2 or above to sacrum) to help achieve a solid fusion at the lumbosacral junction, to avoid sacral insufficiency fractures, and to protect the fixation at S1. Recent advances allow iliac screw fixation via percutaneous minimally invasive techniques.[29] Another option is to place S2-AI screws as described by Kebaish.[30] Alternatively, Anand and colleagues[31] have reported on their use of the presacral minimally invasive approach to provide additional support and avoid pelvic

fixation, although the long-term efficacy of this strategy has not yet been elucidated.

MiSLAT levels I to IV include deformity patterns that are amenable to current MIS techniques. Principles of proximal and distal fusion levels established for open surgery are also applicable to minimally invasive deformity surgery, with the exception of the choice of the upper-instrumented vertebrae. Because the soft tissue overlying the spine is preserved with minimally invasive approaches, typical cranial stopping points for multilevel lumbar instrumentation in MiSLAT IV treatments may vary from T10 to L2.

MiSLAT Treatment Levels V and VI

For patients with claudication-radicular symptoms, back pain, lumbar hypolordosis/kyphosis, and global sagittal imbalance (SVA >5 cm), standard open approaches are preferred, because current minimally invasive techniques often do not permit the achievement of the treatment goals (restoration of overall spinal balance). MiSLAT level V treatment (**Fig. 5**), which refers to open surgery with fusion extending to the T-spine with/without osteotomies, is suitable for these patients if they also show thoracic hyperkyphosis. MiSLAT VI treatment (**Fig. 6**), which involves open surgery with various osteotomies, is suitable for those patients with global sagittal imbalance and stiff, decompensated deformities (eg. iatrogenic flatback syndrome).

Patients with level V disease present with significant coronal and sagittal imbalance in addition to back and leg pain. The deformity remains flexible but extends to the upper thoracic spine and requires thoracic and lumbar realignment to achieve the desired postoperative outcomes. Patients with level VI disease have a fixed deformity such as iatrogenic flatback deformity with over 5 cm of sagittal imbalance, frequently requiring 3-column osteotomy for realignment. Level VI cases do not need fixation to the upper thoracic spine. Because these deformities are more extensive, standard open approaches are preferred, because current minimally invasive techniques do not predictably achieve the intended goals of the surgery. Osteotomies are covered in detail elsewhere in this issue.

Schwab and colleagues[32] recently updated the previous published Scoliosis Research Society (SRS)-Schwab classification to incorporate spinopelvic parameters, which are highly correlated with health-related quality-of-life scores. The classification comprises curve type, which is aimed at describing the relevant coronal aspects of the deformity; and 3 modifiers to characterize sagittal components of the deformity. The interrater and intrarater reliability and interrater agreement for the updated classification are excellent. When it comes to using minimally invasive procedures to treat patients classified with the SRS-Schwab classification, the patients with PI-LL modifier + or ++ (ie, PI-LL value is greater than 20°), or global alignment modifier + or ++ (ie, SVA >40 mm) are typically not suitable for a minimally invasive approach. These patients need more extensive releases or osteotomies to achieve spinopelvic balance.[33]

Recently, the use of a mini-open pedicle subtraction osteotomy (PSO) has been proposed.

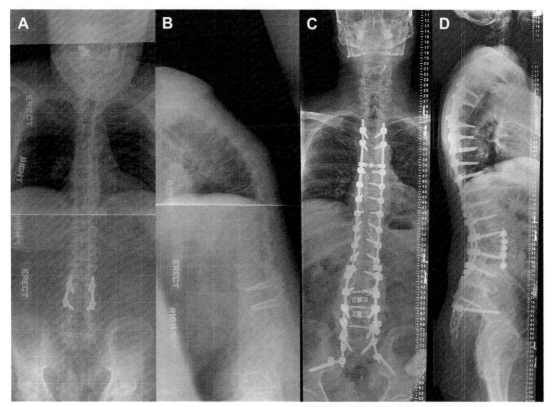

Fig. 5. A 50-year-old man presented with radicular right leg pain, low back pain, and inability to maintain erect posture. (*A, B*) 91.44-cm (36-in) radiographs show severe sagittal imbalance (SVA 21.2 cm) and thoracic hyperkyphosis. (*C, D*) Postoperative 91.44-cm (36-in) radiographs after L3 pedicle subtraction osteotomy, T6 to 8 Smith-Peterson Osteotomy (SPOs), T3-pelvis posterior fusion and staged L2 to 3, 3 to 4 anterior lumbar interbody fusions (MiSLAT V treatment).

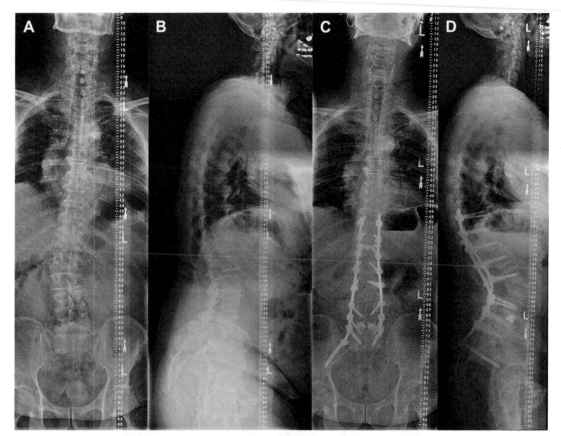

Fig. 6. A 64-year-old man presented with low back pain and inability to stand upright for long. (*A, B*) His 91.44-cm (36-in) radiographs showed significant sagittal imbalance (SVA = 8.5 cm). (*C, D*) Postoperative 91.44-cm (36-in) radiographs after an L3 pedicle subtraction osteotomy with T10 to S1 pedicle screw fixation and extension to right pelvic (MiSLAT VI treatment).

Initial laboratory investigations with cadavers showed the use of bilateral tubular retractors to perform the necessary bone removal.[34] However, in clinical application, the blood loss associated with PSO techniques, the possibility of neural compression during osteotomy closure, and the need for control of the spinal column during deformity correction have limited this MIS application. There is no long-term follow-up on the use of MIS techniques for PSO. We do not use MIS techniques for PSO. We prefer to perform open surgery to complete a PSO.

Rehabilitation and Recovery

Deep vein thrombosis (DVT) prophylaxis is an essential part of postoperative management in patients who have undergone spinal surgery. Sequential compression devices and stockings should be used throughout the postoperative period. Perioperative anticoagulation with low-molecular-weight heparin is mandatory in patients with high risk of thrombosis (excluding those with history of DVT, with acute DVT, having older mechanical valve, or with hypercoagulable status) in addition to the compression stockings. Early mobilization should be encouraged if it is not contraindicated. Rehabilitation is beneficial for patients with focal motor weakness, impairment in motion coordination, and impaired sensory functions.

The length of hospital stay for minimally invasive spinal deformity surgery may be 3 to 5 days, depending on the extent of procedures. Patients can return to regular daily activity in 3 to 4 weeks and are allowed full participation in 3 to 6 months depending on their activities.

CLINICAL RESULTS IN THE LITERATURE

The clinical results of selected references are summarized in **Table 1**.

SUMMARY

Recent advances in minimally invasive access to the spine have empowered spine surgeons to apply these techniques to patients with spinal deformity. However, regardless of technique, it is imperative that the principles of deformity correction are adhered to. These principles include thorough decompression for neurologic symptoms, stabilization of the deformity with pedicle screws, arthrodesis via interbody techniques, and maintenance or correction of the sagittal and coronal global malalignment. We present an established algorithm (MiSLAT) for adult spinal deformity with minimally invasive applications. Our recommendation is to treat levels I to IV with minimally invasive techniques; however, we believe that level V and VI deformities require more traditional open approaches to reliably correct the deformity.

REFERENCES

1. Glassman SD, Bridwell K, Dimar JR, et al. The impact of positive sagittal balance in adult spinal deformity. Spine 2005;30:2024–9.
2. Yadla S, Maltenfort MG, Ratliff JK, et al. Adult scoliosis surgery outcomes: a systematic review. Neurosurgical focus 2010;28(3):E3.
3. Acosta FL, McClendon J, O'Shaughnessy BA, et al. Morbidity and mortality after spinal deformity surgery in patients 75 years and older: complications and predictive factors. Journal of neurosurgery. Spine 2011;15(6):667–74.
4. Mummaneni P, Smith J, Shaffrey C, et al. Risk factors for major perioperative complications in adult spinal deformity surgery. 79th AANS Annual Scientific Meeting. Denver, April 9-13, 2011.
5. Schwab FJ, Hawkinson N, Lafage V, et al. Risk factors for major peri-operative complications in adult spinal deformity surgery: a multi-center review of 953 consecutive patients. Eur Spine J 2012;21: 2603–10.
6. Silva FE, Lenke LG. Adult degenerative scoliosis: evaluation and management. Neurosurg Focus 2010;28:E1.
7. Kelleher MO, Timlin M, Persaud O, et al. Success and failure of minimally invasive decompression for focal lumbar spinal stenosis in patients with and without deformity. Spine 2010;35:E981–7.
8. Yamada K, Matsuda H, Nabeta M, et al. Clinical outcomes of microscopic decompression for degenerative lumbar foraminal stenosis: a comparison between patients with and without degenerative lumbar scoliosis. Eur Spine J 2011;20:947–53.
9. Anand N, Rosemann R, Khalsa B, et al. Mid-term to long-term clinical and functional outcomes of minimally invasive correction and fusion for adults with scoliosis. Neurosurg Focus 2010;28:E6.
10. Tormenti MJ, Maserati MB, Bonfield CM, et al. Complications and radiographic correction in adult scoliosis following combined transpsoas extreme lateral interbody fusion and posterior pedicle screw instrumentation. Neurosurg Focus 2010;28:E7.
11. Dakwar E, Cardona RF, Smith DA, et al. Early outcomes and safety of the minimally invasive, lateral retroperitoneal transpsoas approach for adult degenerative scoliosis. Neurosurg Focus 2010;28:E8.
12. Wang MY, Mummaneni PV. Minimally invasive surgery for thoracolumbar spinal deformity: initial clinical experience with clinical and radiographic outcomes. Neurosurg Focus 2010;28:E9.
13. Isaacs RE, Hyde J, Goodrich JA, et al. A prospective, nonrandomized, multicenter evaluation of extreme lateral interbody fusion for the treatment of adult degenerative scoliosis: perioperative outcomes and complications. Spine 2010;35:S322–30.
14. Scheufler KM, Cyron D, Dohmen H, et al. Less invasive surgical correction of adult degenerative scoliosis. Part II: Complications and clinical outcome. Neurosurgery 2010;67:1609–21 [discussion: 1621].
15. Scheufler KM, Cyron D, Dohmen H, et al. Less invasive surgical correction of adult degenerative scoliosis, part I: technique and radiographic results. Neurosurgery 2010;67:696–710.
16. Acosta FL, Liu J, Slimack N, et al. Changes in coronal and sagittal plane alignment following minimally invasive direct lateral interbody fusion for the treatment of degenerative lumbar disease in adults: a radiographic study. J Neurosurg Spine 2011;15: 92–6.
17. Mundis GM, Akbarnia BA, Phillips FM. Adult deformity correction through minimally invasive lateral approach techniques. Spine 2010;35:S312–21.
18. Berjano P, Lamartina C. Far lateral approaches (XLIF) in adult scoliosis. Eur Spine J 2012. http://dx.doi.org/10.1007/s00586-012-2426-5.
19. Bess S, Boachie-Adjei O, Burton D, et al. Pain and disability determine treatment modality for older patients with adult scoliosis, while deformity guides treatment for younger patients. Spine 2009;34: 2186–90.
20. Glassman SD, Hamill CL, Bridwell KH, et al. The impact of perioperative complications on clinical outcome in adult deformity surgery. Spine 2007;32: 2764–70.
21. Lafage V, Schwab F, Patel A, et al. Pelvic tilt and truncal inclination: two key radiographic parameters in the setting of adults with spinal deformity. Spine 2009;34:E599–606.
22. Schwab FJ, Smith VA, Biserni M, et al. Adult scoliosis: a quantitative radiographic and clinical analysis. Spine 2002;27:387–92.
23. Deukmedjian AR, Le TV, Dakwar E, et al. Movement of abdominal structures on magnetic resonance imaging during positioning changes related to lateral lumbar spine surgery: a morphometric

study: Clinical article. Journal of neurosurgery. Spine 2012;16(6):615–23.

24. Mummaneni PV, Wang MY, Silva FE, et al. Minimally invasive evaluation and treatment for adult degenerative deformity–using the MiSLAT algorithm. SRS E-Text: Scoliosis Research Society; 2012.

25. Taub JS, Dhall SS, Mummaneni PV. Mini-open technique for pedicle cannulation, TLIF, and decompression. In: Wang MY, Anderson DG, Ludwig SC, et al, editors. Handbook of minimally invasive and percutaneous spine surgery. St Louis (MO): Quality Medical Publishing; 2011. p. 45–60.

26. Neubauer PR, Dibra FF, Anderson DG. Pedicle cannulation with true anteroposterior fluoroscopic imaging. In: Wang MY, Anderson DG, Ludwig SC, et al, editors. Handbook of minimally invasive and percutaneous spine surgery. St Louis (MO): Quality Medical Publishing; 2011. p. 21–35.

27. Lafage V, Ames C, Schwab F, et al. Changes in thoracic kyphosis negatively impact sagittal alignment after lumbar pedicle subtraction osteotomy: a comprehensive radiographic analysis. Spine 2012;37:E180–7.

28. Schwab F, Patel A, Ungar B, et al. Adult spinal deformity-postoperative standing imbalance: how much can you tolerate? An overview of key parameters in assessing alignment and planning corrective surgery. Spine 2010;35:2224–31.

29. Wang MY, Ludwig SC, Anderson DG, et al. Percutaneous iliac screw placement: description of a new minimally invasive technique. Neurosurg Focus 2008;25:E17.

30. O'Brien JR, Yu WD, Bhatnagar R, et al. An anatomic study of the S2 iliac technique for lumbopelvic screw placement. Spine 2009;34:E439–42.

31. Anand N, Baron EM. Minimally invasive approaches for the correction of adult spinal deformity. European spine journal: official publication of the European Spine Society, the European Spinal Deformity Society, and the European Section of the Cervical Spine Research Society. 2012.

32. Schwab F, Ungar B, Blondel B, et al. Scoliosis Research Society-Schwab adult spinal deformity classification: a validation study. Spine 2012;37(12):1077–82.

33. Mummaneni PV, Dhall SS, Ondra SL, et al. Pedicle subtraction osteotomy. Neurosurgery 2008;63:171–6.

34. Voyadzis JM, Gala VC, O'Toole JE, et al. Minimally invasive posterior osteotomies. Neurosurgery 2008;63:204–10.

Assessment and Treatment of Cervical Deformity

Justin K. Scheer, BS[a], Christopher P. Ames, MD[b],
Vedat Deviren, MD[c],*

KEYWORDS

- Cervical deformity • Cervical spine osteotomy • Cervical alignment • Pedicle subtraction osteotomy

KEY POINTS

- The significant mass of the head is supported by the cervical spine, and significant deviation from normal alignment increases cantilever loads and muscular activity. In addition, the flexible, mobile cervical segment is connected to the relatively fixed thoracic spine.
- The T1 inclination will determine the amount of subaxial lordosis required to maintain the center of gravity of the head in a balanced position and will vary depending on global spinal alignment as measured by the sagittal vertical axis (SVA) and by inherent upper thoracic kyphosis.
- The radiographic parameters that effect health-related quality of life scores are not well defined in comparison with global/pelvic parameters in thoracolumbar deformity. Chin-brow vertical angle, cervical SVA (C2 SVA), and regional cervical lordosis should all be considered in preoperative planning strategies involving standing 3-ft radiographs in which the external auditory canal (approximation of head center of mass) to femoral heads are visible.
- At the craniocervical junction, an anterior approach with initial anterior linear osteotomy, posterior release and reduction of facet-joint subluxation, and segmental stabilization may be used. A SmithPetersen osteotomy, a pedicle subtraction osteotomy, or a circumferential osteotomy may be used at the mid cervical to cervicothoracic junction to achieve the desired correction.
- Intraoperative imaging guidance systems and intraoperative neuromonitoring can help prevent complications related to the osteotomy. Furthermore, all-posterior approaches may reduce, but do not eliminate, swallowing dysfunction.
- 360 and 540 techniques are best for restoring mid subaxial lordosis while C7 pedicle subtraction osteotomy is best for correction of cervical sagittal imbalance.

INTRODUCTION

The cervical spine is complex, supports the mass of the head, and also allows the widest range of motion relative to the rest of the spine.[1-5] Because of this complexity, the cervical region is susceptible to a variety of disorders and complications, which may lead to malalignment causing significant deformity that may warrant surgical consideration. Abnormalities of the cervical spine can be very debilitating and can induce adverse effects on the overall functioning and health-related quality of life (HRQoL) of the patient.

Indications for surgery to correct cervical malalignment are not well defined and there is no set

Disclosures: None.
[a] University of California, San Diego School of Medicine, 9500 Gilman Drive, La Jolla, CA 92093, USA;
[b] Department of Neurosurgery, University of California, San Francisco, Medical Center, 400 Parnassus Avenue, A850, San Francisco, CA 94143, USA; [c] Department of Orthopaedic Surgery, University of California, San Francisco, Medical Center, 400 Parnassus Avenue, San Francisco, CA 94143, USA
* Corresponding author.
E-mail address: devirenv@orthosurg.ucsf.edu

standard to address the amount of correction to be achieved. Furthermore, classifications of cervical deformity have yet to be fully established, and treatment options defined and clarified. Therefore, this article focuses on normal cervical parameters, deformity evaluation and examination, and treatment options for the proper management of cervical deformity.

NORMAL CERVICAL ALIGNMENT

The cervical spine is primarily responsible for the location of the head over the body as well as the level of horizontal gaze. The center of mass of the head in the sagittal plane directly overlies the occipital condyle approximately 1 cm above and anterior to the external auditory canal (**Fig. 1**),[6] and any deviations from the normal alignment of the mass of the head result in an increase in cantilever loads, which subsequently induces an increase in muscular energy expenditure. The weight of the head is borne through the condyle to the lateral masses of C1 and then to the C1-C2 joint. This load is then divided via the C2 articular pillars into the anterior column and C2-C3 disc, and posterior column and C2-C3 facet.[7] The load distribution of the cervical spine is primarily in the posterior columns, with 36% in the anterior column and 64% in the 2 posterior columns,[7] in contrast to the lumbar spine where the anterior loads (67%–82%) have been reported as higher than the posterior loads (18%–33%).[8,9] The natural curvature of the cervical spine maintains a lordotic shape[10] as a result of the wedge-shaped cervical vertebrae and the need to compensate for the kyphotic curvature of the thoracic spine.[10] This thoracic kyphosis permits expanded lung volumes in the normal range and has been shown to increase with age. The caudal end of the lordotic cervical spine joins the rigid kyphotic thoracic inlet at the cervicothoracic junction (CTJ). Deviations from this curvature, such as a loss of lordosis or the development of cervical kyphosis, are associated with pain and disability.[1,10–13]

Because the cervical spine is the most mobile part of the spinal column, a wide range of normal alignment has been described (**Table 1**).[1,12,14,15]

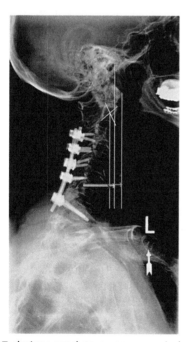

Fig. 1. Technique used to measure cervical sagittal vertical axis (SVA). The green arrow represents C1-C7 SVA (distance between plumb line dropped from anterior tubercle of C1 and posterior superior corner of C7), the red arrow represents C2-C7 SVA (distance between plumb line dropped from centroid of C2 and posterior superior corner of C7), and the yellow arrow represents center of gravity–C7 SVA (distance between plumb line dropped from anterior margin of external auditory canal and posterior superior corner of C7).

Table 1
Normal cervical spinal values in asymptomatic adults from the literature

Segmental Cervical Angles[1]	
Level	Angle (°)
C0-C1	2.1 ± 5.0
C1-C2	−32.2 ± 7.0
C2-C3	−1.9 ± 5.2
C3-C4	−1.5 ± 5.0
C4-C5	−0.6 ± 4.4
C5-C6	−1.1 ± 5.1
C6-C7	−4.5 ± 4.3
C2-C7	−9.6
Total (C1-C7)	−41.8

Cervical Sagittal Vertical Axis[1]	
Odontoid marker at C7	15.6 ± 11.2 mm
Odontoid marker at sacrum	13.2 ± 29.5 mm

C2-C7 Lordosis[14]		
Age Group (y)	Men (°)	Women (°)
20–25	16 ± 16	15 ± 10
30–35	21 ± 14	16 ± 16
40–45	27 ± 14	23 ± 17
50–55	22 ± 15	25 ± 11
60–65	22 ± 13	25 ± 16

Values are presented as the mean ± standard deviation, and the negative sign indicates lordosis in the segmental values.

In asymptomatic normal volunteers, a large percentage of cervical standing lordosis (approximately 75%–80%) is localized to C1-C2[1,16] and relatively little lordosis exists on the lower cervical levels. Similarly the majority of lumbar lordosis is at the caudal end, with L5-S1 having the largest segmental lordotic angle.[17] That the majority of cervical lordosis is localized to C1-C2 may be explained by the finding of Beier and colleagues[6] that the center of gravity of the head sits almost directly above the centers of the C1 and C2 vertebral bodies. The mean total cervical lordosis is approximately −40°, with, on average, the occiput-C1 segment being kyphotic.[1] Only 6° (15%) of lordosis occurs at the lowest 3 cervical levels (C4-C7).[1] The loss of subaxial lordosis has been reported in occipital-C2 fusions whereby excessive hyperlordosis is created at occipital-C2.[18,19] This type of unfavorable reciprocal change is also seen in lumbar and thoracic osteotomy, and has been reported by Lafage and colleagues.[20] Furthermore, in total cervical lordosis there is no difference between asymptomatic men and women, and there is a positive correlation with cervical lordosis and increasing age.[1,14] The average odontoid-C7 plumb-line distance ranges from 15 to 17 ± 11.2 mm.[1] Normal chin-brow vertical angle (CBVA) (**Fig. 2**) has not been characterized, but postoperative values of +10° to −10° have been well tolerated in patients.[21–26]

Cervical lordosis may be dependent on the anatomy of the CTJ, which typically involves the C7 and T1 vertebrae, the C1-C7 disc, and the associated ligaments. This definition may extend to T2 and T3 in terms of osteotomy planning.[27] The CTJ also includes the thoracic inlet, a fixed bony circle that is composed of the T1 vertebral body, the first ribs on both sides, and the upper part of the sternum. Biomechanically, the CTJ is a region where highly mobile cervical spine, which supports the head (average weight 4.5 kg),[28] transitions into the fairly rigid thoracic spine whose mobility is significantly reduced by the rib cage. Furthermore, the CTJ is the site at which the lordosis of the cervical spine changes to kyphosis in the thoracic spine. This change in curvature causes a significant amount of stress at the CTJ, in both the static and dynamic states.[27,29]

The sagittal alignment of the cranium and cervical spine may be influenced by the shape and orientation of the thoracic inlet to maintain a balanced, upright posture and horizontal gaze, similar to the relationship between the pelvic incidence and lumbar lordosis.[30] Lee and colleagues[30] found significant correlations between the thoracic inlet angle and both the cranial offset and craniocervical alignment. The relative contributions of

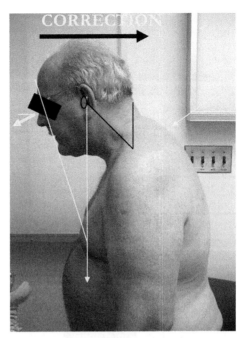

Fig. 2. Chin-brow vertical angle (CBVA) measurement method portrayed on a clinical photograph of a patient standing with hips and knees extended while his neck is in a neutral or flexed position. CBVA is defined as the angle subtended between a line drawn from the patient's chin to brow and a vertical line. Surgical correction of CBVA requires extension of the cervical spine.

the C0-C2 angle and the C2-C7 angle to the overall cervical lordosis have been reported to be 77% and 23%, respectively, in asymptomatic individuals.[30] The relative contributions of cervical tilting and cranial tilting to the overall angle of the occipital-cervical region have been reported to be 70% and 30%, respectively, in asymptomatic individuals.[30]

In the study by Lee and colleagues,[30] neck tilting was maintained around 45° to minimize energy expenditure of the neck muscles. These results indicate that a small thoracic inlet angle creates a small T1 slope and small cervical lordosis angle to maintain the physiologic neck tilting, and vice versa. According to the study, the thoracic inlet angle and T1 slope may be used as parameters to evaluate sagittal balance, predict physiologic alignment, and guide deformity correction of the cervical spine.[30] The T1 inclination will determine the amount of subaxial lordosis required to maintain the center of gravity of the head in a balanced position, and will vary depending on global spinal alignment as measured by SVA and by inherent upper thoracic kyphosis. In patients with scoliosis, the T1 sagittal angle (tilt, **Fig. 3**) has been shown

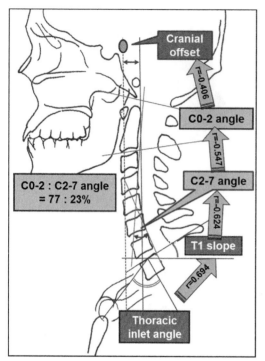

Fig. 3. Sequential linkage of significant correlation from the thoracic inlet angle to the cranial offset and craniocervical alignment. The *r* values within the arrows between each segment illustrate the Pearson correlation coefficient between the two segments. The sequential correlations between adjacent segments link the correlation between the thoracic inlet angle and the cranial offset. (*From* Lee SH, Kim KT, Seo EM, et al. The influence of thoracic inlet alignment on the craniocervical sagittal balance in asymptomatic adults. J Spinal Disord Tech 2012;25:E41–7; with permission.)

to correlate directly with SVA measured from the C2 dens plumb line to provide a measure of overall sagittal alignment (see **Fig. 3**; **Fig. 4**).[31]

ASSESSMENT OF CERVICAL DEFORMITY

Deformities of the cervical spine present many challenges to the surgeon, one of which is determining the ideal treatment option. The most common type of cervical spine deformity occurs in the sagittal plane (**Fig. 5**), malalignment in the coronal plane being much less common.[32–34] Furthermore, the most common type of cervical kyphotic deformity occurs as iatrogenic, specifically after multilevel laminectomy, with an incidence of 20%.[34–36] The primary goal of the various treatment options is restore cervical sagittal alignment, thus to improve horizontal gaze, reduce neck pain and, if the deformity is

severe enough, improve swallowing and respiration.[2,32]

The primary goal during the preoperative assessment of a patient with a cervical kyphotic deformity is to determine the ideal amount of correction and where along the spine the correction needs to be applied. At present, there exist no clear indications for the correct amount of cervical lordosis to be obtained postoperatively; however, a general rule of completely correcting the cervical kyphosis to neutral has been accepted.[34] Current research is likely to define cervical sagittal parameters similar to C7 SVA but instead measured on standing 36-in (91.5-cm) films measured from C2 or head center of mass (see **Fig. 1**; **Fig. 6**). The initial evaluation of the patient includes a complete medical history and physical examination. Many of these patients are high-risk surgical patients, and pertinent history (ie, smoking, use of nonsteroidal anti-inflammatory drugs, and so forth) can be used to tailor treatment. The physical-examination component should include assessing the patient standing upright with hips and knees fully extended, and in the sitting and supine positions. Sitting position will remove the effect of lumbar and pelvic/hip deformity, and the supine position can be used to assess the rigidity of semirigid curves under the direct effect of gravity. CBVA is measured before surgery and after surgery using the CBVA method (see **Fig. 2**). This angle is measured between the chin-brow line and the vertical line with the patient standing with hips and knees extended and the neck in its neutral or fixed position. Based on this angle, the size of the wedge to be removed posteriorly can be determined. Despite lying flat, patients with fixed primary cervical deformity have persistent cervical flexion (**Fig. 7**), whereas patients with thoracic, lumbar, or hip deformities correct in the sitting or supine positions.

Following the physical examination, initial radiographic evaluation includes 36-in standing plain radiograph films and dynamic flexion/extension cervical plain radiograph films (**Fig. 8**). The 36-in standing film allows for global spinal assessment while the dynamic films aid in determining the presence of any atlantoaxial instability and the relative flexibility of the spine.

Further radiographic studies such as computed tomography (CT) and magnetic resonance imaging (MRI) are usually performed to assess osseous landmarks for instrumentation and spinal cord tethering or impingement. CT scans are used to determine the extent of facet fusion and osteophytic bridging at disc to assess the need for osteotomy anteriorly and posteriorly in fixed deformity.

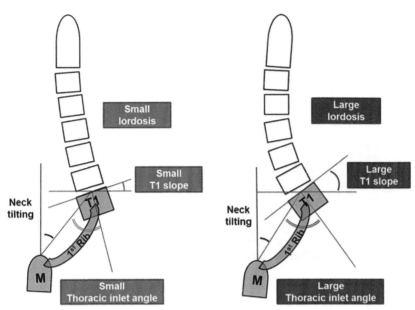

Fig. 4. Relationship between thoracic inlet angle, T1 slope, and cervical lordosis. A small thoracic inlet angle yields a low T1 slope, therefore less cervical lordosis is required to balance the head over the thoracic inlet and trunk. Conversely, a large thoracic inlet angle yields a greater T1 slope so that a greater magnitude of cervical lordosis is required to balance the head over the thoracic inlet and trunk. (*From* Lee SH, Kim KT, Seo EM, et al. The influence of thoracic inlet alignment on the craniocervical sagittal balance in asymptomatic adults. J Spinal Disord Tech 2012;25:E41–7; with permission.)

TREATMENT OF CERVICAL DEFORMITY
Conservative Management

The patient may attempt several conservative treatment options before considering surgical intervention. Conservative treatment of cervical deformity is primarily aimed at reducing symptoms, usually targeting pain. Some options include physical therapy, chiropractic care, cervical traction, brace therapy, steroid injections, and nonsteroidal anti-inflammatory agents. Surgical treatment may be indicated in patients with severe mechanical neck pain, neurologic compromise, and progressive deformity causing significant disability such as dysphagia or loss of horizontal gaze.

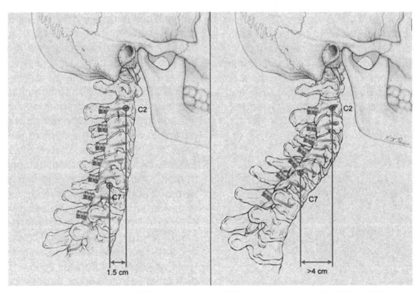

Fig. 5. (*Left*) Normal cervical lordosis, highlighting a small difference between the C2 and C7 plumb lines. (*Right*) cervical sagittal malalignment, highlighting a large difference in the C2 and C7 plumb lines.

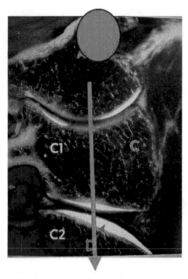
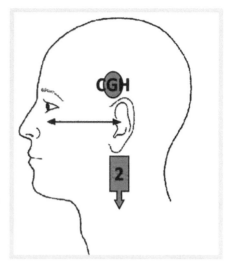

Fig. 6. (*Left*) Sagittal cut through a cadaver cervical spine, illustrating the center of gravity of the head (CGH; *blue oval*) being transmitted through C1 and C2 (*blue plumb line*). (*Right*) Location of the CGH in relation to the ear and C2 plumb line.

Patients who present with cervical camptocormia (head ptosis or neck drop) have a flexible deformity of the spine in the sagittal plane that is corrected on laying supine.[37] The various causes of camptocormia include amyotrophic lateral sclerosis (ALS), different myopathies, parkinsonism disorders, and idiopathic origins.[37] Thus, the initial workup a patient with camptocormia (or other flexible deformity) should include appropriate electromyography and nerve-conduction studies to rule out a primary myopathy or ALS. Furthermore, they should be referred to physical therapy before considering treating with surgical correction and fusion.

Cervical traction may be used to attempt deformity correction before surgical intervention. In general, 3 to 5 days of traction may be sufficient to reduce the deformity.[34] If the deformity is not reduced following 5 days of traction, further traction is unlikely to benefit the patient. In addition

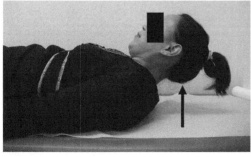

Fig. 7. The supine physical examination component, demonstrating a patient with fixed cervical kyphosis.

to the traction, muscle relaxants may also be used to aid in the reduction. If successful reduction of the cervical kyphosis does occur, posterior fixation and fusion may be used to prevent the deformity from progressing.

Surgical Management

Evaluation of the flexibility of the cervical spine may determine the surgical intervention needed. If the spine is flexible, an anterior-only or posterior-only correction strategy may be used. If the spine is rigid without ankylosed facets, an anterior-only strategy may be used. If the spine is rigid with ankylosed facets, a combination of anterior and posterior strategies may be used to correct the deformity.

The anterior-only strategy allows for correction of the deformity as well as instrumentation to maintain the correction, using both posture and biomechanics to obtain the cervical lordosis needed. The patient is placed in the supine position with the head slightly extended. After exposure, anterior release including disc and osteophytes is performed, and distraction pins are placed in the vertebral bodies to allow for segmental extension of the vertebral bodies and, thus, cervical lordosis. Anterior release is usually by means of a discectomy, as multiple lordosing discectomies are generally more effective than a single long corpectomy at creating lordosis. Following release and distraction, struts and/or lordotic cages or grafts may be placed to facilitate bone fusion. Lastly, a plate is contoured to the desired lordosis and

A   B   C

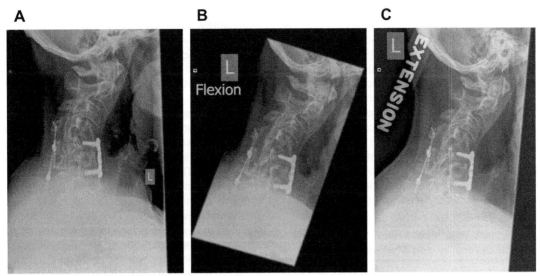

Fig. 8. (*A*) Preoperative lateral radiograph of a patient with fixed cervical kyphosis. Dynamic radiographs assess the extent of rigidity by (*B*) flexion and (*C*) extension.

fixated anteriorly to the cervical spine. Lordotic plates can be used to generate additional lordosis using a 3-point bending technique to "pull" the spine up to the plate once the plate is fixated at the ends. This technique relies on the spine being flexible after discectomy and anterior osteotomy.

When the cervical deformity is rigid with ankylosed facets, a combined anterior-posterior strategy may be used.[38] The side of correction is chosen first and the contralateral side is then released. In general, the posterior strategy is performed first with placement of screws and facetectomy and Smith-Peterson osteotomy. The patient is then turned to the supine position and disc release, anterior osteotomy, and lordotic plating are performed. The patient is then turned prone, and instrumentation and posterior compression applied. In certain cases with significant fixed subaxial kyphosis it may be advantageous to perform an anterior osteotomy first, including release of the vertebral arteries from the foramen transversarium followed by posterior osteotomy and correction using head manipulation after circumferential release. For this technique, the authors prefer the halo ring over the Mayfield clamp to allow a better grip on the head during manual reduction. Usually more lordosis is possible using an anterior release followed by posterior correction than with a posterior release followed by an anterior fixation, as generally it is possible to generate more lordosis from the posterior position.

If the cervical deformity is very kyphotic and rigid with ankylosed facets, an osteotomy or combination of osteotomies may be used to correct the

deformity. Traditionally the Smith-Petersen osteotomy has been used to correct cervical spinal deformities in the sagittal plane. This type of osteotomy may be used in cases where less than 30° of correction is needed.[39] The Smith-Petersen osteotomy does have a few significant limitations. First, there may be a need for multiple osteotomies at different levels to obtain the desired correction. Having multiple osteotomies increases the risk for pseudarthrosis. Second, there is a need for a flexible anterior column (or the creation of an anterior osteotomy) to obtain complete closure, which generally requires an anterior-posterior approach unless osteoclasis is possible, as in cases of ankylosing spondylitis. Simmons popularized the Smith-Petersen osteotomy (opening wedge) allowing for a posterior-only approach in patients with ankylosing spondylitis.[40,41] In patients with anterior bridging osteophytes and a calcified anterior longitudinal ligament, such as with ankylosing spondylitis, controlled anterior osteoclasis, creating an opening wedge in addition to the modified Smith-Petersen osteotomy, may be performed.[40,41] This technique is frequently used for chin-on-chest deformities in ankylosing spondylitis.[40,41]

If the patient has a rigid deformity and requires greater than 15° correction and correction of cervical sagittal imbalance, a cervical or cervicothoracic pedicle subtraction osteotomy (PSO) may be used.[21,42] PSO is becoming increasingly used and has the ability to correct large kyphotic deformities. PSO is a posterior-only approach allowing for all 3 spinal columns to make contact on closure of the osteotomy, thus increasing the likelihood of successful fusion as well as biomechanical stability.[21,43] PSO also can be used in nonankylosed patients in whom anterior osteoclasis is not likely to occur. Furthermore, PSO allows for a controlled closure. If neurologic injury is a concern, PSO may be an appropriate option. However, it is a technically demanding procedure.

Coronal cervical deformities may be isolated or in combination with sagittal deformities. Patients with fixed multiplanar deformities (**Figs. 9** and **10**) may require large 3-column osteotomies to correct the spine in both planes and decompress the cord and nerves. A 540° circumferential osteotomy or, possibly, a cervical vertebral column resection may be used.[44]

Cervical Deformity and Myelopathy

It is worth mentioning the relationship between cervical deformity and myelopathy and surgical considerations regarding treatment. Progressive cervical kyphosis has also been associated with myelopathy. The deformity leads to draping of the spinal cord against the vertebral bodies and anterior abnormality, increasing the longitudinal cord tension caused by the cord being tethered by the dentate ligaments and cervical nerve roots (**Fig. 11**).[35,45] As the curve becomes more pronounced over time, the spinal cord becomes compressed and flattened.[46] The anterior and posterior margins of the cord compress while the lateral margins expand. Tethering of the cord can produce increased intramedullary pressure.[47–49] This compression leads to neuronal loss and demyelination of the cord.[46] Furthermore, there

are significant adverse angiogenic effects of the mechanical compression. The small feeder blood vessels on the cord become flattened, leading to reduced blood supply. There is a large reduction in the number of vessels and the network size, as well as interruption and abnormal arrangement of the blood vessels.[46] As the kyphotic angle increases these changes become greater, especially on the anterior side that is exposed directly to the mechanical compression.[46] Greater cord tension increases intramedullary cord pressure,[47–50] and has been shown to lead to apoptosis in animal models.[46] Shimizu and colleagues[46] induced cervical kyphosis is small game fowls, and quantitatively analyzed the severity of demyelination and neuronal degeneration in histologic sections of the spinal cords. These investigators found a significant correlation between the degree of kyphosis and the amount of cord flattening. Moreover, demyelination of the anterior fasciculus as well as neuronal loss and atrophy of the anterior horn was observed, with the extent of demyelination progressing as the kyphosis became greater.[46] The pattern of demyelination began with the anterior fasciculus but then progressed to the lateral and posterior fasciculi. Further analysis with angiography demonstrated that the vascular supply to the anterior portion of the cords was decreased.[46] Thus, sagittal alignment of the cervical spine may play a substantial role in the development of cervical myelopathy.

The current literature is filled with controversy surrounding the best surgical approach to correct cervical spondylotic myelopathy.[51] Surgical considerations and options for cervical myelopathy

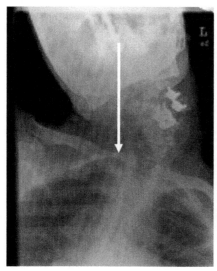
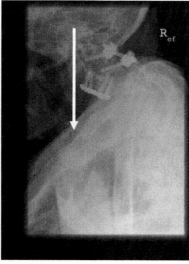

Fig. 9. (*Left*) Anterior-posterior radiograph showing coronal malalignment. (*Right*) Lateral radiograph showing sagittal malalignment.

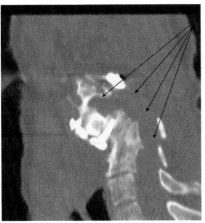
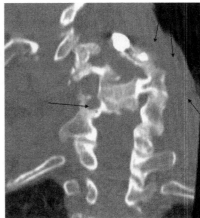

Fig. 10. (*Left*) Sagittal computed tomography (CT) image showing severe cervical sagittal malalignment (*arrows*). (*Right*) Anterior-posterior CT image showing severe coronal malalignment (*arrows*).

must take into account the sagittal alignment of the cervical spine, as it affects the approach to as well as the etiology and progression of myelopathy. Decompression alone, even ventral decompression, which does not decrease cord tension induced by kyphosis, may therefore not result in optimal outcomes.[46]

When correcting cervical myelopathy without sagittal malalignment, the surgeon should consider the possible future development of postlaminectomy kyphosis, which is the most common cause of cervical spine deformity.[35,45,52] As already mentioned, the natural biomechanics of the spine rely on a lordotic curve to distribute most of the load posteriorly. Thus, the posterior neural arch is

responsible for most of the load transmission down the cervical spine, and removal of it causes a significant loss of stability. Initially, performing extensive multilevel laminectomies may not immediately destabilize an intact spine. However, the added instability on losing the posterior arch-facet complex tends to cause a shift in load bearing from the posterior column to the anterior column. Over time, this shift places added stress on the cervical musculature, requiring constant contraction to maintain an upright head posture, which results in fatigue and pain. Cervical kyphosis occurs as the load is shifted anteriorly and, as the discs and vertebral bodies become wedged, it progresses to greater sagittal malalignment. This

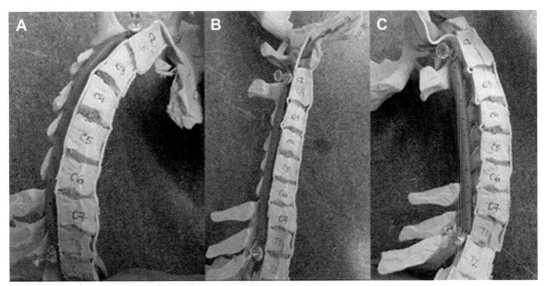

Fig. 11. Sagittal cervical spine model demonstrating spinal cord tension and length changes in response to sagittal alignment. The distance between marks (*black dots*) on the cord were measured and were 1.2 cm for kyphosis (*A*), 1.1 cm for the neutral position (*B*), and 1.0 cm for the cervical lordosis with C3-C5 laminectomy (*C*).

kyphosis can then lead to cervical myelopathy resulting from the curve of the spine as discussed earlier, thus creating worsened myelopathy from a surgical treatment that was intended to treat myelopathy. The kyphosis can then simultaneously contribute to the development of adult spinal deformity caused by the increased loads and pressure anteriorly, possibly adversely affecting the discs.

Furthermore, it is not always possible to correct cervical lordotic alignment in the subaxial spine above C7 through a posterior approach alone. An anterior approach with reconstruction using lordotic interbody spacers may be needed to restore the natural lordotic curve of the cervical spine. If the cervical spine is fused in the kyphotic position or posterior decompression alone is undertaken, this may lead to future myelopathy and/or adult spinal deformity attributable to the reasons discussed. Recent data have shown that patients who underwent 1- or 2-level corpectomies for cervical spondylotic myelopathy had positive long-term outcomes in terms of HRQoL and maintenance of their regional cervical lordosis.[53]

SURGICAL OSTEOTOMIES FOR CERVICAL DEFORMITY

Surgical intervention should be considered if the patient does not respond to a conservative treatment protocol or shows evidence of deteriorating myelopathy, radiculopathy, or functional impairment, such as inability to achieve horizontal gaze, swallowing dysfunction related to head position, tension/kyphosis-induced myelopathy, or neck pain due to head imbalance.[21,32,54–56] The spinal cord may be decompressed effectively by an anterior, posterior, or combined approach, but full decompression may require deformity correction as in cases of kyphosis. Supplemental posterior fixation minimizes the risk of anterior dislodgment of the graft even in the presence of solid anterior fixation.[57] Treatment of these complex cervical deformities is challenging and requires a clear understanding of the disease and the patient. Surgeons must be comfortable with remobilization of the spinal column anteriorly and posteriorly, vertebral artery anatomy, and methods of anterior and posterior correction.

Significant, irreducible deformity of the cervical spine may be sufficient to require corrective osteotomy. At the craniocervical junction, neurologic or functional impairment associated with the deformity may be best managed by osteotomy and fixation. Rigid deformities of the cervical spine below the craniocervical junction are more likely to require some kind of osteotomy to correct the deformity and restore horizontal gaze.

This section details the preoperative considerations and surgical procedures of 4 cervical osteotomies: (1) craniocervical junction osteotomy using sequential anterior-posterior approaches, (2) Smith-Petersen osteotomy, (3) CTJ PSO, and (4) cervical circumferential osteotomy.

Preoperative Considerations in Rigid Cervical Deformity

History
Patients may give a history of past trauma, sometimes associated with intercurrent illness of ankylosing spondylitis or rheumatoid arthritis as well as previous cervical spine surgery, degenerative disorders, and neoplastic disorders.

Signs and symptoms
Symptoms may include suboccipital headache and neck stiffness, occipital neuralgia, symptoms of myelopathy, or progressive deformity leading to functional impairment, such as difficulty with looking forward or with eating and drinking. Patients may complain of low back pain and standing fatigue caused by the use of compensatory muscles to elevate pelvic tilt in order to alter gaze angle.

Physical examination
It is critical to obtain 36-in radiographs and to examine patients while standing. Occasionally lumbar sagittal deformities will need to be corrected first. Correction of lumbar imbalance will alter head position substantially, especially in rigid deformities like ankylosing spondylitis. However, all corrective lumbar osteotomies will change the T1 slope angle to some extent, and therefore will change cervical alignment and often cervical C2 SVA. Signs of myelopathy may be evident in relation to past injury, compression, or cord tension due to stretch induced by kyphosis.

Imaging
The deformity should be evaluated by anterior/posterior and lateral cervical radiographs along with dynamic lateral flexion/extension views. The deformity is then accurately measured (ie, sagittal angle determination) and any other abnormalities noted (eg, subluxation and pseudarthrosis).[32,33,58] It is important to obtain full-length posteroanterior and lateral 36-in scoliosis radiographs to examine overall sagittal and coronal balance in these patients.[32,33,59] The authors assess cervical, thoracic, and lumbar sagittal alignment individually and lobally, and define the effect of regional imbalance on cervical balance and determine whether it is a primary, secondary, or compensatory cervical deformity. The degree of required correction

depends on the angle of the cervical deformity (the CBVA), the C2 plumb line, and the desired final lordosis.[21,25,33,40,60] The goal of treatment is to obtain balance, horizontal gaze, and cord decompression, and to normalize cord tension. Dynamic (ie, flexion/extension) radiographs permit an assessment of the overall flexibility of the cervical spine, which is paramount when designing a treatment strategy. CT scans of the cervical spine are also useful in determining the presence of fusion or ankylosis of the facet joints and discs, and allow assessment of fixation points such as C2 and upper thoracic pedicles.

All patients should be evaluated with preoperative MRI or CT myelography. These imaging modalities permit the evaluation of compressive abnormality. If significant ventral compressive abnormality (disc, osteophyte) is present, a ventral decompressive procedure may first be performed before the correction of the deformity.

Decision for planning of osteotomy

It is important when planning deformity surgery for cervical kyphosis to consider whether the deformity is rigid or fixed and whether there are neurologic symptoms. **Fig. 12** depicts the surgical-decision making process in cervical deformity osteotomy. In the craniocervical junction, osteotomy is indicated when the deformity is irreducible and sufficient to result in severe pain, and functional or neurologic impairment that cannot be relieved with a surgical decompression and/or stabilization procedure alone. In the

flexible subaxial deformity, a posterior stabilization (usually C2-T2) is advocated; when deformity is semirigid, Smith-Petersen osteotomy should be considered.

However, in the clinical setting of rigid cervical kyphosis (high to mid cervical kyphosis) with neurologic symptoms, the spinal cord is usually tethered over the subaxial kyphotic segment, leading to neurologic symptoms and myelopathy; therefore, segmental kyphosis correction (circumferential osteotomy) is mandatory to untether and decompress the spinal cord. In the setting of a rigid cervical kyphosis in mid to low cervical spine with cervical sagittal imbalance, a C7 or T1 PSO may be sufficient.

Craniocervical Junction Osteotomy

At the craniocervical junction it is unusual for an osteotomy to be required, and little has been published on the subject in the surgical literature.[61] However, cases exist, usually in the posttraumatic setting and in association with other conditions such as ankylosing spondylitis or end-stage rheumatoid arthritis with fixed atlantoaxial deformity, whereby the neurologic or functional impairment associated with the deformity may be best managed by osteotomy and fixation.

Indications and contraindications

Osteotomy is indicated when the deformity is irreducible (possibly following a trial of traction) and sufficient to result in severe pain and functional

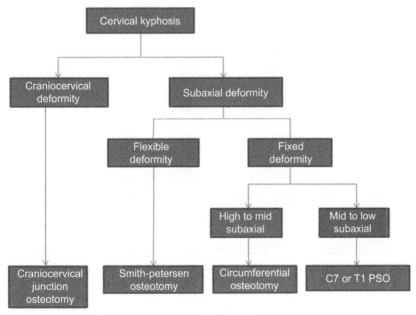

Fig. 12. The surgical decision-making process in cervical kyphosis.

or neurologic impairment that cannot be relieved with a surgical decompression and/or stabilization procedure alone. The procedure is contraindicated in the presence of significant osteoporosis or debilitating comorbidities.

Fig. 13 illustrates a case example of craniocervical junction osteotomy. Plain radiographs at the atlantoaxial level reveal substantial kyphotic deformity, possibly in the presence of an old odontoid fracture, with subluxation or dislocation of the C1/C2 joints (see **Fig. 13**). There may be bony union across the subluxed joints or involving other elements of the atlantoaxial complex.

Surgical technique

1. The ease of surgical access to the ventral aspect of C2 is an important consideration when choosing between an anterior/posterior or posterior-only approach. Grundy and Gill[61] have described a posterior-only approach in cases where the anticipated anterior access

may be difficult. Preoperative planning of the intended osteotomy orientation is also important when considering the type of anterior approach. An osteotomy, which is oriented obliquely backward and upward from the base of C2 (**Fig. 14A**), will enable satisfactory exposure through a high anterior retropharyngeal approach. This approach is described here.

2. The patient will usually require awake endoscopic intubation and is positioned supine for the first (anterior) stage of the surgery. It is preferable to use an operating table such as the Jackson table (Mizuho OSI, Union City, CA), which will enable rotation of the patient to the prone position for the second surgical stage, and to secure the head in a Mayfield 3-point head-holder. Access for adjustment of the head and neck position should be maintained throughout the procedure. Intraoperative image-guided surgical navigation, such as with an O-Arm/Stealth (Medtronic, Dallas, TX), Iso-C (Siemens, Erlangen, Germany), or

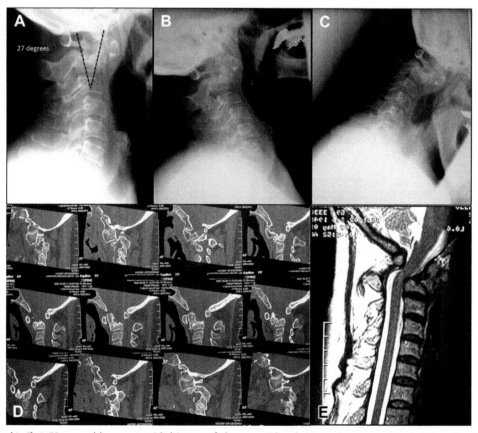

Fig. 13. (*A–E*) A 59 year-old woman with history of rheumatoid arthritis and severe suboccipital neck pain and early signs of myelopathy, 6 months following a motor vehicle accident resulting in type III odontoid fracture, managed conservatively in SOMI (sternal occipital mandibular immobilizer) brace. Plain radiographs, CT scans, and magnetic resonance imaging (MRI) show (*A–C*) development of fixed 27° kyphotic deformity, (*D*) bilateral facet joint dislocations, and (*E*) spinal cord compression.

A

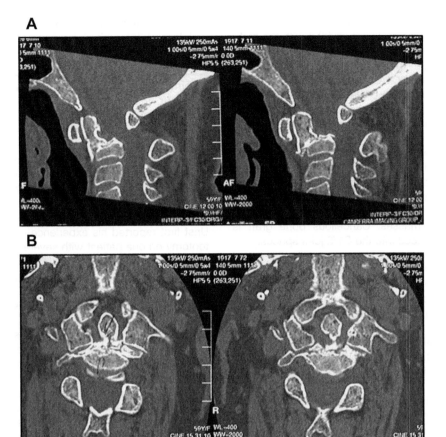

B

Fig. 14. CT scan of sagittal and coronal reconstructions showing (*A*) orientation of planned osteotomy and (*B*) bilateral extent of base of osteotomy.

similar system may facilitate surgeon orientation and placement of the osteotomy. Intraoperative neuromonitoring may be helpful during the deformity reduction.

3. A high, anterolateral skin incision is made for a retropharyngeal approach to the C2 vertebral body.

a. Retropharyngeal approach to the ventral aspect of C2 vertebral body with fluoroscopic confirmation of position.

b. Mobilization of longus coli muscles, bilaterally.

c. Identify the old fracture line (when present). Define the bilateral extents of the fracture line and endeavor to dissect upwards to define the lateral aspects of the odontoid process, bilaterally (**Fig. 14**B); this is important to completely mobilize the odontoid with the osteotomy and to avoid injury to the vertebral arteries.

d. Make the osteotomy through the old fracture line using a high-speed drill with a small cutting burr. Frequent position/orientation checks are made with fluoroscopic or image

guidance. The osteotomy is extended through to back of the odontoid and bilaterally. Take care not to venture too widely, to avoid injury to the vertebral arteries. If necessary, navigation may be used.

e. Depending on whether there is bony union of the posterior elements of the C1/C2 complex, an attempt may be made at this stage to open up the fracture line and correct the deformity using intervertebral spreaders.

f. The anterior wound is then closed over a suction drain before turning the patient to the prone position.

g. Through a midline suboccipital incision, a subperiosteal dissection of the posterior elements of C1-C3 is performed with identification of the C2 nerve roots.

h. While controlling any hemorrhage from the venous plexus around the C2 nerve roots, the superior articular surfaces of C2 are exposed and the posterior edges of the C1 lateral masses, adjacent to the inferior joint surfaces, are defined on each side. If there has been any bony union between the C1 and C2 joints, this is divided with the high-speed drill or osteotome (**Fig. 15**). Dissectors are then carefully inserted into the dislocated C1/C2 joints and used to gently lever back the C1 lateral masses onto C2, while the surgical assistant and anesthesiologist adjust the head position in the Mayfield head-holder.

i. It is helpful to remove the articular cartilage from the C2 joint surfaces before reducing the dislocation. Subsequently, the articular cartilage is removed with a small angled curette from the inferior surface of the C1 lateral masses. Cancellous bone graft is then placed into the C1/2 joint spaces.

j. Depending on surgeon preference and the vertebral artery anatomy, the C1/C2 segment is then stabilized using either transarticular screws (with additional posterior wiring) or a C1 lateral mass and C2 pars screw construct.[62–64]

k. Further bone graft is placed over the decorticated posterolateral elements before posterior wound closure, in layers, over a vacuum drain.

4. Depending on how the patient is tolerating the procedure and the time available, the patient may be repositioned supine immediately or later, as a delayed procedure, for placement of bone graft into the anterior osteotomy site. This site will have opened up into a wedge-shaped defect following the posterior deformity correction (**Fig. 16**A). Suitably fashioned allograft or iliac crest autograft is inserted into the wedge-shaped osteotomy site and secured with a small locking plate (**Fig. 16**B). Subsequent, standard postoperative care follows segmental atlantoaxial stabilization and fusion (**Fig. 17**).

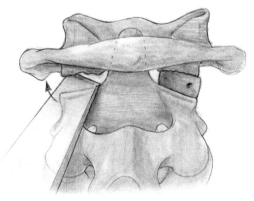

Fig. 15. An osteotome may be used to mobilize the C1-C2 joint space from the anterior or posterior approach in cases of fixed atlantoaxial deformity.

5. The patient is then returned, ventilated, to the intensive care unit.

Smith-Petersen Osteotomy

Semirigid deformity (eg, spondylitic joints and discs but no segmental bridging bone in a patient with good bone quality)

The Smith-Peterson extension osteotomy technique, described in 1945, has been used extensively and was previously considered the prototype procedure for reconstruction of sagittal imbalance in patients with deformity above the thoracolumbar junction.[65] Inspired by the lumbar osteotomy performed by Smith-Petersen, in 1958 Urist first reported his experience of cervical osteotomy on one patient with severe flexion deformity of ankylosing spondylitis.[66] It is important to distinguish between opening wedge osteotomy (the classic Smith-Peterson osteotomy used for ankylosing spondylitis patients at C7) and the procedure involving complete facet removal and posterior closure over a mobile disc space, which is more commonly used for semirigid cervical deformity and sometimes more appropriately called the cervical Ponte osteotomy.

If the deformity is partially correctable with traction or posture (ie, neck extension), a dorsal-only Smith-Petersen osteotomy/Ponte strategy may be used.[40,41,67] Traction may be used to reduce the deformity, and then may be continued in the operating room. Because this osteotomy uses some cantilever force on the pre-bent rod to achieve lordosis and segmental osteotomy closure, a stiffer cobalt-chrome rod is recommended in preference to a 3.5-mm titanium rod. Usually these cases involve fusion from C2-T2/T3 (see case example, **Figs. 18** and **19**).

Ankylosing spondylitis may produce an extreme fixed flexion deformity at the CTJ. This extreme deformity may place the chin in close proximity to the chest, which may interfere with eating and respiration. Some have advocated treating this deformity by Smith-Petersen osteotomy with anterior osteoclasis, with gentle extension of neck intraoperatively, resulting in the classic opening wedge.[40,41,60,67]

Ankylosing spondylitis (opening wedge osteotomy)

Indications and contraindications Severe flexion deformities of the cervical spine, whereby there is loss of horizontal gaze, difficulty with personal hygiene and function, and dysphagia, are corrected by traction or neck extension. Ankylosing spondylitis with fixed deformity is treated with Smith-Petersen osteotomy with anterior osteoclasis. Standing 36-in films are critical in

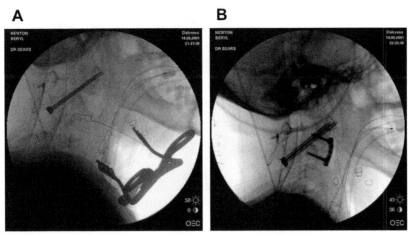

Fig. 16. Intraoperative fluoroscopic images showing (*A*) anterior wedge defect following posterior relocation of dislocated facet joints and transarticular screw fixation, and (*B*) following anterior bone grafting and plate fixation.

deterring whether lumbar or thoracic kyphosis also exists. If so, and global imbalance is present, the thoracolumbar deformity should be corrected first, as this by itself usually may restore horizontal gaze. If lumbar sagittal deformity is present and the cervical osteotomy is performed first, secondary lumbar correction may lead to an unacceptably high (gaze on the ceiling) issue and flexion osteotomy may then be needed.

Surgical technique The surgical technique for C7 Smith-Petersen osteotomy with anterior osteoclasis for fixed low cervical deformity in ankylosing spondylitis is as follows.

1. Classically the patient is positioned sitting. However, at their institution the authors position the patients prone in a halo ring. The kyphotic head position is accommodated by additional rolls and pads as needed to elevate the patient's thorax. Transcortical motor evoked potentials (MEP), somatosensory evoked potentials (SSEP), and electromyography (EMG) are used.

2. An incision is made posteriorly and the paraspinous muscles are dissected in a subperiosteal fashion, exposing the spinous processes, laminar facets, and lateral processes of C4-T2. If the bone is very soft, fixation is extended to bicortical C2 screws. Preoperative standing films will allow determination of the apex of the upper thoracic kyphosis, and the fixation is extended below this apex as needed.

3. After exposure, the osteotomy is performed. A complete C7 laminectomy and partial C6 and T1 laminectomies are performed. The resection is carried laterally to include the removal of the C7 pedicle with rongeurs. All resected bone is saved for reuse later to create the bone graft.

4. The residual portions of the C6 and T1 laminae need to be carefully beveled and undercut to avoid any impingement or kinking of the spinal

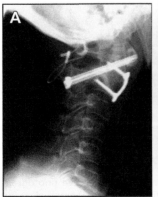
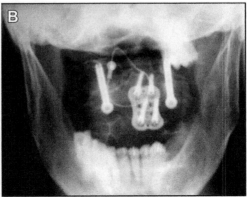

Fig. 17. Six-month postoperative lateral (*A*) and anterior-posterior (*B*) plain radiographs.

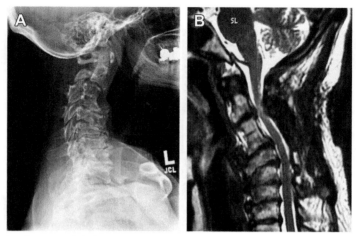

Fig. 18. Case example of semirigid deformity that was treated with Smith-Petersen osteotomy (SPO) and cobalt chromium rods. (*A*) Preoperative lateral radiograph showing cervical kyphosis. (*B*) Preoperative sagittal MRI showing spinal stenosis.

cord on closure of the osteotomy. Furthermore, the area near the C8 nerve root is curved to provide ample room for the nerve root on closure.

5. The surgeon grasps the halo and extends the neck gradually with closure of the osteotomy posteriorly as the osteoclasis across C7-T1 occurs anteriorly. An audible snap and sensation of the osteoclasis is usually heard (**Fig. 20**A). Also at this time, correction of rotation malalignment and lateral tilt is carried out.

6. The pre-bent rod is placed and locked down. The C8 foramen is inspected to make sure the nerve is free after complete closure. At the C7-T1 area, the posterior aspects of the spine may then be decorticated. The autologous

bone graft from the resection is packed bilaterally onto the decorticated areas.

Cervicothoracic Junction PSO (Dorsal Approach)

For patients with fixed cervicothoracic kyphosis, a 360° release and fusion or an osteotomy typically is used to correct the kyphosis.[21] Such cervical osteotomies are performed at C7 or T1 because of the absence of the vertebral artery at this level. Preoperative CT angiography is performed to rule out an aberrant vertebral artery position at C7.

Several investigators have reported successful results for a single-level dorsal decancellation osteotomy, also known as the "eggshell" procedure

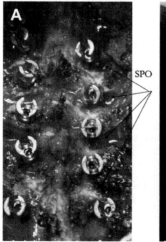
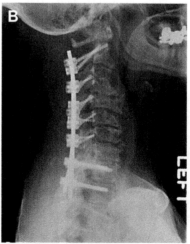

Fig. 19. Case example of semirigid deformity treated with SPO. (*A*) Intraoperative photograph showing the cervical kyphotic correction using multiple SPOs. (*B*) Postoperative lateral radiograph showing correction of the cervical kyphosis and use of a cobalt chromium rod.

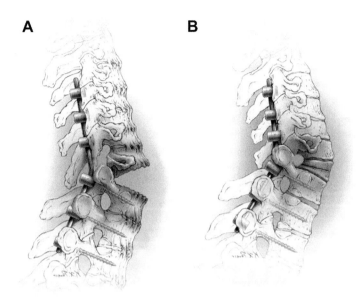

A   **B**

Fig. 20. Correction of kyphosis in Classic SPO. (*A*) Opening wedge for flexion deformity in ankylosing spondylitis. (*B*) Pedicle subtraction osteotomy (PSO). (*From* Scheer JK, Tang JA, Buckley JM, et al. Biomechanical analysis of osteotomy type and rod diameter for treatment of cervicothoracic kyphosis. Spine (Phila Pa 1976) 2011;36:E519–23; with permission.)

or PSO.[21,25,68,69] Once closed, there is bone contact in both columns and the spinal canal is effectively shortened (**Fig. 20**B). Thus the PSO procedure can provide excellent sagittal correction while simultaneously forming a stable construct and minimizing neural compression.

Indications
Indications are fixed sagittal malalignment of the cervical spine (mid to low subaxial cervical spine) affecting horizontal gaze, persistent pain related to cervical sagittal imbalance despite conservative treatment, high pelvic tilt causing low back pain driven by cervical deformity.

Surgical technique
The surgical technique for C7 PSO is as follows (**Fig. 21**).

1. The patient is positioned prone in a halo ring.
2. Transcortical MEP and SSEP as well as EMG neuromonitoring is used.
3. A standard posterior surgical approach is made to the cervical spine, creating an incision from C2 to T3/T5 depending on the location of the kyphotic apex.
4. A posterior incision is made from C2 to T3/T5, and is taken sharply through the skin and down to the fascia. The paraspinous muscles are dissected in a subperiosteal fashion, exposing

the spinous processes, laminar facets, and lateral processes of the cervical spine, and transverse processes in the thoracic spine.

5. After exposure, the spine is instrumented accordingly (C2 bicortical pedicle screws, cervical lateral mass screws, and thoracic pedicle screws). It is preferable to extend the fixation to C2 to obtain bicortical screw placement for a stronger fixation point than at the lateral masses of the inferior vertebrae. Furthermore, it is preferable to have the caudal extent of the fusion terminate at either T3 or T5 depending on the extent of thoracic kyphosis to ensure the apex is within the fusion. Depending on surgeon preference, various types of fusion rods may be used such as stainless steel and titanium; however, cobalt-chrome rods are preferred.
6. The osteotomy begins with release and removal of the facets of C6-C7 as well as C7-T1 (**Fig. 21**I).The nerve roots at C7 and C8 are then identified and followed out of the foramen while carrying out the osteotomy, completely isolating the C7 pedicle (**Fig. 22**).
7. After the bilateral facetectomies and isolation of the C7 pedicle, the C7 pedicle is skeletonized and removed with Lempert rongeurs. Sequential lumbar or custom wedge-shaped spinal taps are used to decancellate the C7

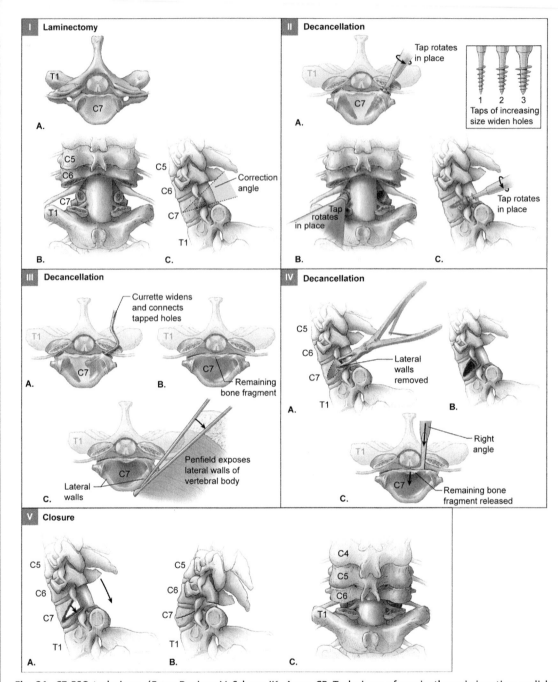

Fig. 21. C7 PSO technique. (*From* Deviren V, Scheer JK, Ames CP. Technique of cervicothoracic junction pedicle subtraction osteotomy for cervical sagittal imbalance: report of 11 cases. J Neurosurg Spine 2011;15:174–81; with permission.)

vertebral body (**Fig. 23**) combined with osteo-tomes and down-pushing curettes to attempt a 30° wedge (**Fig. 21**II and III).

8. The lateral wall of the C7 vertebral body is then dissected out with a Penfield 1 retractor and visualized (**Fig. 21**III, **Fig. 24**). The C7 lateral wall is removed with needle-nose rongeurs and osteotomes via the pedicle hole reamed

out by the taps, followed by removal of the medial column (**Fig. 21**IV).

9. After completion of the osteotomy the head is loosened from the table, and the halo ring is used to extend the head and close the osteot-omy (**Fig. 21**V, **Fig. 25**).

10. The wound is closed and the patient is taken to the surgical intensive care unit.

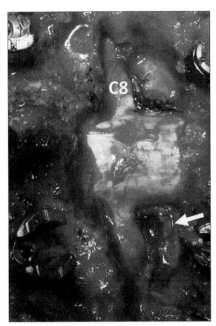

Fig. 22. Intraoperative photograph during C7 pedicle subtraction osteotomy showing isolation of the C7 pedicle and C8 nerve root.

Results

The PSO at the CTJ has 2 key benefits compared with the traditional Smith-Petersen osteotomy (see **Fig. 18**). First, The PSO results in greater biomechanical stability (producing a mechanically stiffer result) than that obtained with the Smith-Petersen osteotomy.[43,70] The Smith-Petersen osteotomy generally results in disc disruption or, in cases of ankylosing spondylitis, osteoclasis through a fused disc space or the anterior cortex of the vertebral body, causing a significant anterior gap in which the anterior longitudinal ligament is completely torn or the autofused anterior bridging osteophyte is fractured. The PSO leaves the anterior longitudinal ligament intact. In addition, the PSO has a wedge component that cleaves the vertebral body, creating a larger bone-on-bone load-bearing interface even when compared with a Smith-Petersen osteotomy that is fully closed posteriorly. This greater bone-on-bone contact significantly increases stiffness, especially in compression, and may provide better fusion rates in patients who do not have ankylosing spondylitis, as the PSO provides a substantial load-bearing surface area in the uniting of the anterior, middle, and posterior columns on closure.[43,70] No secondary anterior grafting is required. Second, The PSO results in a more controlled closure than does the Smith-Petersen osteotomy, because no sudden osteoclastic fracture is necessary.

In their surgical series of 11 patients who received cervicothoracic PSO, the authors found that this procedure results in excellent correction of cervical kyphosis and CBVA with a controlled closure, and improvement in HRQoL measures even at early time points.[21] The mean preoperative and immediate postoperative values (±standard deviation) for cervical sagittal imbalance were 7.9 ± 1.4 cm and 3.4 ± 1.7 cm. The mean overall correction was 4.5 ± 1.5 cm (42.8%), the mean PSO correction 19.0°, and the mean CBVA correction 36.7°. There was a significant decrease in both the Neck Disability Index (51.1–38.6, $P = .03$) and visual analog scale scores for neck pain (8.1–3.9, $P = .0021$). The SF-36 physical-component summary scores increased by 18.4% (30.2–35.8), without neurologic complications.

Complications

Because of the recent advances in surgical technique, anesthesia, and intraoperative neuromonitoring, CTJ PSO has been considered a safe, reproducible, and effective procedure for the management of cervicothoracic kyphotic deformities.[21] Cervicothoracic PSO has reported complications that include neurologic deficits, sudden subluxation, and even death.[40,59,67] Daubs and colleagues[71] found that increasing age was a

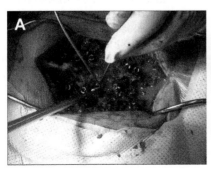
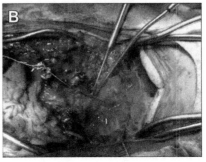

Fig. 23. Intraoperative photographs during C7 pedicle subtraction osteotomy showing 2 different views (*A* and *B*) of using lumbar taps to decancellate the C7 vertebral body.

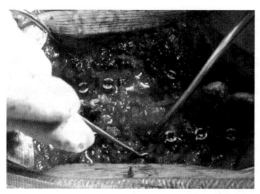

Fig. 24. Intraoperative photograph during C7 pedicle subtraction osteotomy showing the use of a Penfield retractor to expose the lateral wall of C7.

significant factor in predicting a complication for patients older than 60 years; however, in the authors' series 8 of 11 patients were older than 60, among whom there were no perioperative neurologic deficits, with perioperative medical complications in only 2 of the 11 cases. The lower medical complication rate and decreased incidence of dysphagia may be due to the all-posterior nature of this technique. Posterior-only deformity corrections have also been associated with lower complication rates in thoracolumbar surgery in comparison with staged anterior-posterior procedures (**Table 2**).

Cervical Circumferential Osteotomy

In the clinical setting of rigid cervical kyphosis with neurologic symptoms, the spinal cord is usually tethered over the subaxial kyphotic segment, leading to neurologic symptoms and myelopathy. Therefore, segmental kyphosis correction is needed to untether and decompress the spinal

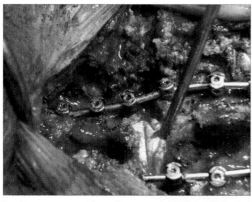

Fig. 25. Intraoperative photograph during C7 pedicle subtraction osteotomy showing closure of the osteotomy.

cord in the mid subaxial region. This technique is in 3 stages: posterior, anterior, posterior (**Figs. 26–28**).

These stages can be carried out during a single anesthesia or in a delayed fashion according to the extension of the planned procedure and the condition of the patient. All stages are performed under general anesthesia with neuromonitoring using standard motor and sensory evoked potentials.

1. First stage (see **Fig. 26**): A standard posterior approach (laminectomy, facetectomy, and insertion of pedicle screw and lateral mass screw) to the cervical spine is performed for the predetermined levels.
2. Second stage (see **Fig. 27**): Anterior approach to the anterior cervical vertebrae for the decompression and remobilizing the cervical spine.
3. Third stage (see **Fig. 28**): The patient is again positioned prone and the previous posterior incision reopened. Final correction of deformity is gained.

Indications and contraindications

Fixed mid subaxial kyphotic deformity results from degenerative or inflammatory conditions or, often, from previous fixation in a kyphotic position (**Fig. 29A**). Cervical sagittal imbalance secondary to failed anterior procedures as a result of nonunions or graft subsidence is increasingly common. It is important to achieve enough correction of sagittal imbalance and regional lordosis to allow dorsal cord migration and decreased cord tension.

Surgical procedure

1. First stage
   a. After a standard posterior cervical approach, previous instrumentation can be removed and the fusion mass explored, searching for any sites of nonunion.
   b. Laminectomies can be done as needed, especially around the apex of the deformity to allow for free movement of the spinal cord after the correction of the deformity. Previous laminectomy scar is removed down to the dura.
   c. Through the same approach, the necessary foraminotomies are performed, dictated by the patient's preoperative clinical and radiographic status. Bilateral osteotomies, including the cephalad part of the superior facet and caudad aspect of the inferior facet, are performed at the apical levels of the kyphosis. Care must be taken to carry the resection lateral enough to release all the fusion mass or facets and generously

Table 2
Demographic data including patient age, cause of deformity, comorbidities, radiographic results, and complications

Case No.	Age (y), Sex	Diagnosis	Operation	Complications
1	70, M	Chin-on-chest deformity	C7 PSO	Pneumonia
2	56, M	Cervical kyphosis and cervical myelopathy	C7 PSO	
3	82, F	Chin-on-chest deformity	C7 PSO	
4	80, M	Chin-on-chest deformity	C7 PSO	Pneumonia
5	73, F	Fixed coronal and sagittal plane cervical deformity	C6 and C7 PSO	
6	69, M	Cervical kyphosis	C7 PSO	Dysphagia/PEG
7	59, F	Chin-on-chest deformity	C7 PSO	
8	75, M	Cervical kyphosis	C7 PSO	
9	94, F	Chin-on-chest deformity	T1 PSO	
10	63, M	Chin-on-chest deformity	C7 PSO	Rod fracture at 4 mo
11	52, M	Chin-on-chest deformity	C7 PSO	

Abbreviations: PEG, percutaneous endoscopic gastrostomy; PSO, pedicle subtraction osteotomy.

decompress the exiting nerve root (see **Fig. 26**).

d. Segmental instrumentation is placed in the form of lateral mass or pedicle screws, depending on the level and surgeon's preference.

e. The incision is closed in the standard fashion postoperatively; the patient can be mobilized with the use of a hard collar until the next stage.

2. Second stage

a. The patient is turned to the supine position and an anterior cervical approach is taken

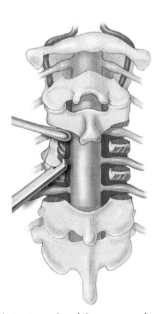

Fig. 26. First stage involving removal of previous instrumentation, central and foraminal decompressions, multiple posterior osteotomies, and posterior reinstrumentation (not depicted here). This procedure is known as the cervical Ponte osteotomy, which can be performed in a single stage to loosen semirigid deformities with mobile discs.

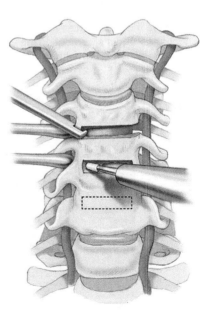

Fig. 27. Anterior second stage with multiple osteotomies/discectomies involving resection of the uncovertebral joints and protection of the vertebral artery. An anterior, overcontoured plate can also be used to produce anterior translation at the apex of the deformity (not depicted here).

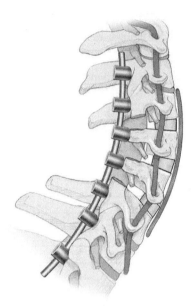

Fig. 28. Final correction after the third stage and rod placement.

through previously operated tissue planes. Any anterior instrumentation used in prior surgeries can be removed at this time.

   b. Anteriorly based osteotomies are performed as needed depending on the presence of ankylosed/fused segments, the necessity of anterior decompression, and the overall deformity. For improved correction, the osteotomies must be performed lateral to the uncovertebral joints, protecting the vertebral artery from the burr with a Penfield #4 dissector[38] (see **Fig. 27**).

   c. After complete release, lordosing distraction is applied at each osteotomy site with Caspar pins, and a laminar spreader is inserted in the disc space.

   d. Interbody lordotic grafting (autograft, allograft, or cages as preferred) is performed.

   e. A plate spanning the osteotomies is overcontoured (**Fig. 30**) and fixed initially at the apical level by parallel screws, conforming the apical segment into more lordosis as the screws are tightened and the spine is sequentially reduced to the plate.

   f. The rest of the screws are placed and secured, and the incision is closed in the standard fashion.

3. Third stage

   a. The patient is again positioned prone and the previous posterior incision reopened.

   b. Bony surfaces are decorticated with bone grafting and rod placement (see **Figs. 28** and **29B**). Compression at the osteotomies may be performed if deemed necessary.

   c. Following closure, the patient is immobilized in a hard cervical collar. Placement of a feeding tube can be done at the end of the procedure if problems with swallowing are anticipated.

   d. The patient is kept intubated and nursed in a head-up position to reduce postoperative pharyngeal edema until it is considered safe to remove the endotracheal tube.

Results

A gradual and acceptable correction is achieved through the summation of correct positioning,

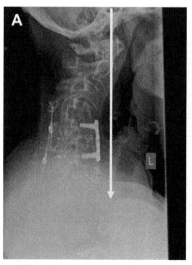
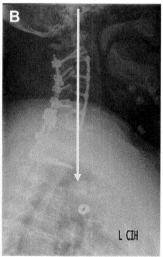

Fig. 29. Preoperative (*A*) and postoperative (*B*) lateral radiographs demonstrating a case example of a 540° circumferential procedure.

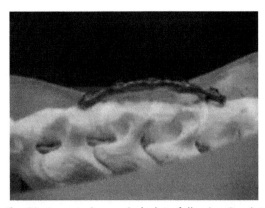

Fig. 30. An anterior cervical plate following 3-point bending resting on top of a model cervical spine for comparison of the curvature obtained from the bending.

multiple osteotomy sites, plated anterior segmental translation, and posterior instrumented compression.

In the authors' 14 cases of surgical experience, osteotomies were performed at 3.9 (range 3–6) levels anteriorly and 6.6 (range 3–18) levels posteriorly. The estimated blood loss was on average 1484 mL (range 400–4600 mL). The average stay in the hospital was 19 days (range 3–55 days) and stay in the intensive care unit 6.2 days (range 0–15 days). Days intubated averaged 3.8 (range 0–15 days).

The average C2-C7 angle changed from 12.4° of kyphosis (range 58° of kyphosis to 30.9° of lordosis) to an average of 14.9° of lordosis after surgery (range 9.4° of kyphosis to 35.1° of lordosis). The average angular correction was

Table 3
Major complications for the various osteotomies

Technique	No. of Patients	Overall Complication Rate	Mortality Rate	Neurologic Complication Rate	Complications
PSO: Deviren et al[21]	11	4/11	0	0	1 dysphagia/PEG, 1 rod fracture, 2 pneumonia
360°: Nottmeier et al[72]	41	2/41	0	2/41	1 quadriparesis, 1 C8 radiculopathy
540°: Acosta et al[44]	14	5/14	0	1/14	1 incidental durotomy, 1 persistent CSF leak, 1 superficial wound infection, 1 infection at iliac bone harvest site, 1 C5 palsy
Circumferential: Mummaneni et al[73]	30	11/30	2/30	0	2 wound infections, 1 fall with fracture of C6, 1 plate dislodgment, 1 transient dysphonia, 1 intraoperative CSF leak, 3 perioperative tracheostomy and gastrostomy, 2 deaths
OWO: Simmons et al[40]	131	55/131	4/131	21/131	2 intraoperative neurologic, 1 hemiparesis, 16 C8 radiculopathy, 2 C8 nerve root irritations, 6 pseudarthrosis, 5 pneumonia, 4 deep vein thrombosis with pulmonary embolism, 15 halo pin infections, 4 deaths
Anterior-posterior: O'Shaughnessy et al[74]	20	7/20	0	4/20	2 durotomy, 3 transient C5 palsy, 1 head-holder failure with resultant quadriplegia, 1 late progression of deformity at the caudal junctional end

Abbreviations: CSF, cerebrospinal fluid; OWO, opening wedge osteotomy; PEG, percutaneous endoscopic gastrostomy; PSO, pedicle subtraction osteotomy.

27.7° (range 1.9°–74.6°). The average preoperative C2-C7 translation improved from 46.9 mm (range 86–2 mm) to 26 mm (range 57 to −3 mm) for an average 20.8 mm of correction.

Complications

In the authors' surgical series, there was 1 case of incidental durotomy that was repaired during the same surgery. One patient had persistent cerebrospinal fluid leak postoperatively and was taken back to the operation room for repair. There was 1 superficial wound infection and 1 infection at the iliac crest bone harvest site. The former resolved with irrigation and debridement and oral antibiotics. The latter was managed with a wound vacuum system and oral antibiotics. Other complications not directly related to surgery were 1 acute subdural hematoma that required craniotomy and 1 pneumothorax secondary to line placement. Regarding neurologic complications, 1 patient had postoperative right C5 palsy interpreted to be secondary to root stretching after deformity correction. Complications from the literature regarding the osteotomies discussed are presented in **Table 3**.

REFERENCES

1. Hardacker JW, Shuford RF, Capicotto PN, et al. Radiographic standing cervical segmental alignment in adult volunteers without neck symptoms. Spine (Phila Pa 1976) 1997;22:1472–80 [discussion: 1480].
2. Glassman SD, Bridwell K, Dimar JR, et al. The impact of positive sagittal balance in adult spinal deformity. Spine (Phila Pa 1976) 2005;30:2024–9.
3. Pichelmann MA, Lenke LG, Bridwell KH, et al. Revision rates following primary adult spinal deformity surgery: six hundred forty-three consecutive patients followed-up to twenty-two years postoperative. Spine (Phila Pa 1976) 2010;35:219–26.
4. Schwab F, Farcy JP, Bridwell K, et al. A clinical impact classification of scoliosis in the adult. Spine (Phila Pa 1976) 2006;31:2109–14.
5. Schwab FJ, Smith VA, Biserni M, et al. Adult scoliosis: a quantitative radiographic and clinical analysis. Spine (Phila Pa 1976) 2002;27:387–92.
6. Beier G, Schuck M, Schuller E, et al. Determination of physical data of the head I. Center of gravity and moments of inertia of human heads. Arlington (VA): Office of Naval Research; 1979. p. 44.
7. Pal GP, Sherk HH. The vertical stability of the cervical spine. Spine (Phila Pa 1976) 1988;13:447–9.
8. Lorenz M, Patwardhan A, Vanderby R Jr. Load-bearing characteristics of lumbar facets in normal and surgically altered spinal segments. Spine (Phila Pa 1976) 1983;8:122–30.
9. Nachemson A. Lumbar intradiscal pressure. Experimental studies on post-mortem material. Acta Orthop Scand Suppl 1960;43:1–104.
10. Gay RE. The curve of the cervical spine: variations and significance. J Manipulative Physiol Ther 1993;16:591–4.
11. McAviney J, Schulz D, Bock R, et al. Determining the relationship between cervical lordosis and neck complaints. J Manipulative Physiol Ther 2005;28:187–93.
12. Gore DR. Roentgenographic findings in the cervical spine in asymptomatic persons: a ten-year follow-up. Spine (Phila Pa 1976) 2001;26:2463–6.
13. Tang JA, Scheer JK, Smith JS, et al. The impact of standing regional cervical sagittal alignment on outcomes in posterior cervical fusion surgery. Neurosurgery 2012;71:662–9.
14. Gore DR, Sepic SB, Gardner GM. Roentgenographic findings of the cervical spine in asymptomatic people. Spine (Phila Pa 1976) 1986;11:521–4.
15. Blondel B, Schwab F, Ames CP, et al. Age related cervical and spino-pelvic parameters variations in a volunteer population. Spine, in press.
16. Jackson RP, McManus AC. Radiographic analysis of sagittal plane alignment and balance in standing volunteers and patients with low back pain matched for age, sex, and size. A prospective controlled clinical study. Spine (Phila Pa 1976) 1994;19:1611–8.
17. Bernhardt M, Bridwell KH. Segmental analysis of the sagittal plane alignment of the normal thoracic and lumbar spines and thoracolumbar junction. Spine (Phila Pa 1976) 1989;14:717–21.
18. Yoshida G, Kamiya M, Yoshihara H, et al. Subaxial sagittal alignment and adjacent-segment degeneration after atlantoaxial fixation performed using C-1 lateral mass and C-2 pedicle screws or transarticular screws. J Neurosurg Spine 2010;13:443–50.
19. Yoshimoto H, Ito M, Abumi K, et al. A retrospective radiographic analysis of subaxial sagittal alignment after posterior C1-C2 fusion. Spine (Phila Pa 1976) 2004;29:175–81.
20. Lafage V, Ames C, Schwab F, et al. Changes in thoracic kyphosis negatively impact sagittal alignment after lumbar pedicle subtraction osteotomy: a comprehensive radiographic analysis. Spine (Phila Pa 1976) 2012;37:E180–7.
21. Deviren V, Scheer JK, Ames CP. Technique of cervicothoracic junction pedicle subtraction osteotomy for cervical sagittal imbalance: report of 11 cases. J Neurosurg Spine 2011;15:174–81.
22. Kim KT, Lee SH, Son ES, et al. Surgical treatment of "chin-on-pubis" deformity in an ankylosing spondylitis patient: a case report of consecutive cervical, thoracic and lumbar corrective osteotomies. Spine (Phila Pa 1976) 2012;37:E1017–21.
23. Kim KT, Suk KS, Cho YJ, et al. Clinical outcome results of pedicle subtraction osteotomy in

ankylosing spondylitis with kyphotic deformity. Spine (Phila Pa 1976) 2002;27:612–8.

24. Pigge RR, Scheerder FJ, Smit TH, et al. Effectiveness of preoperative planning in the restoration of balance and view in ankylosing spondylitis. Neurosurg Focus 2008;24:E7.

25. Suk KS, Kim KT, Lee SH, et al. Significance of chin-brow vertical angle in correction of kyphotic deformity of ankylosing spondylitis patients. Spine (Phila Pa 1976) 2003;28:2001–5.

26. Wang Y, Zhang Y, Mao K, et al. Transpedicular bivertebrae wedge osteotomy and discectomy in lumbar spine for severe ankylosing spondylitis. J Spinal Disord Tech 2010;23:186–91.

27. Wang VY, Chou D. The cervicothoracic junction. Neurosurg Clin N Am 2007;18:365–71.

28. Yoganandan N, Maiman DJ, Guan Y, et al. Importance of physical properties of the human head on head-neck injury metrics. Traffic Inj Prev 2009;10:488–96.

29. An HS, Vaccaro A, Cotler JM, et al. Spinal disorders at the cervicothoracic junction. Spine (Phila Pa 1976) 1994;19:2557–64.

30. Lee SH, Seo EM, Suk KS, et al. The influence of thoracic inlet alignment on the craniocervical sagittal balance in asymptomatic adults. J Spinal Disord Tech 2012;25(2):E41–7.

31. Knott PT, Mardjetko SM, Techy F. The use of the T1 sagittal angle in predicting overall sagittal balance of the spine. Spine J 2010;10:994–8.

32. Chi JH, Tay B, Stahl D, et al. Complex deformities of the cervical spine. Neurosurg Clin N Am 2007;18: 295–304.

33. Mummaneni PV, Deutsch H, Mummaneni VP. Cervicothoracic kyphosis. Neurosurg Clin N Am 2006; 17:277–87, vi.

34. Steinmetz MP, Stewart TJ, Kager CD, et al. Cervical deformity correction. Neurosurgery 2007; 60:S90–7.

35. Albert TJ, Vacarro A. Postlaminectomy kyphosis. Spine (Phila Pa 1976) 1998;23:2738–45.

36. Kaptain GJ, Simmons NE, Replogle RE, et al. Incidence and outcome of kyphotic deformity following laminectomy for cervical spondylotic myelopathy. J Neurosurg 2000;93:199–204.

37. Umapathi T, Chaudhry V, Cornblath D, et al. Head drop and camptocormia. J Neurol Neurosurg Psychiatry 2002;73:1–7.

38. Wang VY, Aryan H, Ames CP. A novel anterior technique for simultaneous single-stage anterior and posterior cervical release for fixed kyphosis. J Neurosurg Spine 2008;8:594–9.

39. Gill JB, Levin A, Burd T, et al. Corrective osteotomies in spine surgery. J Bone Joint Surg Am 2008;90: 2509–20.

40. Simmons ED, DiStefano RJ, Zheng Y, et al. Thirty-six years experience of cervical extension osteotomy in

ankylosing spondylitis: techniques and outcomes. Spine (Phila Pa 1976) 2006;31:3006–12.

41. Simmons EH. The surgical correction of flexion deformity of the cervical spine in ankylosing spondylitis. Clin Orthop Relat Res 1972;86:132–43.

42. Samudrala S, Vaynman S, Thiayananthan T, et al. Cervicothoracic junction kyphosis: surgical reconstruction with pedicle subtraction osteotomy and Smith-Petersen osteotomy. Presented at the 2009 Joint Spine Section Meeting. Clinical article. J Neurosurg Spine 2010;13:695–706.

43. Scheer JK, Tang JA, Buckley JM, et al. Biomechanical analysis of osteotomy type and rod diameter for treatment of cervicothoracic kyphosis. Spine (Phila Pa 1976) 2011;36:E519–23.

44. Acosta FL Jr, McClendon J Jr, O'Shaughnessy BA, et al. Morbidity and mortality after spinal deformity surgery in patients 75 years and older: complications and predictive factors. J Neurosurg Spine 2011;15:667–74.

45. Deutsch H, Haid RW, Rodts GE, et al. Postlaminectomy cervical deformity. Neurosurg Focus 2003; 15:E5.

46. Shimizu K, Nakamura M, Nishikawa Y, et al. Spinal kyphosis causes demyelination and neuronal loss in the spinal cord: a new model of kyphotic deformity using juvenile Japanese small game fowls. Spine (Phila Pa 1976) 2005;30:2388–92.

47. Jarzem PF, Quance DR, Doyle DJ, et al. Spinal cord tissue pressure during spinal cord distraction in dogs. Spine (Phila Pa 1976) 1992;17:S227–34.

48. Tachibana S, Kitahara Y, Iida H, et al. Spinal cord intramedullary pressure. A possible factor in syrinx growth. Spine (Phila Pa 1976) 1994;19:2174–8 [discussion: 2178–9].

49. Iida H, Tachibana S. Spinal cord intramedullary pressure: direct cord traction test. Neurol Med Chir (Tokyo) 1995;35:75–7.

50. Kitahara Y, Iida H, Tachibana S. Effect of spinal cord stretching due to head flexion on intramedullary pressure. Neurol Med Chir (Tokyo) 1995;35:285–8.

51. Klineberg E. Cervical spondylotic myelopathy: a review of the evidence. Orthop Clin North Am 2010;41:193–202.

52. Uchida K, Nakajima H, Sato R, et al. Cervical spondylotic myelopathy associated with kyphosis or sagittal sigmoid alignment: outcome after anterior or posterior decompression. J Neurosurg Spine 2009;11:521–8.

53. Andaluz N, Zuccarello M, Kuntz C. Long-term follow-up of cervical radiographic sagittal spinal alignment after 1- and 2-level cervical corpectomy for the treatment of spondylosis of the subaxial cervical spine causing radiculomyelopathy or myelopathy: a retrospective study. J Neurosurg Spine 2012;16:2–7.

54. Epstein NE. Evaluation and treatment of clinical instability associated with pseudoarthrosis after

anterior cervical surgery for ossification of the posterior longitudinal ligament. Surg Neurol 1998; 49:246–52.

55. Hilibrand AS, Carlson GD, Palumbo MA, et al. Radiculopathy and myelopathy at segments adjacent to the site of a previous anterior cervical arthrodesis. J Bone Joint Surg Am 1999;81:519–28.

56. Mason C, Cozen L, Adelstein L. Surgical correction of flexion deformity of the cervical spine. Calif Med 1953;79:244–6.

57. Chapman JR, Anderson PA, Pepin C, et al. Posterior instrumentation of the unstable cervicothoracic spine. J Neurosurg 1996;84:552–8.

58. Edwards CC 2nd, Riew KD, Anderson PA, et al. Cervical myelopathy. Current diagnostic and treatment strategies. Spine J 2003;3:68–81.

59. Mummaneni PV, Mummaneni VP, Haid RW Jr, et al. Cervical osteotomy for the correction of chin-on-chest deformity in ankylosing spondylitis. Technical note. Neurosurg Focus 2003;14:e9.

60. Belanger TA, Milam RA, Roh JS, et al. Cervicothoracic extension osteotomy for chin-on-chest deformity in ankylosing spondylitis. J Bone Joint Surg Am 2005;87:1732–8.

61. Grundy PL, Gill SS. Odontoid process and C1-C2 corrective osteotomy through a posterior approach: technical case report. Neurosurgery 1998;43: 1483–6 [discussion: 1486–7].

62. Goel A, Laheri V. Plate and screw fixation for atlanto-axial subluxation. Acta Neurochir (Wien) 1994;129: 47–53.

63. Harms J, Melcher RP. Posterior C1-C2 fusion with polyaxial screw and rod fixation. Spine (Phila Pa 1976) 2001;26:2467–71.

64. Jeanneret B, Magerl F. Primary posterior fusion C1/2 in odontoid fractures: indications, technique, and results of transarticular screw fixation. J Spinal Disord 1992;5:464–75.

65. Smith-Petersen MN, Larson CB, Aufranc OE. Osteotomy of the spine for correction of flexion deformity in rheumatoid arthritis. Clin Orthop Relat Res 1969; 66:6–9.

66. Urist MR. Osteotomy of the cervical spine; report of a case of ankylosing rheumatoid spondylitis. J Bone Joint Surg Am 1958;40:833–43.

67. McMaster MJ. Osteotomy of the cervical spine in ankylosing spondylitis. J Bone Joint Surg Br 1997; 79:197–203.

68. Danisa OA, Turner D, Richardson WJ. Surgical correction of lumbar kyphotic deformity: posterior reduction "eggshell" osteotomy. J Neurosurg 2000; 92:50–6.

69. Kim YJ, Bridwell KH, Lenke LG, et al. Results of lumbar pedicle subtraction osteotomies for fixed sagittal imbalance: a minimum 5-year follow-up study. Spine (Phila Pa 1976) 2007;32: 2189–97.

70. Scheer JK, Tang JA, Deviren V, et al. Biomechanical analysis of cervicothoracic junction osteotomy in cadaveric model of ankylosing spondylitis: effect of rod material and diameter. J Neurosurg Spine 2011;14:330–5.

71. Daubs MD, Lenke LG, Cheh G, et al. Adult spinal deformity surgery: complications and outcomes in patients over age 60. Spine (Phila Pa 1976) 2007; 32:2238–44.

72. Nottmeier EW, Deen HG, Patel N, et al. Cervical kyphotic deformity correction using 360-degree reconstruction. J Spinal Disord Tech 2009;22: 385–91.

73. Mummaneni PV, Dhall SS, Rodts GE, et al. Circumferential fusion for cervical kyphotic deformity. J Neurosurg Spine 2008;9:515–21.

74. O'Shaughnessy BA, Liu JC, Hsieh PC, et al. Surgical treatment of fixed cervical kyphosis with myelopathy. Spine (Phila Pa 1976) 2008;33:771–8.

Management of High-Grade Spondylolisthesis

Manish K. Kasliwal, MD, MCh[a], Justin S. Smith, MD, PhD[a],*,
Adam Kanter, MD[b], Ching-Jen Chen, BA[a],
Praveen V. Mummaneni, MD[c], Robert A. Hart, MD[d],
Christopher I. Shaffrey, MD[a]

KEYWORDS

- Adolescents • Adult spondylolisthesis • Classification • High-grade spondylolisthesis
- Management • Surgery • Complications

KEY POINTS

- Management of high-grade spondylolisthesis (HGS) remains challenging and is associated with significant controversies.
- Symptomatic patients presenting with intractable pain, neurologic deficits, or global deformity are often considered candidates for surgery.
- The best surgical procedure still remains debatable, considering the absence of high-quality studies in the literature demonstrating superiority of one approach over another.
- Recognition of the importance of overall spinopelvic alignment and global deformity has provided strong rationale for at least partial slip reduction.
- Complications associated with operative management of HGS still remains the key factor dictating the selection of surgical approach.

INTRODUCTION

The term spondylolisthesis is derived from the Greek words, *spondylos,* meaning "vertebrae" and *olisthesis,* meaning "to slip." High-grade spondylolisthesis (HGS) is defined as greater than 50% slippage of a spinal vertebral body relative to an adjacent vertebral body as per Meyerding classification, and most often affects the alignment of the L5 and S1 vertebral bodies (**Fig. 1**).[1] Although more than 50% of linear translation in the sagittal plane is used to define HGS, it is the associated rotational component that often plays a greater role in prognosis and overall management.[2,3] The treatment of high-grade lumbosacral spondylolisthesis differs from that of low-grade slips, and operative management remains challenging and is associated with significant controversies in terms of the optimal surgical technique.[4–7] This review highlights the pathophysiology, classification, clinical presentation, and management controversies of HGS in light of recent advances in our understanding of the importance of sagittal spinopelvic alignment and technologic advancements.

PATHOPHYSIOLOGY OF DEVELOPMENT OF HIGH-GRADE SPONDYLOLISTHESIS

The clinical syndrome of spondylolisthesis was first described in 1782 by the Belgian obstetrician Herbiniaux, long before an understanding of its pathophysiology, when he reported a bony

Funding: No funding was received in support of this study.
[a] Department of Neurosurgery, University of Virginia, PO Box 800212, Charlottesville, VA 22908, USA; [b] Department of Neurosurgery, University of Pittsburgh Medical Center, UPMC Presbyterian, Suite A-402, 200 Lothrop Street, Pittsburgh, PA 15213, USA; [c] Department of Neurosurgery, University of California San Francisco, 400 Parnassus Avenue, San Francisco, CA 94143, USA; [d] Department of Orthopaedic Surgery, Oregon Health Sciences University, 3303 SW Bond Ave #12, Portland, OR 97239, USA
* Corresponding author. Department of Neurosurgery, University of Virginia Medical Center, PO Box 800212, Charlottesville, VA 22908.
E-mail address: Jsmith1enator@gmail.com

Neurosurg Clin N Am 24 (2013) 275–291
http://dx.doi.org/10.1016/j.nec.2012.12.002
1042-3680/13/$ – see front matter © 2013 Elsevier Inc. All rights reserved.

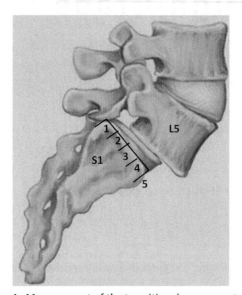

Fig. 1. Measurement of the transitional component of spondylolisthesis per Meyerding grade.

prominence anterior to the sacrum that created an impediment to vaginal delivery in a cohort of his patients. Spondylolisthesis shows a strong familial association, with an incidence in first-degree or second-degree relatives of approximately 25% to 30%.[8] A radiographic study by Wynne-Davies and Scott[9] showed that dysplastic spondylolisthesis has a familial incidence of 33%, whereas the isthmic variant has a familial incidence of 15%, with a multifactorial autosomal dominant pattern of inheritance with incomplete penetrance. Although the etiology of the condition is not completely understood, the evidence available thus far suggests that factors beyond developmental susceptibilities may play a significant role in the development of HGS. Activities that involve hyperextension and persistent lordosis such as gymnastics, weightlifting, diving, football, and volleyball increase shear stresses at the neural arch and have been implicated as causative factors in the development of spondylolysis, with subsequent development of spondylolisthesis in a subset of patients.[10] The majority of HGS cases are of the isthmic or dysplastic variety.[11] The presence of a congenitally dysplastic lumbosacral segment with incompetent posterior elements cannot withstand typical forces associated with maintenance of an upright posture; this often leads to development of a slip, which over time can result in an HGS.

Variations in the cross-sectional anatomy of the pars at each level in the lumbar spine likely contribute to the increased incidence of isthmic spondylolisthesis in more caudal segments, especially at the L5/S1 level. The pars is fairly large in diameter in the upper lumbar vertebra and relatively thin at the L5 level.[12] Fredrickson and colleagues[13] prospectively followed 500 elementary students and found a 4.4% incidence of spondylolysis at the age of 6 years, which increased to 6% in adulthood. Of note, the same investigators also evaluated 500 newborns and found no evidence of spondylolysis/spondylolisthesis, suggesting that development of a pars defect with subsequent development of spondylolisthesis is an acquired phenomenon.

Sagittal sacropelvic morphology and orientation modulate the geometry of the lumbar spine and, consequently, the mechanical stresses at the lumbosacral junction. There have been recent attempts to quantify the relation between the lumbosacral spine and the pelvis by means of various geometric parameters in an effort to better understand the development of spondylolisthesis.[3,14–16] These parameters include sacral slope (SS), pelvic tilt (PT), and pelvic incidence (PI). Multiple studies have demonstrated the importance of harmonious alignment among pelvic and spinal parameters with regard to standardized measures of health-related quality of life (HRQOL).[17–19] Various sagittal lumbosacral spine and spinopelvic parameters are illustrated in **Fig. 2** and are further described in **Table 1**.

Labelle and colleagues[20] found that PI, SS, PT, and LL (lumbar lordosis) measurements were significantly higher in subjects with spondylolisthesis than in controls. These investigators further demonstrated that the values increased with the severity of the spondylolisthesis, leading them to conclude that PI (and thus pelvic anatomy) influences the development of spondylolisthesis, and that an increased PI may be a risk factor for the development and progression of developmental spondylolisthesis.[20] Other reports have contributed increasing evidence that in high-grade L5-S1 spondylolisthesis, the sacropelvic morphology is abnormal and that, combined with the presence of a local lumbosacral deformity and dysplasia, it can result in an abnormal sacropelvic orientation and disturbed global sagittal alignment of the spine.[3,15,16,21,22] These findings have important implications for the evaluation and treatment of patients with HGS and have been the basis of recent spondylolisthesis classifications.[23–25] These data also provide a compelling rationale to reduce and realign the deformity in order to restore global spinopelvic alignment and improve the biomechanical environment for fusion.[26]

CLASSIFICATION OF HIGH-GRADE SPONDYLOLISTHESIS

The classification systems described by Wiltse and by Marchetti and Bartolozzi have remained the most

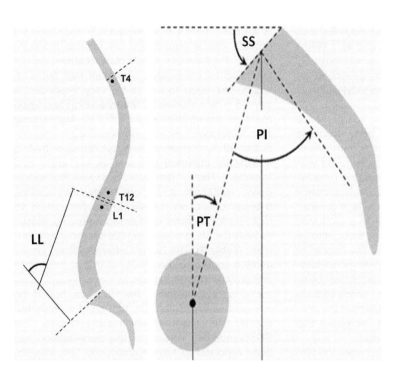

Fig. 2. Sagittal pelvic parameters assessed from the standing lateral radiograph. The pelvic incidence (PI) is always equal to the sum of the sacral slope (SS) and the pelvic tilt (PT). LL, lumbar lordosis.

Table 1
Description of various radiographic parameters used to define spondylolisthesis and sagittal spinopelvic alignment

Boxall slip angle (BSA)	The angle subtended by the inferior endplate of L5 with a line perpendicular to the posterior aspect of S1
Dubousset lumbosacral angle (Dub-LSA)	The angle subtended by the superior endplate of L5 with the posterior aspect of S1
Sacral slope (SS)	The angle between the horizontal line and the cranial sacral endplate tangent
Pelvic tilt (PT)	The angle between the vertical line and the line joining the middle of the sacral plate to the center of the bicoxofemoral axis
Pelvic incidence (PI)	The angle between the line perpendicular to the middle of the cranial sacral endplate and the line joining the middle of the cranial sacral endplate to the center of the bicoxofemoral axis
Sagittal vertical axis (SVA)	The horizontal offset between the C7 plumb line and the posterior superior aspect of the S1 vertebral body. Positive and negative values of SVA reflect cases in which the C7 plumb line falls anterior or posterior, respectively, to the posterosuperior corner of the S1 vertebral body
Lumbar lordosis (LL)	Cobb Angle measured from the superior endplate of L1 to the superior endplate of S1
C7 Plumb line	Vertical line drawn from the center of C7 vertebrae on a radiograph. Often used as a reference line for measuring sagittal balance. The distal reference point for this parameter is the posterosuperior corner of the sacrum

commonly used classifications for spondylolisthesis over the last few decades (**Figs. 3** and **4**).[27] Wiltse provided a classification based on etiology. By contrast, the classification system described by Marchetti and Bartolozzi divides spondylolisthesis into two types, developmental and acquired, with the distinction between them being the presence of either a high or low amount of bony dysplasia with developmental spondylolisthesis and lack of such dysplasia with the acquired type.[27] The vast majority of HGS seen in either pediatric or adult patients occurs in patients with developmental spondylolisthesis, particularly with a high amount of dysplasia. In general, progression of an acquired spondylolisthesis to high-grade slip is thought to be relatively uncommon.[22] The greater the degree of dysplasia present in a developmental spondylolisthesis, the greater the amount of secondary bony changes and slippage that occur, which include a rounding off of the sacrum, angulation of the inferior endplate of L5 (trapezoid L5), increased slip angle, and verticalization of the sacrum.

Although Marchetti and Bartolozzi were the first to introduce the concept of low-dysplastic and high-dysplastic developmental spondylolisthesis, they did not include strict criteria to differentiate these two subtypes. Another limitation of their classification system is a lack of consideration of spinopelvic alignment, which recently has been shown to differ significantly between high-grade and low-grade HGS, and even within HGS between the high-dysplastic and low-dysplastic cases.[22] Although rare, acquired spondylolisthesis may progress to high grades of slippage. Most are iatrogenic following a destabilizing surgical procedure of the underlying soft tissue including the disc, facet capsules, musculature, and ligaments. This type of HGS is more similar to posttraumatic kyphosis than to the dysplastic developmental types of spondylolisthesis, and reduction of an iatrogenic postsurgical acquired spondylolisthesis seems to have a lower risk of neurologic injury than developmental types of slippage.[28]

Although these classification systems have been popular for several years, there are substantial limitations; perhaps most notably they do not provide useful information on clinical management.[27] Furthermore, these classifications do not take sagittal sacropelvic alignment into account, which has been found to be very important in several recent studies for the evaluation and treatment of spondylolisthesis.[3,15,20,22,29] Mac-Thiong and colleagues[25] recently proposed a new classification of lumbosacral spondylolisthesis that is specifically intended to guide its evaluation and treatment. This system incorporates sagittal sacropelvic alignment and morphology, and defines 8 types based on the slip grade (low-grade vs high-grade), degree of dysplasia (low-dysplastic vs high-dysplastic), and sagittal sacropelvic alignment (**Table 2**). The Spine Deformity Study Group (SDSG) confirmed the validity of this classification and provided modifications, further dividing lumbosacral spondylolisthesis into 6 types based on 3 important characteristics that can be easily assessed from preoperative imaging studies. The SDSG-modified version of the classification has been reported to have significantly less interobserver and intraobserver variability in assessment of the grade of slip, the sacropelvic balance, and the global spinopelvic balance (**Table 3**).[24]

For the SDSG classification system modified from that of Mac-Thiong, first the degree of slip is quantified from the lateral radiograph, to determine if it is low grade (grades 0, 1, and 2, or <50% slip) or high-grade (grades 3, 4, and spondyloptosis, or ≥50% slip). Next, the sagittal alignment is measured by determining sacropelvic and global spinopelvic alignment, using measurements of PI, SS, PT, and the C7 plumb line. In HGS, sacropelvic alignment is assessed based on the SS and PT.[26,30] Each subject is classified as high SS/low PT (balanced sacropelvis) or low SS/high PT (unbalanced sacropelvis) (**Fig. 5**). Patients with low-grade spondylolisthesis can be subdivided into 3 types based on their sacropelvic balance : type 1, the nutcracker type, a subgroup with low PI <45°; type 2, a subgroup with normal PI (between 45°, and 60°); and type 3, the shear type, a subgroup with high PI (≥60°) (see **Table 3**). Patients with

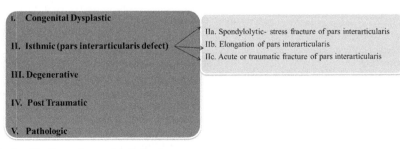

Fig. 3. Wiltse's classification of spondylolisthesis.

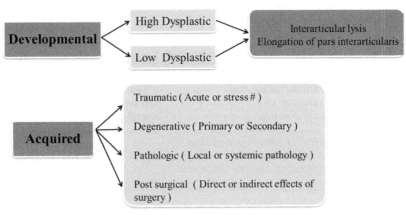

Fig. 4. Spondylolisthesis classification by Marchetti and Bartolozzi.

Table 2
Original classification system of lumbosacral spondylolisthesis as proposed by Mac-Thiong and Labelle

Grade	Dysplasia	Sacropelvic Balance	Example
Low grade (<50% slip)	Low-Dysplastic Minimal lumbosacral kyphosis Almost rectangular L5 Minimal sacral doming Relatively normal sacrum Minimal posterior elements dysplasia (eg, spina bifida occulta) Relatively normal transverse processes	Low PI/Low SS Sacral slope <40°	Type 1
		High PI/High SS Sacral slope >40°	Type 2
	High-Dysplastic Lumbosacral kyphosis Trapezoidal L5 Sacral doming Sacral dysplasia and kyphosis Posterior elements dysplasia Small transverse processes	Low PI/Low SS Sacral slope ≤40°	Type 3
		High PI/High SS Sacral slope >40°	Type 4

(continued on next page)

Table 2
(continued)

Grade	Dysplasia	Sacropelvic Balance	Example
High grade (≥50% slip)	Low-Dysplastic Minimal lumbosacral kyphosis Almost rectangular L5 Minimal sacral doming Relatively normal sacrum Minimal posterior elements dysplasia (eg, spina bifida occulta) Relatively normal transverse processes	High SS/Low PT (balanced pelvis) Balanced sacrum Sacral slope ≥50° Pelvic tilt ≤35°	Type 5
		Low SS/High PT (unbalanced pelvis) Vertical sacrum Sacral slope <50° Pelvic tilt ≥25°	Type 6
	High-Dysplastic Lumbosacral kyphosis Trapezoidal L5 Sacral doming Sacral dysplasia and kyphosis Posterior elements dysplasia Small transverse processes	High SS/Low PT (balanced pelvis) Balanced sacrum Sacral slope ≥50° Pelvic tilt ≤35°	Type 7
		Low SS/High PT (unbalanced pelvis) Vertical sacrum Sacral slope <50° Pelvic tilt ≥25°	Type 8

Abbreviations: PI, pelvic incidence; PT, pelvic tilt; SS, sacral slope.
Reprinted form Mac-Thiong JM, Labelle H, Parent S, et al. Reliability and development of a new classification of lumbosacral spondylolisthesis. Scoliosis 2008;3:19; with permission from SpringerOpen.

a high PI have a high shear stress across the lumbosacral junction and a higher likelihood of their spondylolisthesis progressing to a high grade. Patients with a low PI, on the other hand, have low shear stress across the lumbosacral junction and less chance of progression of their spondylolisthesis to a high grade.[20] Finally, global spinopelvic alignment is determined using the C7 plumb line. If this line falls over or behind the femoral heads the spine is aligned, whereas if it lies in front of both femoral heads the spine is malaligned.

CLINICAL PRESENTATION

Although HGS can often be asymptomatic, those who do become symptomatic usually present with back pain, leg pain, or a combination of these.[2,13,14,31–33] Complaints of back pain with activity that are relieved with recumbency are often described. The leg pain, which may also include numbness or paresthesias, described by symptomatic patients is predominately dermatomal in distribution, and often related to the nerve(s) being compressed in the lateral recess at the level of the pars defect. The leg symptoms are described as sclerodermal if they are referred into the broad region of the buttock or posterior thigh, which usually occurs as a result of the disc degeneration that often accompanies the pars defect. In addition, the postural changes associated with HGS in adults can lead to low back pain, tight hamstrings, and postural deformity.[34]

Table 3
SDSG classification of lumbosacral spondylolisthesis

Slip Grade	Sacropelvic Balance	Spinopelvic Balance	Spondylolisthesis Type
Low grade	Nutcracker (PI < 45°)		Type 1
	Normal pelvic incidence (60° > PI ≥ 45°)	—	Type 2
	High pelvic incidence	—	Type 3
	PI ≥ 60°		
High grade	Balanced	—	Type 4
	Unbalanced	Balanced	Type 5
		Unbalanced	Type 6

On clinical examination, palpation of the spine may elicit midline tenderness, and a step-off of the spinous processes may be felt above the level of the slip. There will often be limited flexion of the lumbar spine caused by paraspinal spasm as those muscles attempt to prevent shear forces across the affected segment. There can be presence of trunk foreshortening, and hamstring tightness may be noted, with compensatory hyperlordosis above the slip and a waddling gait. Patients may have a classically described Phalen-Dickson sign (ie, a knee-flexed, hip-flexed gait). Neurologically, deficits may include motor weakness and/or sensory deficits depending on the degree of nerve compression in the lateral recess, which typically occurs as a result of the fibrocartilaginous mass or Gill lesion. Cauda equina syndrome is rare because of a relative enlargement of the canal that occurs as the cephalad vertebra slips anterior to the caudal vertebra, leaving the separated posterior elements of the cephalad vertebra in a posterior position. Unlike low-grade slips, whose manifestations are typically limited to painful segmental instability or neural compromise at the affected level, high-grade slips invariably provoke secondary changes in the regional pelvic anatomy, and thus contribute to global sagittal deformity.[15,20] Historically the cosmetic deformity

of HGS has been underappreciated or considered to be of secondary importance to symptoms of pain. The local deformity of the high-grade slip invariably induces compensatory changes in the regional pelvic anatomy, forcing the patient into positive sagittal malalignment.[33] The body's attempts to restore alignment via tonic activation of the paraspinous (eg, erector spinae) muscles, and progressive retroversion of the pelvis (increased PT) is typically accompanied by clinical sequelae of low back pain (presumably caused by chronic paraspinous muscle activation and/or segmental instability), tight hamstrings, and postural deformity.[22,24–26,35] The presence of this global deformity contributes to the complexity of surgical management of HGS.

RADIOLOGY OF HIGH-GRADE SPONDYLOLISTHESIS

Radiographic evaluation should consist of anteroposterior and lateral flexion-extension radiographs. This combination allows the determination of translational instability. However, radiologic evaluation of HGS is no longer limited to assessment of the degree of translational slip alone. Long cassette scoliosis radiographs should also be evaluated to assess for overall sagittal alignment. Computed

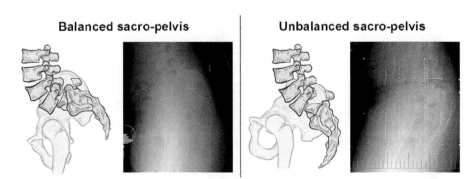

Balanced sacro-pelvis   **Unbalanced sacro-pelvis**

Fig. 5. Schematic figure demonstrating balanced versus unbalanced spinopelvis. (*Reprinted from* Mac-Thiong JM, Labelle H, Parent S, et al. Reliability and development of a new classification of lumbosacral spondylolisthesis. Scoliosis 2008;3:19; with permission from SpringerOpen.)

tomography scans provide excellent bony details of the pathologic status, and magnetic resonance imaging can give much better delineation of the soft-tissue abnormalities. **Table 1** summarizes key radiographic parameters used to characterize HGS. In spondylolisthesis, there are 2 primary components involved in the underlying deformity: translational and angular.[1,36,37] The diagnosis of HGS is overt even on plain radiographs, obviating any need of oblique radiographs to demonstrate the pars defect seen in spondylosis. Measurement of slip grade as per Meyerding classification clearly confirms the diagnosis of high-grade spondylolisthesis by grading the translational component of the deformity (see **Fig. 1**). By contrast, there are multiple techniques to measure angular deformity.[37] Normally the junction between the fifth

lumbar and the first sacral vertebrae is lordotic. However, as the degree of slip progresses to higher grades, this relationship tends to become kyphotic in nature. Studies have suggested a role of lumbosacral kyphosis (LSK) in determining the risk of slip progression,[2,33,37,38] and have also suggested the importance of correcting LSK because this helps to restore global spinal alignment, enhances the biomechanics of fusion, and can protect against stretch of the L5 nerve root. The Boxall slip angle and lumbosacral angle (LSA) provide assessment of the angular component of deformity associated with HGS (**Fig. 6**).[39,40] With progression of slippage, the inferior endplate of L5 tends to become dysplastic and the L5 vertebral body may adopt a trapezoidal shape.[41–43] Moreover, remodeling of the S1 endplate can occur, referred to as sacral

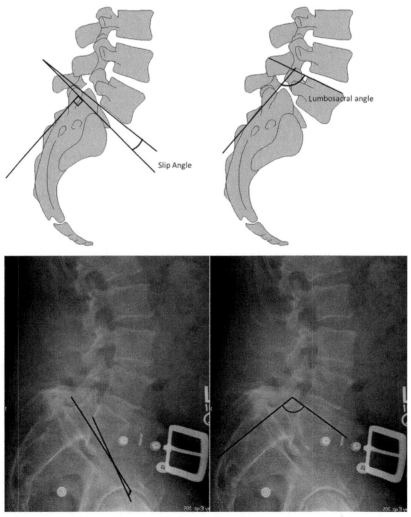

Fig. 6. Schematic diagram and lateral radiograph demonstrating measurement of Dubousset lumbosacral angle (*upper and lower right*) and Boxall slip angle (*upper and lower left*).

doming or rounding.[44] These changes can make the identification of the inferior endplate of L5 and superior endplate of S1 difficult, as can be observed in the radiograph shown in **Fig. 6**, favoring evaluation of the LSK based on the LSA rather than the slip angle. Positive and negative values of the sagittal vertical axis reflect cases whereby the C7 plumb line falls anterior or posterior, respectively, to the posterosuperior corner of the S1 vertebral body (**Fig. 7**).

NATURAL HISTORY: TO OPERATE OR NOT TO OPERATE?

Symptomatic high-grade isthmic spondylolisthesis in children and adolescents has an unfavorable natural history, with a high risk of progression and low likelihood of symptomatic relief. Conservative treatment is generally not recommended in symptomatic patients, who constitute the majority of patients with high-grade slips in this age group.[45,46] Pizzutillo and colleagues[47] found that only 1 of 11 symptomatic patients treated conservatively had significant pain relief at long-term follow-up. Asymptomatic patients can be treated

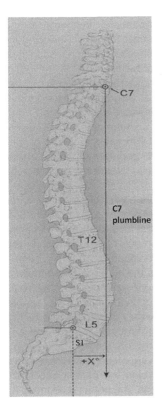

Fig. 7. Measurement of spinal vertical axis. The sagittal vertical axis is measured as the distance from the posterior superior corner of the sacrum to a vertical plumb line dropped from the C7 centroid (C7 plumb line).

with observation, and if symptoms do develop surgery is generally recommended. Some investigators have recommended surgical treatment for these patients regardless of symptoms, because of the high risk of progression.[46] However, Harris and Weinstein[5] reported that 10 of 11 patients with high-grade slips who were treated nonoperatively remained active and required only minor modifications in activity.

In contrast to children or adolescents, adults with high-grade slips have often reached a stable position and typically do not experience progression, making slip progression less of a concern. Autofusion or ankylosis of the slipped level can occur. Some of these patients are asymptomatic or minimally symptomatic, and can be successfully treated with physical therapy and selective nerve-root injections if radicular symptoms are present. If conservative treatment fails, surgery is recommended in adult patients who have high-grade slips with back pain and/or radicular symptoms. Unlike low-grade slips, whose manifestations are typically limited to painful segmental instability or neural compromise at the affected level, high-grade slips invariably provoke secondary changes in the regional pelvic anatomy and can thus produce global sagittal deformity with clinical manifestations of intractable back pain or deformity, which might be another indication for surgery.[33]

INDICATIONS FOR SURGERY: WHEN TO OPERATE?

1. *Slip progression.* Progression is more common in skeletally immature patients who have not reached the adolescent growth spurt. The higher the grade of slip, the more likely it is to progress. Slip progression rarely occurs in adults. Although asymptomatic progression alone may be considered an indication for surgery, patients with progressive slips frequently have significant pain that does not respond to conservative treatment.
2. *Sagittal alignment.* High-grade slip with significant lumbosacral kyphotic deformity causing sagittal spinopelvic malalignment.
3. *Neurologic deficit.* In most cases of neurologic deficit, the L5 nerve root is involved. Objective weakness is not common in this condition, but if present, surgery should be strongly considered to relieve nerve-root compression.
4. *Back pain.* Low back pain unresponsive to a prolonged course of conservative treatment.
5. *Leg symptoms.* Radicular pain with associated nerve-root compression on imaging studies that is not responsive to conservative treatment.

PEDIATRIC VERSUS ADULT HGS: ARE THEY THE SAME?

There are several important differences between the pediatric and adult population regarding the overall approach to the management of HGS.

1. With degenerative changes contributing to nerve-root compression, adults are more likely to require direct neural decompression. Even in the presence of radicular symptoms, pediatric and adolescent patients often experience symptom relief with fusion alone when a hypermobile segment is stabilized.

2. Considering the higher risk of pseudarthrosis in adults secondary to smoking, poor general health, and secondary comorbidities, instances whereby a posterior-only approach may be suitable for adolescents may not be appropriate in the adult, in whom a circumferential fusion may be advisable to increase the likelihood of fusion success.

3. Reduction of high-grade slips is generally more difficult in adults because of the increased rigidity of the deformity and stiffness across the lumbosacral junction. Because of the presence of secondary degenerative changes in adults, the deformity tends to be less mobile.

4. Risk of progression is higher in children and adolescents than in adults. The younger the patient is at the time of diagnosis, the greater the risk of progression, because the deformity is likely to progress during periods of active spinal growth. For this reason, slip progression is a more common indication for surgery in children and adolescents with high-grade slips. Progression is uncommon in adults, and surgery is rarely indicated for this reason in the adult patient. Most adults with high-grade slips who need surgery have pain or radicular symptoms that have not responded to conservative treatment or are secondary to the chronic deformity attributable to HGS.

TO REDUCE OR NOT TO REDUCE: WHAT IS THE PROBLEM WITH REDUCTION?

Although slip reduction was contemplated as early as 1921, associated unacceptably high rates of neurologic injury made many experts believe that in situ fusion was safer and produced acceptable results. As recently as 1976, Nachemson and Wiltse[48] stated without equivocation that in situ fusion worked so well that reduction was rarely warranted, citing an increased risk of neurologic complications, longer operative time, and greater blood loss with reduction. Nevertheless, some surgeons continued to pursue reduction, believing that correction of the underlying deformity was supported by sound mechanical principles and, in the right hands, could be safely accomplished. Over the last quarter-century, tremendous advances have been made in surgical techniques, particularly in the realm of spinal instrumentation, with the result that reduction can now be accomplished more safely and effectively than ever before. Along with the importance of restoring the sagittal alignment, this has once again rekindled the discussions between proponents of reduction and advocates of in situ fusion. Unfortunately, no randomized controlled trials exist to definitively answer the question of whether one of these approaches is superior, and most of the available evidence in favor of reduction or use of anterior column support has been from retrospective studies and case series.[4,14,31,35,39,49–66]

The primary rationale behind a reduction maneuver in severe slips is to correct the lumbosacral kyphotic deformity to improve the sagittal malalignment and the patient's ability to stand upright, with a secondary advantage of a reduction procedure being an improvement in fusion rate.[3,15,16,22,26,67,68] From a biomechanical standpoint, an in situ fusion performed in the setting of severe lumbosacral kyphosis is subjected to significant shear forces.[68] Reducing the lumbosacral kyphosis should improve the biomechanical environment for a fusion by converting the shear forces to compressive forces and reducing the risk of further progression of deformity. In contemporary surgical practice, the understanding of complex deformity often associated with HGS and its secondary effects on pelvic version and global sagittal alignment have reignited enthusiasm in reconsidering the role of reduction.[14,15,20,24,25,39,41,57,68] First, high-grade slips almost invariably have a dysplastic component,[29] with implications for the feasibility of fixation and posterolateral fusion; and the slip angle becomes a greater source of deformity than the degree of forward translation.[2,3,20,39] Second, the local deformity of the high-grade slip invariably induces compensatory changes in the regional pelvic anatomy—changes that are propagated up the spinal column, ultimately producing a global postural deformity.[33] As L5 slips anteriorly and then inferiorly on the sacrum, the mass gravity line (and with it the trunk and head) is drawn forward, forcing the patient into positive sagittal malalignment. The postural changes (tonic activation of the paraspinous muscles, retroversion of the pelvis, external rotation of hip, knee flexion) secondary to this represent the end stage of severe lumbosacral spondylolisthesis and are typically accompanied by clinical sequelae of low back pain, tight hamstrings, postural deformity, and in some cases radiculopathy or even cauda equina syndrome. Although proponents of in situ fusion have argued that good results are predictably obtained simply through the elimination of abnormal segmental motion, reduction offers several benefits over in situ fusion. First, in situ fusion has been consistently associated with higher rates of nonunion, up to 44% in some series, presumably attributable to the continued presence of powerful shear forces acting at the lumbosacral junction and to a decrease in available surface area for fusion, specifically as a result of significant dysplastic changes associated with HGS.[29,45,55] The troublesome phenomenon of slip progression despite solid fusion, which has been reported after in situ fusion in up to 26% of cases, is further testament to the perils of leaving the kyphotic deformity of severe lumbosacral spondylolisthesis uncorrected.[45,55] Labelle and colleagues[16] have shown that whereas sacropelvic shape (PI), which is an anatomic parameter, is unaffected by attempts at surgical reduction, proper repositioning of L5 over S1 through partial or complete reduction significantly improves sacropelvic alignment and the orientation of the lumbar spine in developmental spondylolisthesis. Their results also emphasize the importance of subdividing subjects with HGS into types 4, 5, and 6, and further support the contention that reduction techniques might preferably be considered for SDSG types 5 and 6, as has been suggested in other studies also.[25,26] Finally, although some patients may not express dissatisfaction with their appearance, there are many patients for whom cosmetic concerns remain paramount. For this subset of patients, surgery that does not incorporate some element of reduction will inevitably produce an inferior result.

Historically the principal argument against reduction has been focused on the associated unacceptably high rate of neurologic deficit. It must be emphasized, however, that iatrogenic neurologic deficit is not a constant finding after reduction, and that when neurologic deficits do occur they are typically transient, with rates of permanent neurologic deficit after reduction averaging 5% and rarely exceeding 10%.[69] Moreover, in situ fusion is not completely innocuous, and deficits have also been reported after in situ fusion.[63] In 1988, the Scoliosis Research Society (SRS) morbidity and mortality report indicated no difference in the rates of neurologic deficit after reduction and in situ fusion in this patient population. This finding was subsequently echoed in another report by Kasliwal and colleagues[69] from

the most recent SRS database on complication rates following surgery specifically for HGS. This report again demonstrated no difference in rates of neurologic deficits in patients with or without reduction of HGS. The existence of several series in which patients underwent reduction without neurologic complication is testament to the fact that, through adherence to the principles of wide decompression and judicious correction, reduction of high-grade lumbosacral spondylolisthesis can be achieved safely.[6,39,50,59] Moreover, partial reduction of the deformity, which also leads to correction of slip angle, may be adequate as opposed to full reduction, because slip angle has been correlated better than the degree of slip in predicting the risk of progression of spondylolisthesis.[39] Moreover, as studies have shown that most of the total L5 nerve strain occurs during the second half of reduction, attempting a partial reduction may be safer than total reduction, with the benefit of increasing the fusion rate and correcting overall deformity.[70]

Despite the facts that reduction offers overwhelming biomechanical advantages and that procedures not incorporating some degree of correction are at risk of providing an inferior result because of persistent physical deformity or construct failure, due in large part to the rarity of high-grade lumbosacral spondylolisthesis, no prospective studies exist comparing reduction with fusion in situ. A formal review of the literature by Transfeldt and Mehbod[7] found no randomized controlled trials or comparative prospective studies comparing fusion in situ versus reduction and fusion for HGS. In their analysis they found 5 comparative retrospective studies, none of which showed any benefit to reduction.[49,52,60,61,71] Of interest, Poussa and colleagues[49] found that in patients with HGS, the in situ fusion group performed better than the reduction group. However, there is ample evidence in the literature, mostly from retrospective studies and case series, reporting the safety of reduction procedures in HGS.[22,39,50,52,60,64,68,72–74]

In summary, at least partial reduction of the lumbosacral deformity should be considered in cases of HGS. Reducing the percentage of translation of L5 on S1 is of secondary importance because it is the lumbosacral kyphosis that is primarily responsible for the sagittal malalignment. Therefore, improvement of the slip angle should be the primary goal of any reduction attempt, and it has been recognized that partial reduction of the slip angle is the key to restoring sagittal alignment.[39] In situ fusion may be an option and may be preferred in the instance when the patient: (1) presents with back pain in the absence of radicular complaints, neurologic deficit, or cosmetic deformity; (2) has adequate neural foraminal space; and (3) has acceptable global sagittal spinopelvic alignment and good sagittal alignment of the proximal instrumented vertebra.

ANTERIOR COLUMN SUPPORT

Regardless of patient age, HGS creates increased shear stress at the lumbosacral junction. Various studies have reported high rates of pseudarthrosis and progression of the postoperative slip after posterior in situ fusion.[71,75] The addition of anterior column structural support not only provides greater stability at the lumbosacral junction but also, more importantly, leads to higher fusion rates because of the greater surface area available with an interbody fusion. Presence of significant dysplasia often associated with HGS leads to a reduction in the posterior surface area available for fusion, and hence lowers fusion rates in comparison with patients treated for low-grade slips.[29] If reduction is performed for HGS, circumferential fusion and stable fixation with iliac screws should be considered to prevent slip progression and pseudarthrosis. This aspect may be particularly relevant in patients with a high PI who have additional shear forces at the lumbosacral junction. If the severity of the slip precludes interbody fusion, a transsacral approach as described by Bohlman and Cook[76] can be used to provide anterior fixation, or the use of transvertebral fibular dowel and/or screws might be an option, as discussed next.[6,54,73]

SURGICAL OPTIONS
Basic Surgical Principles and Pearls

Irrespective of the surgical technique used, there are inherent principles that should be adhered to in order to maximize the chances of a successful outcome following the surgical treatment of HGS.

- The role of instrumentation is less controversial with high-grade slips. Instrumentation is recommended in patients who undergo in situ posterolateral fusion from L4 to S1.
- Partial reduction (particularly of slip angle) offers significant biomechanical advantages, whereas complete (anatomic) reduction though desirable is rarely necessary (**Fig. 8**).
- Wide decompression of the neural elements with particular attention to compressive dysmorphic elements (eg, fibrocartilaginous pars, sacral dome), in addition to judicious distractive reduction under direct visualization of the neural elements, is essential to avoid iatrogenic neural injury.
- Interbody fusion, whether performed from an anterior or posterior approach, may substantially improve the long-term success of the final construct.
- Consideration should be given to incorporating supplemental fixation such as iliac screws, S2 pedicle screws, and/or L4 pedicle screws to protect the construct from the powerful shear forces acting at the lumbosacral junction, especially if anatomic reduction is not performed. Extending the fusion proximally to L4 should be considered in HGS, especially if instability

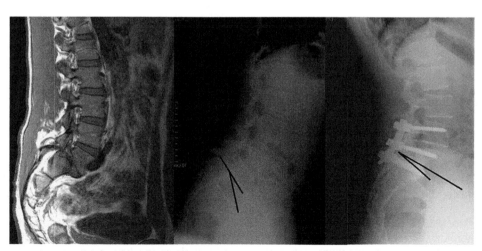

Fig. 8. Lateral parasagittal T1-weighted magnetic resonance image (*left*) and lateral standing radiograph (*middle*) of a 21-year-old male patient with intractable back pain and high-grade spondylolisthesis (grade IV). (*Right*) Postoperative radiograph demonstrating L4-S1 posterior segmental instrumentation and partial reduction of HGS to grade I with correction of the slip angle.

is present at the L4-L5 segment, if the L5 transverse processes are very small with minimal area for a fusion mass, or in the presence of degenerative changes/stenosis at the L4-L5 level that may be contributing to the patient's symptoms. In a high-grade slip, fusion from L5 to sacrum creates a horizontally oriented fusion, which is under high shear stress and prone to failure. Inclusion of L4 improves the mechanical advantage by creating a more vertical fusion. Another difficulty with fusion of L5 to sacrum in a high-grade slip is the anterior position of the L5 transverse processes in relation to the sacral ala, which makes fusion technically challenging.

- Consider transsacral, transvertebral fibular dowel and/or screws when anatomic reduction is not performed.[6,7,54,66,73,76]
- Consider using the Gaines method when reduction of spondyloptosis is deemed necessary.[77]

SURGICAL TECHNIQUES

The various surgical techniques for the management of HGS can be summarized as follows.

1. Posterolateral instrumented in situ fusion (with or without decompression)
2. Posterior reduction of spondylolisthesis, decompression, and instrumented posterolateral fusion
3. Posterior reduction of spondylolisthesis, decompression, and circumferential fusion
4. Transsacral fibular dowel graft supplemented with posterolateral instrumented fusion (no reduction attempt)
5. Spondylectomy for spondyloptosis

Posterior In Situ Fusion

Historically, the mainstay for HGS surgery in both adolescents and adults has been posterior in situ arthrodesis, and this approach has been recommended by many investigators. In light of the limitations associated with noninstrumented posterolateral fusions, most proponents of in situ arthrodesis now recommend the addition of instrumentation to the posterior in situ arthrodesis for adolescents and adults. Although the pendulum for management of HGS seems to be shifting more toward some attempt at reduction, in situ fusion with instrumentation may still be preferred in patients with grade 3 or 4 lumbosacral spondylolisthesis who (1) present with back pain in the absence of radicular complaints, neurologic deficit, or cosmetic deformity; (2) have adequate neural

foraminal space; and (3) have acceptable overall sagittal alignment and good sagittal alignment of the proximal instrumented vertebra.

Posterior Reduction of Spondylolisthesis, Decompression, and Instrumented Posterolateral Fusion

To avoid the neurologic risks associated with reduction procedures and the high pseudarthrosis rates seen with posterior in situ arthrodesis without instrumentation, it has been generally accepted that posterior spinal fusion with instrumentation has become the standard for patients with higher-grade spondylolisthesis. However, there has been mounting evidence recently in favor of the safety and efficacy of posterior reduction of spondylolisthesis, decompression, and instrumented posterolateral fusion. Hu[67] attempted to use autogenous iliac or fibular struts to provide anterior column support in HGS following partial reduction. However, often the severity of high-grade slips can make an anterior interbody approach extremely challenging. In the modern era, pedicle screw-rod fixation remains the most common instrumentation; however, considering the challenges associated with transpedicular screws into the listhesed L5 pedicles associated with HGS, transvertebral screws, in which transsacral S1 pedicle screws are extended across the sacral promontory into the slipped L5 vertebral body, may be successfully used in these cases, and not only provide support for the L5 body anterior to the sacrum but achieve tricortical bony purchase through the sacrum and L5 body. Fibular dowels and various cage implants have also been inserted through the sacrum into the L5 body through a posterior approach with good results, providing another option in patients who are difficult to reduce (see **Fig. 1**). As the L5 vertebral body slips anterior to the sacrum, a fibular strut can be inserted through the sacrum into the body of L5 through a reamed canal. Despite the perceived difficulty in this procedure, there is a general lack of reports of neurologic injury associated with this technique.

Posterior Reduction of Spondylolisthesis, Decompression, and Circumferential Fusion

In general, the use of interbody support is recommended for HGS to aid in deformity correction, provide greater stability at the lumbosacral junction, and facilitate higher fusion rates. Regardless of patient age, HGS creates increased shear stress at the lumbosacral junction, with multiple studies reporting high rates of pseudarthrosis and progression of the postoperative slip after posterior in situ fusion.[38,45,55,76,78] This situation arises because a posterior fusion mass in HGS is exposed to high tensile forces. Anterior interbody arthrodesis can be performed through separate anterior and posterior approaches or through a posterior approach alone (PLIF or TLIF). Molinari and colleagues[51] reported higher fusion rates following anterior support and arthrodesis when compared with posterior lateral fusion alone. Although there is absence of high-quality evidence to enable definitive recommendations, if reduction is performed, circumferential fusion should be strongly considered to improve the overall biomechanics for fusion and greater stability. This procedure may be particularly relevant in patients with a high PI who have additional shear forces at the lumbosacral junction. Also, the presence of significant dysplasia often associated with HGS leads to a reduction in the surface area available for fusion, and hence lowers fusion rates in comparison with patients with low-grade slips in the absence of anterior column support.[29]

Transsacral Fibular Dowel Graft Supplemented with Posterolateral Instrumented Fusion (No Reduction Attempt)

Methods that can be used to obtain a circumferential fusion include staged anterior and posterior approaches, a posterior (or transforaminal) lumbar interbody approach, and the transsacral approach. If the severity of the slip precludes interbody fusion, a transsacral approach as described by Bohlman and Cook[76] can be used to provide anterior fixation.[76] The angle of the lumbosacral disc space in HGS can make discectomy and arthrodesis difficult, requiring osteotomizing the anterior inferior corner of L5 to allow exposure of the L5-S1 disc space during an anterior approach. With severe slips an interbody fusion may not be possible, owing to minimal bony contact between the L5 and S1 vertebral bodies. Therefore, other methods of anterior column fusion can be pursued, which may involve either a transsacral approach using a fibular dowel or using transvertebral screws as described earlier.[6,73,76] Although reduction is not necessary with this technique, some investigators have performed a partial reduction followed by transsacral fusion with resection of the dome of the sacrum if additional lumbosacral kyphosis correction was desired.[54,66] Performance of sacral dome osteotomy, however, can be associated with an increased risk of neurologic deficit and should be kept in mind.[69]

Spondylectomy for Spondyloptosis

The Gaines vertebral resection remains an option for grade 5 spondylolistheses or spondyloptosis.[72,77]

In these higher-grade and optosis deformities, the L5 vertebra is not in bony contact with the superior endplate of the sacrum, making the surgical approach challenging. The L5 vertebral body can be resected through an anterior retroperitoneal spinal approach and the vertebral body of L4, then placed directly superior to the S1 body and secured with pedicle screw-rod instrumentation.

COMPLICATIONS

The main complications associated with the surgical management of adult HGS include neurologic deficits (permanent or temporary), pseudarthrosis, instrumentation failure, accelerated adjacent segment degeneration, durotomy, malposition/failure, and deep wound infection.[69,79] Apart from the experience of the treating surgeon and clinical presentation, the potential for complications often significantly affects the choice of approach for the management of HGS, especially considering that there is currently no definitive literature proving the superiority of one approach over another.[7] Occurrence of new neurologic deficits remains the most common and among the most concerning complications with surgery for HGS, and the overall incidence has been reported to be approximately 10%.[69] Although performance of a reduction maneuver has been traditionally thought of as increasing the chances of neurologic deficit, there are no high-quality data supporting this presumption, and various studies have documented the rates of neurologic deficit being the same irrespective of whether a reduction maneuver is performed.[50,69,74] Anecdotal experience from some surgeons have suggested a role of keeping the patients in bed with knees and hips flexed immediately in the postoperative period following HGS reduction, to decrease stretch on L5 nerves and thus lower the incidence of foot drop. Fortunately many of the postoperative neurologic deficits resolve over time, with reports suggesting that only about 10% (1% overall) may be permanent.[14,41,60,64,69] The use of neuromonitoring during surgery for HGS may reduce the incidence of postoperative neurologic deficits, and its use has become more prevalent, especially when reduction maneuvers are planned. Nevertheless, there is a lack of published high-quality data demonstrating the benefit of neuromonitoring in reducing the incidence of postoperative neurologic deficits. Performance of a sacral dome osteotomy has been shown to be associated with a significantly higher incidence of new neurologic deficits, and caution should be exercised when performing this procedure. Although the addition of instrumentation and anterior interbody structural grafts has improved fusion rates, adjacent segment degeneration has been reported to occur in as many as 35% of cases and may require extension of instrumentation, often including iliac fixation.[80] Although the incidences are generally low, apart from surgical and neurologic complications these patients are prone to develop other complications such as peripheral nerve palsy associated with positioning, respiratory complications including pulmonary embolism, epidural hematoma, deep venous thrombosis, and postoperative visual acuity deficit.[69,79]

SUMMARY

Management of high-grade lumbosacral spondylolisthesis is complex and is associated with significant controversies. Although there is general consensus on the need for surgical treatment of symptomatic patients presenting with severe pain, neurologic deficits, or progressive deformity once symptomatic or progressive, the optimal surgical approach and techniques remain controversial. Recent advances in spinal instrumentation, improved understanding of the pelvic anatomy and its role in determining sagittal spinopelvic alignment, and its influence on the development of HGS have had a significant impact on surgical management of HGS. Although not proven in randomized studies, posterior instrumented fixation and fusion with attempted partial deformity reduction and interbody structural support have been gaining widespread acceptance, and have been shown to provide satisfactory rates of fusion and a good clinical outcome. Regardless of the choice of surgical technique, significant complications can be associated with the surgical treatment of HGS and may dictate the type of surgical approach chosen.

REFERENCES

1. Meyerding HW. Spondylolisthesis; surgical fusion of lumbosacral portion of spinal column and interarticular facets; use of autogenous bone grafts for relief of disabling backache. J Int Coll Surg 1956;26:566–91.
2. Tanguay F, Labelle H, Wang Z, et al. Clinical significance of lumbosacral kyphosis in adolescent spondylolisthesis. Spine 2012;37:304–8.
3. Labelle H, Mac-Thiong JM, Roussouly P. Spinopelvic sagittal balance of spondylolisthesis: a review and classification. Eur Spine J 2011;20(Suppl 5): 641–6.
4. Goyal N, Wimberley DW, Hyatt A, et al. Radiographic and clinical outcomes after instrumented reduction and transforaminal lumbar interbody fusion of mid and high-grade isthmic spondylolisthesis. J Spinal Disord Tech 2009;22:321–7.
5. Harris IE, Weinstein SL. Long-term follow-up of patients with grade-III and IV spondylolisthesis. Treatment with and without posterior fusion. J Bone Joint Surg Am 1987;69:960–9.
6. Lakshmanan P, Ahuja S, Lewis M, et al. Transsacral screw fixation for high-grade spondylolisthesis. Spine J 2009;9:1024–9.
7. Transfeldt EE, Mehbod AA. Evidence-based medicine analysis of isthmic spondylolisthesis treatment including reduction versus fusion in situ for high-grade slips. Spine 2007;32:S126–9.
8. Newman PH. Degenerative spondylolisthesis. Orthop Clin North Am 1975;6:197–8.
9. Wynne-Davies R, Scott JH. Inheritance and spondylolisthesis: a radiographic family survey. J Bone Joint Surg Br 1979;61:301–5.
10. Dietrich M, Kurowski P. The importance of mechanical factors in the etiology of spondylolysis. A model analysis of loads and stresses in human lumbar spine. Spine 1985;10:532–42.
11. Letts M, Smallman T, Afanasiev R, et al. Fracture of the pars interarticularis in adolescent athletes: a clinical-biomechanical analysis. J Pediatr Orthop 1986; 6:40–6.
12. Krenz J, Troup JD. The structure of the pars interarticularis of the lower lumbar vertebrae and its relation to the etiology of spondylolysis, with a report of a healing fracture in the neural arch of a fourth lumbar vertebra. J Bone Joint Surg Br 1973;55:735–41.
13. Fredrickson BE, Baker D, McHolick WJ, et al. The natural history of spondylolysis and spondylolisthesis. J Bone Joint Surg Am 1984;66:699–707.
14. DeWald CJ, Vartabedian JE, Rodts MF, et al. Evaluation and management of high-grade spondylolisthesis in adults. Spine 2005;30:S49–59.
15. Labelle H, Roussouly P, Berthonnaud E, et al. The importance of spino-pelvic balance in L5-s1 developmental spondylolisthesis: a review of pertinent radiologic measurements. Spine 2005;30:S27–34.
16. Labelle H, Roussouly P, Chopin D, et al. Spino-pelvic alignment after surgical correction for developmental spondylolisthesis. Eur Spine J 2008;17: 1170–6.
17. Schwab FJ, Lafage V, Farcy JP, et al. Predicting outcome and complications in the surgical treatment of adult scoliosis. Spine 2008;33:2243–7.
18. Lafage V, Schwab F, Skalli W, et al. Standing balance and sagittal plane spinal deformity: analysis of spinopelvic and gravity line parameters. Spine 2008;33:1572–8.
19. Lafage V, Schwab F, Patel A, et al. Pelvic tilt and truncal inclination: two key radiographic parameters in the setting of adults with spinal deformity. Spine 2009;34:E599–606.
20. Labelle H, Roussouly P, Berthonnaud E, et al. Spondylolisthesis, pelvic incidence, and spinopelvic balance: a correlation study. Spine 2004;29:2049–54.

21. Huang RP, Bohlman HH, Thompson GH, et al. Predictive value of pelvic incidence in progression of spondylolisthesis. Spine 2003;28:2381–5.

22. Lamartina C, Zavatsky JM, Petruzzi M, et al. Novel concepts in the evaluation and treatment of high-dysplastic spondylolisthesis. Eur Spine J 2009; 18(Suppl 1):133–42.

23. Hanson DS, Bridwell KH, Rhee JM, et al. Correlation of pelvic incidence with low- and high-grade isthmic spondylolisthesis. Spine 2002;27:2026–9.

24. Mac-Thiong JM, Duong L, Parent S, et al. Reliability of the Spinal Deformity Study Group classification of lumbosacral spondylolisthesis. Spine 2012;37:E95–102.

25. Mac-Thiong JM, Labelle H, Parent S, et al. Reliability and development of a new classification of lumbosacral spondylolisthesis. Scoliosis 2008;3:19.

26. Hresko MT, Labelle H, Roussouly P, et al. Classification of high-grade spondylolistheses based on pelvic version and spine balance: possible rationale for reduction. Spine 2007;32:2208–13.

27. Hammerberg KW. New concepts on the pathogenesis and classification of spondylolisthesis. Spine 2005;30:S4–11.

28. Hammerberg KW. Spondylolysis and spondylolisthesis. In: DeWald RL, editor. Spinal deformities: the comprehensive text. 1st edition. New York: Thieme; 2003. p. 787–801.

29. Pawar A, Labelle H, Mac-Thiong JM. The evaluation of lumbosacral dysplasia in young patients with lumbosacral spondylolisthesis: comparison with controls and relationship with the severity of slip. Eur Spine J 2012;21(11):2122–7.

30. Hresko MT, Hirschfeld R, Buerk AA, et al. The effect of reduction and instrumentation of spondylolisthesis on spinopelvic sagittal alignment. J Pediatr Orthop 2009; 29:157–62.

31. Agabegi SS, Fischgrund JS. Contemporary management of isthmic spondylolisthesis: pediatric and adult. Spine J 2010;10:530–43.

32. Jones TR, Rao RD. Adult isthmic spondylolisthesis. J Am Acad Orthop Surg 2009;17:609–17.

33. Lenke LG, Bridwell KH. Evaluation and surgical treatment of high-grade isthmic dysplastic spondylolisthesis. Instr Course Lect 2003;52:525–32.

34. Ploumis A, Hantzidis P, Dimitriou C. High-grade dysplastic spondylolisthesis and spondyloptosis: report of three cases with surgical treatment and review of the literature. Acta Orthop Belg 2005;71: 750–7.

35. Li Y, Hresko MT. Radiographic analysis of spondylolisthesis and sagittal spinopelvic deformity. J Am Acad Orthop Surg 2012;20:194–205.

36. Bourassa-Moreau E, Mac-Thiong JM, Labelle H. Redefining the technique for the radiologic measurement of slip in spondylolisthesis. Spine 2010;35:1401–5.

37. Glavas P, Mac-Thiong JM, Parent S, et al. Assessment of lumbosacral kyphosis in spondylolisthesis: a computer-assisted reliability study of six measurement techniques. Eur Spine J 2009;18:212–7.

38. Dubousset J. Treatment of spondylolysis and spondylolisthesis in children and adolescents. Clin Orthop Relat Res 1997;(337):77–85.

39. Sasso RC, Shively KD, Reilly TM. Transvertebral transsacral strut grafting for high-grade isthmic spondylolisthesis L5-S1 with fibular allograft. J Spinal Disord Tech 2008;21:328–33.

40. Mac-Thiong JM, Labelle H. A proposal for a surgical classification of pediatric lumbosacral spondylolisthesis based on current literature. Eur Spine J 2006;15(10):1425–35.

41. Lonstein JE. Spondylolisthesis in children. Cause, natural history, and management. Spine 1999;24: 2640–8.

42. Vialle R, Schmit P, Dauzac C, et al. Radiological assessment of lumbosacral dystrophic changes in high-grade spondylolisthesis. Skeletal Radiol 2005; 34:528–35.

43. Yue WM, Brodner W, Gaines RW. Abnormal spinal anatomy in 27 cases of surgically corrected spondyloptosis: proximal sacral endplate damage as a possible cause of spondyloptosis. Spine 2005; 30:S22–6.

44. Mac-Thiong JM, Labelle H, Parent S, et al. Assessment of sacral doming in lumbosacral spondylolisthesis. Spine 2007;32:1888–95.

45. Boxall D, Bradford DS, Winter RB, et al. Management of severe spondylolisthesis in children and adolescents. J Bone Joint Surg Am 1979;61:479–95.

46. Pizzutillo PD, Hummer CD 3rd. Nonoperative treatment for painful adolescent spondylolysis or spondylolisthesis. J Pediatr Orthop 1989;9:538–40.

47. Pizzutillo PD, Mirenda W, MacEwen GD. Posterolateral fusion for spondylolisthesis in adolescence. J Pediatr Orthop 1986;6:311–6.

48. Nachemson A, Wiltse LL. Editorial: spondylolisthesis. Clin Orthop Relat Res 1976;(117):2–3.

49. Poussa M, Remes V, Lamberg T, et al. Treatment of severe spondylolisthesis in adolescence with reduction or fusion in situ: long-term clinical, radiologic, and functional outcome. Spine 2006;31:583–90 [discussion: 91–2].

50. Ruf M, Koch H, Melcher RP, et al. Anatomic reduction and monosegmental fusion in high-grade developmental spondylolisthesis. Spine 2006;31:269–74.

51. Molinari RW, Bridwell KH, Lenke LG, et al. Anterior column support in surgery for high-grade, isthmic spondylolisthesis. Clin Orthop Relat Res 2002;(394):109–20.

52. Molinari RW, Bridwell KH, Klepps SJ, et al. Minimum 5-year follow-up of anterior column structural allografts in the thoracic and lumbar spine. Spine 1999;24:967–72.

53. Acosta FL Jr, Ames CP, Chou D. Operative management of adult high-grade lumbosacral spondylolisthesis. Neurosurg Clin N Am 2007;18:249–54.

54. Boachie-Adjei O, Do T, Rawlins BA. Partial lumbosacral kyphosis reduction, decompression, and posterior lumbosacral transfixation in high-grade isthmic spondylolisthesis: clinical and radiographic results in six patients. Spine 2002;27:E161–8.

55. Boos N, Marchesi D, Zuber K, et al. Treatment of severe spondylolisthesis by reduction and pedicular fixation. A 4-6-year follow-up study. Spine 1993;18:1655–61.

56. Bridwell KH. Utilization of iliac screws and structural interbody grafting for revision spondylolisthesis surgery. Spine 2005;30:S88–96.

57. Bridwell KH. Surgical treatment of high-grade spondylolisthesis. Neurosurg Clin N Am 2006;17:331–8, vii.

58. Karampalis C, Grevitt M, Shafafy M, et al. High-grade spondylolisthesis: gradual reduction using Magerl's external fixator followed by circumferential fusion technique and long-term results. Eur Spine J 2012;21(Suppl 2):S200–6.

59. Molinari RW, Bridwell KH, Lenke LG, et al. Complications in the surgical treatment of pediatric high-grade, isthmic dysplastic spondylolisthesis. A comparison of three surgical approaches. Spine 1999;24:1701–11.

60. Muschik M, Zippel H, Perka C. Surgical management of severe spondylolisthesis in children and adolescents. Anterior fusion in situ versus anterior spondylodesis with posterior transpedicular instrumentation and reduction. Spine 1997;22:2036–42 [discussion: 43].

61. Poussa M, Schlenzka D, Seitsalo S, et al. Surgical treatment of severe isthmic spondylolisthesis in adolescents. Reduction or fusion in situ. Spine 1993;18:894–901.

62. Remes V, Lamberg T, Tervahartiala P, et al. Long-term outcome after posterolateral, anterior, and circumferential fusion for high-grade isthmic spondylolisthesis in children and adolescents: magnetic resonance imaging findings after average of 17-year follow-up. Spine 2006;31:2491–9.

63. Schoenecker PL, Cole HO, Herring JA, et al. Cauda equina syndrome after in situ arthrodesis for severe spondylolisthesis at the lumbosacral junction. J Bone Joint Surg Am 1990;72:369–77.

64. Shufflebarger HL, Geck MJ. High-grade isthmic dysplastic spondylolisthesis: monosegmental surgical treatment. Spine 2005;30:S42–8.

65. Slosar PJ, Reynolds JB, Koestler M. The axial cage. A pilot study for interbody fusion in higher-grade spondylolisthesis. Spine 2001;1:115–20.

66. Smith JA, Deviren V, Berven S, et al. Clinical outcome of trans-sacral interbody fusion after partial reduction for high-grade L5-S1 spondylolisthesis. Spine 2001;26:2227–34.

67. Hu SS, Bradford DS, Transfeldt EE, et al. Reduction of high-grade spondylolisthesis using Edwards instrumentation. Spine 1996;21:367–71.

68. Martiniani M, Lamartina C, Specchia N. "In situ" fusion or reduction in high-grade high dysplastic developmental spondylolisthesis (HDSS). Eur Spine J 2012;21(Suppl 1):S134–40.

69. Kasliwal MK, Smith JS, Shaffrey CI, et al. Short-term complications associated with surgery for high-grade spondylolisthesis in adults and pediatric patients: a report from the Scoliosis Research Society morbidity and mortality database. Neurosurgery 2012;71:109–16.

70. Petraco DM, Spivak JM, Cappadona JG, et al. An anatomic evaluation of L5 nerve stretch in spondylolisthesis reduction. Spine 1996;21:1133–8 [discussion: 9].

71. Burkus JK, Lonstein JE, Winter RB, et al. Long-term evaluation of adolescents treated operatively for spondylolisthesis. A comparison of in situ arthrodesis only with in situ arthrodesis and reduction followed by immobilization in a cast. J Bone Joint Surg Am 1992;74:693–704.

72. Gaines RW. L5 vertebrectomy for the surgical treatment of spondyloptosis: thirty cases in 25 years. Spine 2005;30:S66–70.

73. Hanson DS, Bridwell KH, Rhee JM, et al. Dowel fibular strut grafts for high-grade dysplastic isthmic spondylolisthesis. Spine 2002;27:1982–8.

74. Sailhan F, Gollogly S, Roussouly P. The radiographic results and neurologic complications of instrumented reduction and fusion of high-grade spondylolisthesis without decompression of the neural elements: a retrospective review of 44 patients. Spine 2006;31:161–9 [discussion: 70].

75. Frennered AK, Danielson BI, Nachemson AL, et al. Midterm follow-up of young patients fused in situ for spondylolisthesis. Spine 1991;16:409–16.

76. Bohlman HH, Cook SS. One-stage decompression and posterolateral and interbody fusion for lumbosacral spondyloptosis through a posterior approach. Report of two cases. J Bone Joint Surg Am 1982;64:415–8.

77. Gaines RW, Nichols WK. Treatment of spondyloptosis by two stage L5 vertebrectomy and reduction of L4 onto S1. Spine 1985;10:680–6.

78. Stanton RP, Meehan P, Lovell WW. Surgical fusion in childhood spondylolisthesis. J Pediatr Orthop 1985;5:411–5.

79. Ogilvie JW. Complications in spondylolisthesis surgery. Spine 2005;30:S97–101.

80. Okuda S, Iwasaki M, Miyauchi A, et al. Risk factors for adjacent segment degeneration after PLIF. Spine 2004;29:1535–40.

Health Economic Analysis of Adult Deformity Surgery

Ian McCarthy, PhD[a,b,*], Richard Hostin, MD[c],
Michael O'Brien, MD[c], Rajiv Saigal, MD[d],
Christopher P. Ames, MD[d]

KEYWORDS

- Spine deformity surgery • Adult spinal deformity • Healthy economics studies
- Health-related quality of life

KEY POINTS

- The last decade has witnessed a substantial increase in the frequency and expense of spine deformity surgeries.
- With increasing economic scrutiny, spine deformity surgeries must be done more efficiently, and maintaining quality of care in the face of such economic pressures requires continued development in health economics research in adult spinal deformity.
- This article reviews the literature on the costs and health-related quality-of-life outcomes after adult deformity surgery, as well as cost effectiveness and decision modeling.
- This article introduces future areas of health economics research in adult spine deformity, including bundled payments and demand for surgical treatment.

INTRODUCTION

Health economics is a broad field, covering a wide range of topics from single-center cost-effectiveness studies to large-scale health services research. The discipline primarily concerns questions of health policy, including the determinants and distribution of health and access to health care, optimal delivery of health care services, and optimal allocation of resources among competing health care uses.[1] The field draws heavily from microeconomic theory as well as applied econometrics and statistics.

When considered in the context of specific medical conditions or treatments, health economics generally takes the form of cost- or comparative-effectiveness studies (including value-based insurance design and cost sharing), utilization and demand analysis, and bundled payment analysis (including calculation and guidance regarding implementation). In the general spine literature, health economics studies have traditionally focused on cost effectiveness and utilization of treatments for low back pain, with particular emphasis on the trends, expense, quality-of-life improvements, and cost effectiveness of spine surgery. However, only recently has health economics made its way to the literature specifically on adult spinal deformity (ASD).

The purpose of this article is 2-fold. First, we hope to introduce areas in which health economics might play some role in future research on ASD. Second, the article provides an update on the current state of health economics studies in the ASD literature. We do not intend for this article to be a comprehensive guide for how to effectively evaluate health care

[a] Institute for Health Care Research and Improvement, Baylor Health Care System, Dallas, TX, USA; [b] Southern Methodist University, Dallas, TX, USA; [c] Baylor Scoliosis Center, Plano, TX, USA; [d] University of California San Francisco, San Francisco, CA, USA
* Corresponding author. Institute for Health Care Research and Improvement, Baylor Health Care System, Dallas, TX.
E-mail address: Ian.McCarthy@baylorhealth.edu

Neurosurg Clin N Am 24 (2013) 293–304
http://dx.doi.org/10.1016/j.nec.2012.12.005
1042-3680/13/$ – see front matter © 2013 Elsevier Inc. All rights reserved.

programs from an economic perspective. We leave this to the many health economics experts and texts that have already laid out such guides in much more detail and accuracy.[1-5]

TRENDS IN SPINAL DEFORMITY SURGERY

From a clinical perspective, ASD is defined simply as an abnormal curvature of the spine in patients who have completed their growth. The condition is distinct from more common spine problems such as lumbar spinal stenosis or herniated discs. However, despite clinical distinctions between ASD and other spine problems, there is some overlap in the treatment of spinal deformity and treatment of more common spine conditions such as herniated discs. In fact, the application of complex spinal fusion surgeries to more common spine problems (eg, incorporating spinal fusions with discectomies for patients with herniated discs and radiculopathy) has been under scrutiny over the last several years.[6,7]

Overlap in treatment complicates the identification of patients with ASD based purely on diagnosis-related groups or procedure codes. To briefly review the trends in spinal deformity surgery, we therefore follow the literature and identify spine deformity surgeries based on the International Classification of Diseases, Ninth Revision, Clinical Modification (ICD-9-CM) principal diagnosis codes.[8]

Fig. 1 presents total discharges by payor type undergoing surgical treatment of spinal deformity from 1993 through 2010. From 2000 to 2010, the figure illustrates a 4-fold increase in the number of spine deformity surgeries for Medicare patients and a 70% increase for managed care patients. The Medicare population, therefore, accounts for most of the growth in spine deformity surgeries of the past decade. Over this same period, the mean length of stay for Medicare patients decreased from 7.4 days to 6.2 days (16%), with a similar 16% decrease in length of stay for managed care patients (from 6.7 to 5.6 days). Yet, despite the apparent increase in efficiency based on reduced length of stay, the average charge per inpatient stay has increased more than 230% for Medicare patients and approximately 190% for managed care patients from 2000 to 2010, as illustrated in Fig. 2.

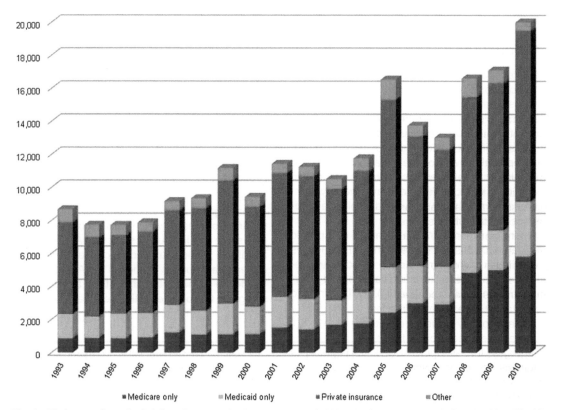

Fig. 1. Discharges for spinal deformity surgeries by payor type (1993–2010). Note: Spine deformity identified by ICD-9-CM principal diagnosis codes 737.0–737.9. (*Data from* Healthcare Cost and Utilization Project (HCUP), National Inpatient Sample. Available at: www.hcupnet.ahrq.gov/. Accessed September 15, 2012.)

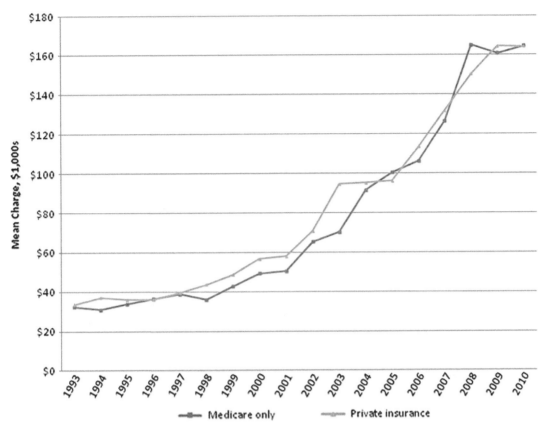

Fig. 2. Average charge for spinal deformity surgery by payor type (1993–2010). Note: Spine deformity identified by ICD-9-CM principal diagnosis codes 737.0-737.9. (*Data from* Healthcare Cost and Utilization Project (HCUP), National Inpatient Sample. Available at: www.hcupnet.ahrq.gov/. Accessed September 15, 2012.)

Combining the average charge figures with the total number of discharges, we estimate total charges for spine deformity surgeries in **Fig. 3.** Over the last decade, total charges for spine deformity surgery for Medicare patients increased from $56 million to more than $958 million, a 16-fold increase, whereas total charges for the managed care population increased nearly 4-fold from $344 million to more than $1.7 billion. Of course, charges are a flawed measure of either costs or payments, but trends in charges over time are still informative and relevant to the growing health economics literature in this area. Together, **Figs. 1–3** indicate a substantial increase in the frequency and expense of spine deformity surgeries over the last 10 years.

As a reference point, the total number of discharges for all spine nondeformity primary diagnosis codes increased from 675,470 in 2000 to 813,849 in 2010 (20% increase). For the Medicare and managed care populations, respectively, total discharges increased from 220,793 to 328,750 (49%) and from 320,274 to 332,935 (4.0%) over the same period. These figures are

dwarfed by the 400% and 70% increase in spine deformity discharges among the Medicare and managed care populations, respectively. Average charges for nondeformity spine surgery have increased more than average charges for deformity surgeries; however, when adjusting for the decrease in length of stay in spine deformity surgeries over the same period, the average charge for deformity surgeries has increased at a faster rate than that for nondeformity surgeries among Medicare patients. These data are summarized in **Table 1.**

HEALTH ECONOMICS RESEARCH IN ASD

Given the intense economic scrutiny placed on spine fusion surgeries in general,[6,8,9] the comparison above is particularly telling—in the likely near future, complex spine deformity surgeries must be done more efficiently, and maintaining quality of care in the face of such economic pressures requires continued development in health economics research in ASD.

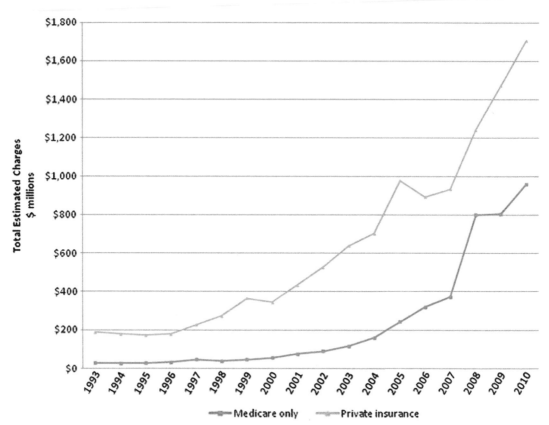

Fig. 3. Total estimated charges for spinal deformity surgery by payor type (1993–2010). Note: Spine deformity identified by ICD-9-CM principal diagnosis codes 737.0-737.9. (*Data from* Healthcare Cost and Utilization Project (HCUP), National Inpatient Sample. Available at: www.hcupnet.ahrq.gov/. Accessed September 15, 2012.)

There are 2 areas in the ASD literature in which health economics research has become relatively standard: (1) analyses of health-related quality-of-life (HRQOL) outcomes after surgery and (2) analyses of the cost of surgical treatment. Two additional areas in which health economics research in ASD is slowly emerging but not yet fully adopted include cost-effectiveness studies and

Table 1
Average charge, length of stay, and charge per day for deformity and nondeformity spine surgeries

	Nondeformity		Deformity	
	Medicare	**Managed Care**	**Medicare**	**Managed Care**
Average Charge				
2000	$15,167	$16,278	$49,399	$56,730
2010	$52,415	$59,133	$164,538	$164,285
Length of Stay				
2000	4.4	2.9	7.4	6.7
2010	4.0	2.9	6.2	5.6
Charge per Day				
2000	$3447	$5613	$6676	$8467
2010	$13,104	$20,391	$26,538	$29,337
% Increase in Charge per Day	280.1	263.3	297.5	246.5

decision modeling. We review the literature in each of these 4 areas in more detail below.

Health-Related Quality-of-Life Outcomes

Of the existing quality-of-life studies on surgical treatment of ASD, authors often compare pre- and postoperative HRQOL measures and analyze whether significant improvements in HRQOL were observed. Common instruments in the spinal deformity literature include the disease-specific 22-item and 30-item Scoliosis Research Society (SRS) questionnaires (SRS-22 and SRS-30, respectively), the regional-specific Oswestry Disability Index (ODI), and Medical Outcomes Study Short Form 36 and 12-item general health questionnaires (SF-36 and SF-12, respectively), all of which have been validated and applied in spinal deformity.[10–17] Adopting these measures, Glassman and colleagues[18] reported a significant improvement in patients' SRS-22, SF-12 Physical Component Scores, and ODI scores after surgery. The authors also found that HRQOL measures improved the most over the first year after surgery, stabilizing thereafter with generally no significant change from 1-year to 2-year follow-up. Many other studies have similarly found significant improvements in HRQOL scores after surgical treatment for ASD.[19–21]

Concerned that improvement in HRQOL scores does not necessarily translate into a clinically discernible qualitative improvement in HRQOL, investigators have also studied the proportion of patients reporting a minimum clinically important difference (MCID) in HRQOL improvement. To this point, however, there is little agreement in the literature regarding the appropriate MCID for different outcome measures. For example, in a comprehensive literature review covering both general spine and spine deformity, Yadla and colleagues[22] cite 15 studies reporting pre- and postoperative ODI scores, with an average improvement of 15.7 points and MCID of 3.1–32.3 points. Bagó and colleagues[23] reported the MCID in SRS scores of 0.6 points in the pain domain, 0.3 points in functional activity, 1.3 points in self-image, and 0.4 points in mental health.

The application of MCID in HRQOL research remains an area of debate, and although the general concept has been around for more than 20 years, much of the literature remains in flux.[24] Conceptually, MCID avoids the use of statistically significant results that are qualitatively meaningless and dovetails with the general distinction between practical relevance and statistical significance. But despite its intuitive appeal, the appropriate estimation and use of MCID remain unclear. At least 2 general estimation strategies have been espoused in the literature: (1) the anchor-based approach and (2) the distributional approach.[25,26] The anchor-based approach uses some external responses, such whether the patient reported feeling better or worse after treatment, and calculates the MCID by comparing the HRQOL of patients in the better group with those of the worse group. Conversely, the distributional approach calculates MCID based on the within-sample change in HRQOL scores relative to some measure of variability in the distribution. The distributional approach, therefore, bases its calculation of MCID on existing HRQOL responses and does not rely on an external criterion.

Each approach carries with it some potential flaws.[24,26] For example, in practice, the external criterion used in the anchor-based approach is often some other subjective questionnaire. In such a case, it can be argued that the MCID is essentially converting one subjective measure to match another. Conversely, the distributional approach attempts to provide a statistical framework around the calculation of the MCID. For example, some investigators estimate MCID as one standard error above the mean score. Far from an alternative to statistical significance, this approach largely amounts to changing the threshold for statistical significance. The point here is not to argue for or against the MCID but rather to discuss some of the potential conceptual problems in its calculation. In spirit, the MCID is an excellent concept and could be an important part of HRQOL research; however, to date, many questions remain regarding how the measure is calculated and ultimately its appropriateness in identifying evidence-based practices.

Although there is increasing awareness in the literature regarding the importance of HRQOL research, few existing studies formally analyze the potential causal factors underlying patients' self-reported HRQOL improvements after ASD surgery.[10,18] The determinants of HRQOL improvements are important given the potential disconnect between common clinical and radiographic outcomes (eg, fusion status) and a patient's quality of life after spine surgery.[18] As such, HRQOL measures may provide clinically relevant information separate from radiographic measurements. A patient-centered, evidence-based decision analysis should, therefore, incorporate not only the standard radiographic measures but also the patient's predicted HRQOL improvement from surgery. Improved HRQOL analyses can also be used to develop more formal cost-effectiveness studies regarding the incremental benefit and costs of surgical versus nonsurgical treatment.

Unfortunately, statistically modeling the causal factors of HRQOL improvements is far from straightforward. One difficulty lies in the multidimensional nature of existing questionnaires used in the ASD literature. For example, the SRS-22/30 questionnaire yields a summary score in each of 5 dimensions (functional activity, self-image, mental health, pain, and satisfaction) in addition to an overall summary score calculated as a weighted average of each individual domain. But an average across domains does not account for patient preference (ie, patient 1 may care only about functional activity and pain, whereas patient 2 may weigh more heavily their self-image and mental health). Researchers are then left to answer, on their own, what does it mean if a surgical patient improves in functional activity but deteriorates in pain? Is this patient better or worse off after surgery?

This problem does not emerge in all HRQOL questionnaires. For example, researchers using the EQ-5D, the SF-6D, or the Health Utilities Index (HUI1, HUI2, or HUI3) have developed scoring algorithms to collapse the HRQOL responses in each dimension into a single index (also termed a *utility score*). Coupled with a time component, the index scores from the SF-6D, EQ-5D, or HUI are used to estimate quality-adjusted life-years (QALYs). As a simple example, assume a study has collected HRQOL responses at 6-month and 1-year follow-up examinations, which yield index scores of 0.66 and 0.75 and a QALY of $(0.66*[6/12] + 0.75*[6/12]) = 0.33 + 0.375 = 0.705$.

The index scores of 0.66 and 0.75 in the above example would be derived from published algorithms to convert HRQOL responses to a single index. These scoring algorithms are generally based on population-level studies, in which individual health states elicited from the HRQOL questionnaire of interest are valued by patients through a series of questions intended to measure patient preferences. The standard gamble (SG), time trade-off (TTO), and visual analog scale are some of the most common methods of measuring preferences over health states used in the literature.[1–5] Economists are generally fonder of the SG or TTO because these methods are choice based, requiring patients to explicitly compare alternative health states with one another.

Most HRQOL questionnaires have far too many possible responses to measure each health profile explicitly. Therefore, many scoring methods culminate in a statistical model that can be used to estimate an index score from all possible responses to the HRQOL questionnaire. Published algorithms are currently available in the literature based on the EQ-5D, the SF-6D (derived from either the SF-36 or the SF-12), and the HUI questionnaires.[1–5] Unfortunately, research in ASD has not consistently relied on generic health-profile questionnaires, such as the EQ-5D or the SF-36,

focusing instead on disease-specific or regional-specific questionnaires, such as the SRS-22/30 or the ODI. Directly valuing responses to these questionnaires using the SG or TTO methods is somewhat unclear because the questionnaires do not elicit a general health profile but rather a specific measure of certain characteristics relevant to the patient population in question. As such, statistical models have been developed to convert ODI scores to SF-6D utility scores.[27]

In applying statistical models to estimate index scores (whether scoring the SF-6D or EQ-5D directly, or converting the ODI to the SF-6D), researchers should be aware of at least 2 important issues:

1. Although there may be exceptions, the standard scoring algorithms in the literature are based on population studies, and the algorithms will generally differ depending on the population for which the algorithm was based. For example, in comparing algorithms derived from a US versus UK population, investigators have found potentially significant differences in the conclusions regarding the estimated treatment effect.[28] Although algorithms for the EQ-5D have been assessed in both US and UK populations, not all HRQOL questionnaires have been separately studied in different countries (including, for example, the SF-6D, for which there is not yet a published algorithm derived from a US population). Similarly, the algorithm developed to convert ODI scores to the SF-6D was not derived solely from spine deformity patients but rather a slightly wider range of patients undergoing lumbar fusion for degenerative disorders.
2. In applying statistical models to estimate index scores, researchers should also take caution in interpreting predicted index scores for a given patient. This is because regression-based models are inherently estimating the conditional mean function and may on average provide accurate predictions, whereas for a given patient provide relatively inaccurate predictions. Researchers are, therefore, encouraged to focus on the average prediction rather than an individual prediction.

In response to these concerns, one additional approach worth mentioning involves the concept of dominant health states.[28] For example, the EQ-5D responses are ranked from 1 to 3 in each of 5 domains, with 1 being no problems, 2 being some problems, and 3 being significant problems. The resulting health state for a given patient can then be easily characterized based on the patient's response to each question (eg, 11211 or 22212, denoting the patient's response of 1, 2, or 3 in each of the 5 domains). These health states can then be ordered, with 11111 dominating 21111. Other comparisons, such as 11211 versus 12111, would be considered unordered health states because both states have 4 responses of no problems and one response of some problems. This method, therefore, avoids assigning weight to each domain and relying on statistical models to estimate a single index, with the downside that many health state comparisons would be indistinguishable.

Still, whether the analysis considers a disease-specific questionnaire such as the SRS-22/30 or a generic profile such as the EQ-5D, the researcher may remain interested in analyzing individual HRQOL domains. Here, the most common statistical tools in current practice may fall short. For example, the EQ-5D responses are inherently discrete, ordered, and likely correlated across domains. With observational data, estimating the effect of surgery on HRQOL will require statistical tools that are robust to the complicated nature of the dependent variable. Although multivariate ordered logit or probit models can be estimated, these tools are not yet part of the standard toolbox for clinical researchers and may be considered unnecessarily complicated by some audiences. Future research in HRQOL may need to embrace these more complicated tools to accurately estimate the effects of interest.

One final point regarding HRQOL: the literature on condition-specific HRQOL questionnaires versus generic health profiles and the distinction between non–preference-based versus preference-based questionnaires is broad and well beyond the scope of this article. For the curious reader, many excellent texts are relevant to this area (often in the context of cost-effectiveness analyses).[2,3,5]

Costs of Surgery

Although there have been several cost studies in the general spine fusion literature, only recently have investigators begun to study the cost of medical treatment of ASD. Glassman and colleagues[29] found that among 68 ASD patients with nonoperative treatment, mean treatment cost over 2 years was $10,815. Mean treatment costs increased with symptoms—$9704 for low-symptom patients, $11,116 for midsymptom patients, and $14,022 for high-symptom patients. In a study of surgical treatment of adolescent idiopathic scoliosis, Kamerlink and colleagues[30] reported mean costs of $32,836. To our knowledge, however, the costs of surgical treatment of ASD have not been reported and analyzed in the literature. Advances in this area

will help determine the predictors of cost for surgical care of spinal deformity and allow comparisons among different centers treating ASD, ultimately identifying best practices in the treatment of ASD.

Because of the highly skewed nature of the distribution of costs for surgical treatment of spinal deformity, an appropriate analysis of the costs of surgery requires a careful statistical approach. The 2 most common statistical approaches to cost analyses include:

1. Analyze a log-transformed model of costs, wherein the costs of surgery (dependent variable) are measured in logs such that the distribution is less skewed and relatively more bell shaped. The intention of such a transformation is to restore homoscedasticity and normality of the residuals. However, one drawback of a log transformation is that coefficients are then interpreted as the estimated effect on the geometric mean cost rather than the arithmetic mean. Although investigators have suggested retransformations that may address this issue, assumptions required for an accurate retransformation are not satisfied in many cases.[31,32]

2. Estimate a generalized linear model (GLM) of costs as a function of other covariates of interest.[33] Unlike ordinary least squares with a log-transformed dependent variable, the use of GLM with log link function preserves the standard interpretation of regression coefficients in terms of the effect of an independent variable on average costs.[4] Extensions to the GLM approach have also been proposed in which the regression and link parameters are estimated semiparametrically.[34] Although more robust, this method carries with it a substantial loss of parity compared with the standard GLM and particularly ordinary least squares; however, the estimation technique proposed by Basu and Rathouz[34] should be considered if one is concerned about assumptions regarding the GLM link function and if advanced econometric tools are appropriate for the intended audience.

Aside from statistical modeling, another difficulty in the area of cost analysis involves how to define cost. Although seemingly simple, this is not a straightforward question. Providers may be most interested in the total or direct costs of surgery. Studies of direct costs may be particularly relevant to compare across hospitals because overhead and other indirect costs are not identified specifically with a given inpatient stay and instead are allocated to inpatient stays using general accounting algorithms. Such an allocation introduces additional noise into the total cost measure that is largely hospital specific and may not be reflective of actual costs incurred for surgical treatment.

Payors may also be interested in observed costs of surgery if they intend to negotiate lower rates; however, payors are generally interested in reimbursements or allowed amounts, because such costs are what the payors actually incur. Reimbursements may also be of interest from a policy standpoint because these amounts represent the dollar amount ultimately spent for the procedure in question.

Charges are sometimes used as a proxy for costs. Although many researchers do not consider charges to be an appropriate proxy for costs, charges still provide some level of information regarding the cost of care. Combined with actual cost data, an analysis of charges may still be useful, for example, as an indicator of a provider's markup on medical devices. And combined with cost and reimbursement data, charges would provide a relatively complete picture of the provider's negotiated rates with suppliers and payors. In a perfectly transparent system, such data would be extremely useful in synchronizing health care prices and reimbursement rates among comparable providers and payors. All measures of cost (direct costs, total costs, charges, or reimbursements), therefore, have some relevant information, particularly if analyzed together across providers.

In practice, researchers rarely have the luxury of choosing which measure of costs to adopt. Costs are instead determined by the best measure available in the data. Sometimes, this means estimating costs based on charges or utilization data, in which case estimating costs often can be done with one of 2 common methods—a bottom-up or a top-down approach. Although a thorough description of different costing methods is beyond the scope of this article, the appropriate estimation of costs is a common concern in large-scale studies (particularly when using publically available or restricted-use datasets), for which the Chapko and colleagues[35] and Tumeh and colleagues[36] studies, among others, should prove as valuable resources.

Cost-Effectiveness Studies

In a general sense, cost effectiveness has become a critical component in the economic evaluation of medical care, demonstrated by numerous initiatives encouraging more cost- and comparative-effectiveness research. For example, the United States recently created the Patient-Centered Outcomes Research Institute (PCORI) as part of the Patient Protection and Affordable Care Act.

PCORI was specifically created to promote and ultimately fund the development of comparative effectiveness research in health care.[37,38] PCORI and other similar initiatives illustrate a general movement toward a value-based health care economy and increasing focus on both costs and patient-reported outcomes in the economic evaluation of health care programs.

Cost effectiveness is generally measured by the dollar value of health care services. Operationally, researchers calculate cost effectiveness as the ratio of costs to some measurable outcome.[2] The outcome of interest is often the improvement in QALYs but may also be some other metric such as symptom-free days or number of positive screenings. Investigators often reserve the term cost-utility analysis (CUA) to describe cost-effectiveness studies with a utility-based outcome measure (e.g., QALYs), as opposed to cost-effectiveness studies with a non–utility-based outcome, such as symptom-free days.[39,40]

Although there is increasing awareness regarding the importance of cost-effectiveness research, few cost-effectiveness studies currently exist in the general spine literature. Of the few studies available, the measure of interest largely involves the cost effectiveness of surgical treatment in the lumbar spine, including disc herniation and degenerative spondylolisthesis. For example, as part of the Spine Patient Outcomes Research Trial study, Tosteson and colleagues[41] studied the cost effectiveness of surgical versus nonoperative treatment of lumbar disc herniation. The authors estimated costs based on patient-reported utilization multiplied by Medicare per-unit allowable payment rates and measured outcomes as QALYs based on the EQ-5D. Based on total costs, the study reported an incremental cost-effectiveness ratio of $69,403 for all patients and a ratio of $34,355 for Medicare patients. Based on direct costs only, the incremental cost-effectiveness ratio increased to $72,181 for all patients and $37,285 for Medicare patients.

Glassman and colleagues[42] analyzed the cost effectiveness of single-level posterolateral lumbar fusion for 93 patients, with cost data based on actual reimbursements from third-party payors and outcomes measured as QALYs based on the SF-6D.[2,43] As part of the cost of surgery, the authors included outpatient visits up to 6 months after surgery. The authors reported an average reimbursement amount per QALY of $164,261 after 1 year and $154,865 after 2 years, although estimates varied depending on the patient cohort of interest.

Although interest in cost-effectiveness research seems to be growing in the spine literature, studies generally do not focus specifically on surgical treatment of ASD and often do not have precise cost information for the episode of surgical care, relying instead on outside data sources, including surveys of the existing literature, high-level Medicare payment rates applied to observed utilization, or total reimbursements from third-party payors. Additional costs incurred after initial treatment should also be considered (eg, costs of revision surgery, follow-up visits) as well as additional so-called indirect benefits, such as improved productivity. These additional considerations, however, are rarely explicitly quantified in existing cost-effectiveness studies. Regardless, the literature on the cost effectiveness of spine deformity surgery is new, and there are significant research opportunities in this area.

Decision Analysis

Decision analysis or decision modeling derives largely from statistical decision theory, drawing from Bayesian statistics as well as expected utility theory.[3] Decision analysis also combines several sources of information (often involving multiple treatment options) into one analysis and is, therefore, distinct from pure cost analyses or cost-/comparative-effectiveness studies. Another area in which decision analysis is distinct from other analyses discussed above is in the explicit consideration of uncertainty and variability (including heterogeneity across patients or patient groups).[2,3,44]

Few decision analysis studies currently exist in the general spine literature. For example, in 2 related studies involving degenerative spondylolisthesis, Kuntz and colleagues[45] studied fusion with and without instrumentation, and Kim and colleagues[46] analyzed decompression with or without fusion. Both studies relied on simulations to form expected benefits and costs of alternative treatments after 10 years. Kuntz and colleagues[45] relied entirely on data collected from the literature, including average complication rates, fusion rates, and costs, whereas Kim and colleagues[46] relied on a combination of observational data and a review of the literature. Both studies measured costs based on total hospital costs, including direct costs, such as implants, as well as indirect costs, such as administration and facility usage.

Kuntz and colleagues[45] reported an incremental cost effectiveness of approximately $3.1 million per additional QALY for instrumented fusion compared with noninstrumented fusion; however, the results were sensitive to assumptions regarding the rate of patients with symptom relief after instrumented fusion. Kim and colleagues[46] reported an incremental cost effectiveness of $185,878 per

additional QALY for decompression with fusion compared with decompression alone, again with significant sensitivity regarding assumptions on the magnitude of QALY improvements over time, costs, and revision rates.

As is clear from the findings discussed above, there is some overlap in the characterization of cost effectiveness and decision analysis. We chose to label the Kuntz and colleagues[45] and Kim and colleagues[46] studies as decision models rather than pure cost-effectiveness studies for 3 primary reasons: (1) both studies relied, at least in part, on additional data from the literature (eg, on the average complication rate after specific types of surgery); (2) both studies considered multiple outcomes after surgery, the associated costs of such outcomes, and the probability associated with each outcome under consideration; and (3) both studies projected costs and benefits 10 years out. These features are fundamental aspects of decision analysis and easily differentiate the studies of Kim and colleagues[46] and Kuntz and colleagues[45] from the cost-effectiveness studies discussed previously.

As with our discussion of cost effectiveness, decision analysis studies remain relatively rare in the spine literature and have not yet caught on in spinal deformity. This is partly because of a lack of data and prior research on which to build an appropriate decision analytic model. For example, most studies of pseudoarthrosis or proximal junctional kyphosis (2 of the more commonly cited concerns among surgeons treating ASD) are still based on small patient cohorts. Progress is being made in this area with the collaboration of multiple centers, including the Spinal Deformity Study Group and the International Spine Study Group, with the goal of collecting data on larger cohorts of patients across several different geographic regions undergoing treatment from several different surgeons. As these datasets continue to grow, we can better estimate the HRQOL outcomes and costs of surgical and nonsurgical treatment for ASD, the rate of different complications after surgical treatment, the costs associated with such complications (eg, revision surgery), and eventually a breakdown of these variables by the type of surgical procedure or technique. Combining all such data would provide a solid foundation for a wide range of decision analytic modeling in spinal deformity.

FUTURE AREAS FOR HEALTH ECONOMICS RESEARCH IN SPINAL DEFORMITY

The above discussion provides an overview of areas in which health economics analysis is currently applied in the spine or spine deformity literature. However, as anyone watching the news can see, US health care is in a seemingly perpetual state of flux and uncertainty. Some of the largest areas of uncertainty relevant to health economics research include health care financing and the demand for health care services (and supply of physicians). These areas, discussed in more detail below, are far from an exhaustive list of important health economics topics. Rather, these areas were chosen largely out of self-interest, applicability to current events, and brevity.

Bundled Payments Analysis

In general, the potential impact of bundled payments to achieve cost reduction through improved incentive alignment has been well documented in the literature. Recent or ongoing initiatives involving bundled payments include:

1. A 2006 Robert Wood Johnson Foundation series of projects to spur the development of bundled payment software through the PROMETHEUS payment project
2. A 2009 Centers for Medicare and Medicaid Services bundled payment pilot program initiative, intended for select joint replacement and cardiovascular acute care episodes
3. A 2011 Center for Medicare and Medicaid Innovation Bundled Payments for Care Improvement initiative.[47]

Existing bundled payment efforts have thus far been limited in 2 important ways. First, calculations have focused on deriving a single value or range of values with which to set a bundled payment amount. This is a good start, but even with some risk adjustment, this approach will likely struggle in its attempt to assign a standardized value to patient-specific care. As found in a recent survey by the Commonwealth Fund, only 1 in 5 hospitals pursuing an Accountable Care Organization model is attempting to use data to predict which patients will actually need more services.[48] Without appropriate detail in the payment formulas, bundled payments and other alternative payment models may systematically under- or overestimate payment amounts. If providers and payors are to embrace the bundled payment or Accountable Care Organization model, payment calculations must be both patient specific and parsimonious.

Second, the inherent uncertainty with the bundled payment model has made many hospitals hesitant to commit to bundled payments in practice and hesitant to take on additional risk.[48] To this end, future research must also include detailed simulation studies of the financial impact of bundled payments, which could ultimately provide a decision tool to assist in the deployment of bundled payments for other providers.

Demand and Utilization of Surgical Treatment

Little is known about the drivers of demand for a patient considering surgical treatment for spinal deformity. For many patients, the decision of whether to have surgery is driven by severe pain and disability, but other factors may also be at play. For example, a patient's insurance plan likely has some impact because of the high cost of spine deformity surgery. This introduces the role of moral hazard, wherein insured patients demand more health care compared with uninsured patients.[49] The supply of physicians may also have some impact on demand for surgical treatment. Such an effect is often referred to as *supplier-induced demand* or simply *inducement*.[50,51]

Ultimately, insurance status, number of physicians, advertising, geography, patient demographics, and severity of disease may all have some impact on the demand for spine deformity surgery. The effects of these variables on the demand for health care services have been well studied in a general practice setting, but we are not aware of any formal studies estimating the impact of such variables on the demand for spine deformity surgery (or many other elective procedures). Although research in this area will require more advanced statistical tools, the findings may be invaluable to payors, providers, and regulators in designing policies to deliver health care to spine deformity patients in a safe, timely, effective, efficient, and equitable manner.

Even still, conditional on the decision to have surgery, what determines a patient's choice of physician? How important is the interaction between the physician and patient in ultimately deciding on (1) surgery and (2) a surgeon? Referrals no doubt have some impact on one's choice of physician, but the interaction of patients and physicians and the resulting shared decision-making process (both before and after surgical treatment) are not well studied in the current literature.

SUMMARY

The purpose of this article was to provide an update on the current state of health economics studies in the literature and to introduce areas in which health economics might play some additional role in future research. Ultimately, spine deformity surgeries (like many other complex, expensive, and highly valuable procedures) must be done more efficiently. Maintaining quality of care in the face of such economic pressures, and formally measuring the value of surgical treatment for ASD, will require continued development in health economics research in ASD. We hope to have convinced the reader of the importance of health economics research in this field and to have spurred interest in areas in which we believe health economics will have a particularly important role going forward.

REFERENCES

1. Glied S, Smith PC. The Oxford Handbook of health economics. New York: Oxford Univ Pr; 2011.

2. Brazier J, Ratcliffe J, Salomon J, et al. Measuring and valuing health benefits for economic evaluation. New York: Oxford University Press, USA; 2007.

3. Drummond MF, Sculpher MJ, Torrance GW. Methods for the economic evaluation of health care programmes. New York: Oxford University Press, USA; 2005.

4. Glick H, Doshi JA, Sonnad S, et al. Economic evaluation in clinical trials. In: Gray A, Briggs A, editors. Handbooks in health economic evaluations series. New York: Oxford University Press; 2007.

5. Gray AM, Clarke PM, Wolstenholme J, et al. Applied methods of cost-effectiveness analysis in healthcare. New York: Oxford Univ Pr; 2011.

6. Deyo RA, Nachemson A, Mirza SK. Spinal-fusion surgery—the case for restraint. N Engl J Med 2004; 350(7):722–6.

7. Deyo RA, Mirza SK. The case for restraint in spinal surgery: does quality management have a role to play? Eur Spine J 2009;18:331–7.

8. Martin BI, Turner JA, Mirza SK, et al. Trends in health care expenditures, utilization, and health status among US adults with spine problems, 1997–2006. Spine (Phila Pa 1976) 2009;34(19):2077.

9. Deyo RA, Mirza SK, Martin BI, et al. Trends, major medical complications, and charges associated with surgery for lumbar spinal stenosis in older adults. JAMA 2010;303(13):1259–65.

10. Burton DC, Glattes RC. Measuring outcomes in spinal deformity. Neurosurg Clin N Am 2007;18(2): 403–5.

11. Asher M, Min Lai S, Burton D, et al. The reliability and concurrent validity of the scoliosis research society-22 patient questionnaire for idiopathic scoliosis. Spine (Phila Pa 1976) 2003;28(1):63.

12. Asher M, Min Lai S, Burton D, et al. Discrimination validity of the scoliosis research society-22 patient questionnaire: relationship to idiopathic scoliosis curve pattern and curve size. Spine (Phila Pa 1976) 2003; 28(1):74.

13. Asher M, Min Lai S, Burton D, et al. Scoliosis research society-22 patient questionnaire: responsiveness to change associated with surgical treatment. Spine (Phila Pa 1976) 2003;28(1):70.

14. Bridwell KH, Cats-Baril W, Harrast J, et al. The validity of the SRS-22 instrument in an adult spinal deformity population compared with the Oswestry and SF-12: a study of response distribution, concurrent validity, internal consistency, and reliability. Spine (Phila Pa 1976) 2005;30(4):455.

15. Bridwell KH, Berven S, Glassman S, et al. Is the SRS-22 instrument responsive to change in adult scoliosis patients having primary spinal deformity surgery? Spine (Phila Pa 1976) 2007;32(20):2220–5.

16. Berven S, Deviren V, Demir-Deviren S, et al. Studies in the modified Scoliosis Research Society Outcomes Instrument in adults: validation, reliability, and discriminatory capacity. Spine (Phila Pa 1976) 2003;28(18): 2164.

17. Schwab F, Dubey A, Pagala M, et al. Adult scoliosis: a health assessment analysis by SF-36. Spine (Phila Pa 1976) 2003;28(6):602.

18. Glassman SD, Schwab F, Bridwell KH, et al. Do 1-year outcomes predict 2-year outcomes for adult deformity surgery? Spine J 2009;9(4):317–22.

19. Albert TJ, Purtill J, Mesa J, et al. Health outcome assessment before and after adult deformity surgery: a prospective study. Spine (Phila Pa 1976) 1995; 20(18):2002.

20. Glassman SD, Hamill CL, Bridwell KH, et al. The impact of perioperative complications on clinical outcome in adult deformity surgery. Spine (Phila Pa 1976) 2007;32(24):2764.

21. Cho SK, Bridwell KH, Lenke LG, et al. Comparative analysis of clinical outcome and complications in primary versus revision adult scoliosis surgery. Spine (Phila Pa 1976) 2012;37(5):393.

22. Yadla S, Maltenfort MG, Ratliff JK, et al. Adult scoliosis surgery outcomes: a systematic review. Neurosurg Focus 2010;28(3):3.

23. Bagó J, Pérez-Grueso FJ, Les E, et al. Minimal important differences of the SRS-22 Patient Questionnaire following surgical treatment of idiopathic scoliosis. Eur Spine J 2009;18(12):1898–904.

24. Jaeschke R, Singer J, Guyatt GH. Measurement of health status: ascertaining the minimal clinically important difference. Control Clin Trials 1989;10(4): 407–15.

25. Copay AG, Subach BR, Glassman SD, et al. Understanding the minimum clinically important difference: a review of concepts and methods. Spine J 2007;7(5):541–6.

26. Beaton DE, Boers M, Wells GA. Many faces of the minimal clinically important difference (MCID): a literature review and directions for future research. Curr Opin Rheumatol 2002;14(2):109.

27. Carreon LY, Glassman SD, McDonough CM, et al. Predicting SF-6D utility scores from the Oswestry disability index and numeric rating scales for back and leg pain. Spine (Phila Pa 1976) 2009;34(19): 2085.

28. Parkin D, Rice N, Devlin N. Statistical analysis of EQ-5D profiles: does the use of value sets bias inference? Med Decis Making 2010;30(5):556–65.

29. Glassman SD, Carreon LY, Shaffrey CI, et al. The costs and benefits of nonoperative management for adult scoliosis. Spine (Phila Pa 1976) 2010;35(5):578–82.

30. Kamerlink JR, Quirno M, Auerbach JD, et al. Hospital cost analysis of adolescent idiopathic scoliosis correction surgery in 125 consecutive cases. J Bone Joint Surg Am 2010;92(5):1097–104.

31. Duan N. Smearing estimate - a nonparametric retransformation method. J Am Stat Assoc 1983;78(383):605–10.

32. Manning WG, Mullahy J. Estimating log models: to transform or not to transform? J Health Econ 2001;20(4):461–94.

33. McCullagh P, Nelder JA. Generalized linear models. 2nd edition. London: Chapman and Hall; 1989.

34. Basu A, Rathouz PJ. Estimating marginal and incremental effects on health outcomes using flexible link and variance function models. Biostatistics 2005;6(1):93–109.

35. Chapko MK, Liu CF, Perkins M, et al. Equivalence of two healthcare costing methods: bottom-up and top-down. Health Econ 2009;18(10):1188–201.

36. Tumeh JW, Moore SG, Shapiro R, et al. Practical approach for using Medicare data to estimate costs for cost–effectiveness analysis. Expert Rev Pharmacoecon Outcomes Res 2005;5(2):153–62.

37. PCORI. Draft national priorities for research and research agenda. Washington, DC: Patient-Centered Outcomes Research Institute; 2012.

38. Selby JV, Beal AC, Frank L. The Patient-Centered Outcomes Research Institute (PCORI) national priorities for research and initial research agenda. JAMA 2012;307(15):1583–4.

39. Walters SJ, Brazier JE. Comparison of the minimally important difference for two health state utility measures: EQ-5D and SF-6D. Qual Life Res 2005;14(6):1523–32.

40. Robinson R. Cost-utility analysis. BMJ 1993;307(6908):859–62.

41. Tosteson AN, Skinner JS, Tosteson TD, et al. The Cost Effectiveness of Surgical versus Non-Operative Treatment for Lumbar Disc Herniation over Two Years: Evidence from the Spine Patient Outcomes Research Trial (SPORT). Spine (Phila Pa 1976) 2008;33(19):2108.

42. Glassman SD, Polly DW, Dimar JR, et al. The cost effectiveness of single-level instrumented posterolateral lumbar fusion at five years after surgery. Spine (Phila Pa 1976) 2012;37(9):769–74.

43. Brazier J, Roberts J, Deverill M. The estimation of a preference-based measure of health from the SF-36. J Health Econ 2002;21(2):271–92.

44. Briggs A, Sculpher M, Claxton K. Decision modelling for health economic evaluation. New York: Oxford University Press; 2006.

45. Kuntz KM, Snider RK, Weinstein JN, et al. Cost-effectiveness of fusion with and without instrumentation for patients with degenerative spondylolisthesis and spinal stenosis. Spine (Phila Pa 1976) 2000;25(9):1132.

46. Kim S, Mortaz Hedjri S, Coyte PC, et al. Cost-utility of lumbar decompression with or without fusion for patients with symptomatic degenerative lumbar spondylolisthesis. Spine J 2012;12(1):44–54.

47. HCI3. Bundled Payment across the U.S. Today: status of implementations and operational finding. Newtown, CT: Healthcare Incentives Improvement Institute; 2012.

48. Audet A, Kenward K, Patel S, et al. Hospitals on the path to accountable care: highlights from a 2011 National Survey of Hospital Readiness to Participate in an Accountable Care Organization. New York: The Commonwealth Fund; 2012.

49. Nyman JA. Is 'moral hazard' inefficient? The policy implications of a new theory. Health Aff 2004;23(5):194–9.

50. Dijk CE, Berg B, Verheij RA, et al. Moral hazard and supplier-induced demand: empirical evidence in general practice. Health Econ 2012. [Epub ahead of print].

51. Richardson J. The inducement hypothesis: that doctors generate demand for their own services. Health, Economics, and Health Economics: Proceedings of the World Congress on Health Economics. Leiden, The Netherlands; 1981;189–214.

Index

Note: Page numbers of article titles are in **boldface** type.

Neurosurg Clin N Am 24 (2013) 305–308
http://dx.doi.org/10.1016/S1042-3680(13)00018-1
1042-3680/13/$ – see front matter © 2013 Elsevier Inc. All rights reserved.

Moving?

Make sure your subscription moves with you!

To notify us of your new address, find your **Clinics Account Number** (located on your mailing label above your name), and contact customer service at:

Email: journalscustomerservice-usa@elsevier.com

800-654-2452 (subscribers in the U.S. & Canada)
314-447-8871 (subscribers outside of the U.S. & Canada)

Fax number: 314-447-8029

Elsevier Health Sciences Division
Subscription Customer Service
3251 Riverport Lane
Maryland Heights, MO 63043

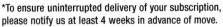

*To ensure uninterrupted delivery of your subscription, please notify us at least 4 weeks in advance of move.

Printed and bound by CPI Group (UK) Ltd, Croydon, CR0 4YY

03/10/2024

01040347-0013